PHYSICAL ASSESSMENT OF THE NEWBORN:

A Comprehensive Approach to the Art of Physical Examination

4th Edition

Ellen P. Tappero, DNP, RN, NNP-BC
Mary Ellen Honeyfield, MS, RN, NNP-BC

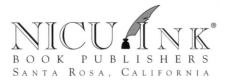
NICU INK®
BOOK PUBLISHERS
SANTA ROSA, CALIFORNIA

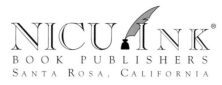

BOOK PUBLISHERS
SANTA ROSA, CALIFORNIA

2220 Northpoint Parkway
Santa Rosa, CA 95407-7398

COPYRIGHT © **2009** BY NICU Ink BOOK PUBLISHERS

Editor-in Chief: Charles Rait, RN, MSEd, PNC
Managing Editor: Suzanne G. Rait, RN
Editorial Coordinator: Tabitha Parker
Continuing Education Course Content: Debbie Fraser Askin, MN, RNC-NIC
Continuing Education Course Reviewers: Jodi Behr, RNC, MSN, JD
Angela Burd, APRN, CCNS
Lori Jackson, DNP, NNP-BC, RNC-NIC
Mary Klawitter, RNC, MSN
Phyllis Lawlor-Klean, RNC, MS
Ruth Snyder, RNC, BSN
Laurel Vessey, RN, BSN
Reviewer: Susan Tucker Blackburn, RN, PhD, FAAN
Editors: Beverley DeWitt, BA
Janine Stanich, RNC, BA
Lynn Stansbury, MD, MPH
Sylvia Stein Wright, BA
Proofreader: Joanne Gosnell, BA
Indexer: Mary Coe, Potomac Indexing, LLC
Illustrator: Elizabeth Weadon Massari

Book design and composition by:
Marsha Godfrey Graphics

LIBRARY OF CONGRESS CATALOGING-IN-PUBLICATION DATA

Physical assessment of the newborn : a comprehensive approach to the art of physical examination / [edited by] Ellen P. Tappero, Mary Ellen Honeyfield. — 4th ed.

p. ; cm.

Includes bibliographical references and index.

ISBN 978-1-887571-17-3 (pbk.)

1. Newborn infants—Medical examinations. 2. Newborn infants—Diseases—Diagnosis. I. Tappero, Ellen P., 1952– II. Honeyfield, Mary Ellen, 1944–

[DNLM: 1. Physical Examination—methods. 2. Infant, Newborn. 3. Neonatal Nursing— methods. WS 420 P5775 2009]

RJ255.5.P435 2009

618.92'01—dc22   2009027488

TABLE OF CONTENTS

CONTRIBUTORS

Debbie Fraser Askin, MN, RNC-NIC
St. Boniface General Hospital
Winnipeg, Manitoba
Athabasca University
Athabasca, Alberta
Canada

Michelle Bennett, MSN, NNP-BC
NNP Services of Colorado, Inc.
Presbyterian/St. Luke's Medical Center
Denver, Colorado

Carol Turnage Carrier, MSN, RN, CNS
Texas Children's Hospital
Houston, Texas

Terri A. Cavaliere, DNP, RN, NNP-BC
Schneider Children's Hospital at North Shore
Manhasset, New York
State University of New York
Stony Brook, New York

Martha Goodwin, MSN, RN, NNP-BC
Children's Mercy Hospital
Kansas City, Missouri

Pamela Dillon Heaberlin, RN, MS, NNP-BC
The Children's Hospital
Aurora, Colorado

Mary Ellen Honeyfield, MS, RN, NNP-BC
NNP Services of Colorado, Inc.
Sedalia, Colorado

Patricia J. Johnson, DNP, MPH, RN, NNP
Maricopa Integrated Health System
Neonatology Associates, Ltd.
Phoenix, Arizona

Kimberly Horns LaBronte, PhD, RN, NNP-BC
College of Nursing and Health Innovation
Arizona State University
Phoenix, Arizona

Jacqueline McGrath, PhD, RN, NNP, FNAP, FAAN
Virginia Commonwealth University
Richmond, Virginia

Susan Meier, MSN, NNP-BC
NNP Services of Colorado, Inc.
Denver, Colorado

Ellen P. Tappero, DNP, RN, NNP-BC
Neonatology Associates, Ltd.
Phoenix, Arizona

Carol Wiltgen Trotter, PhD, RN, NNP-BC
University of Missouri—Kansas City
St. Louis, Missouri

Lyn Vargo, PhD, RN, NNP-BC
St. Luke's Hospital
St. Louis, Missouri

Marlene Walden, PhD, RN, CCNS, NNP-BC
University of Texas School of Nursing
Austin, Texas
Texas Children's Hospital
Houston, Texas

Catherine Witt, RN, MS, NNP-BC
Presbyterian/St. Luke's Medical Center
Denver, Colorado

Foreword

Systematic, accurate, ongoing physical assessment is a critical component of managing neonates across all settings. The purposes of neonatal assessment include identifying influences of the prenatal environment, evaluating transition to extrauterine life, recognizing early the subtle indicators or changes that may be harbingers of serious problems, and evaluating a plethora of clinical findings to distinguish between normal variations and problems. Assessment is an integral part of care planning and parent teaching.

There is a tremendous range of variation even among normal newborns, including differences characteristic of infants in general and traits that are specific and unique within an individual family. Family traits, due to genetic variation, may or may not have pathologic significance. Variations seen in newborns may also be abnormal. Minor or subtle anomalies may be missed unless the practitioner has heightened awareness and skill in assessment and is specifically looking for them during the newborn examination. These subtle alterations are important in that they can provide clues to the presence of internal malformations or syndromes that have significant consequences for the infant and family. In addition, many problems in the neonate, such as infection, metabolic alterations, necrotizing enterocolitis, or changes in skin integrity, can be detected early, long before electronic monitors or other equipment record them, by an astute practioner with good assessment skills. Identification of infant state and behavioral cues is critical in recognizing and reducing stress and in providing individualized care.

Physical Assessment of the Newborn, now in its fourth edition, continues to be a valuable and essential resource for all those involved in neonatal care. Editors Ellen P. Tappero and Mary Ellen Honeyfield have developed a comprehensive text with a wealth of detailed information on assessment of the newborn. The book is an excellent resource for beginning and experienced clinicians on gestational, neurologic, and behavioral assessment, neonatal history, and assessment of the dysmorphic infant, as well as evaluation of individual body systems. Implications of antepartum testing and intrapartum monitoring for the newborn and assessing behavioral organization in term and preterm infants are also included. All of the content has been updated and in some areas expanded and reorganized and provides state-of-the-art knowledge. A valuable and timely addition to this edition is a new chapter on pain assessment. This chapter describes a systematic approach to evaluating the behavioral and physiologic indicators of neonatal pain. Assessment tools and the evidence base for appraising pain in infants of extremely low gestational age, infants with neurologic impairment, infants who are pharmacologically paralyzed or sedated, and others, are discussed.

The numerous tables, figures, and illustrations are a major strength that enhances the book's usefulness as a clinical resource. The many additional color illustrations and photographs in this edition further increase its usefulness. The chapter authors clearly identify areas for assessment, provide the scientific basis for and rationale underlying its various techniques, review standard terminology, and define and exemplify normal and abnormal findings and common variations. The book not only illustrates the skills needed to gather assessment data systematically and accurately, but also provides a knowledge base for interpretation of these data.

The text is both an excellent teaching tool and a resource for anyone who does newborn examinations, including nurses, neonatal and pediatric nurse practitioners, nurse-midwives, physicians, and therapists. It should be a core text for any program preparing individuals for advanced practice roles in neonatal care, and it should be a resource in every setting providing care to neonates. Individual practitioners have varying degrees of familiarity and comfort with the many areas of newborn assessment. This text can serve as an in-depth, systematic introduction to the major components of and techniques for evaluating all the major systems. For more experienced practitioners, it can reinforce, update, and improve knowledge and techniques. At all levels of practice, it serves as a convenient reference to normal parameters, common variations, and less commonly seen abnormalities.

Understanding the unique physical, physiologic, neurologic, and behavioral findings in the neonate helps practitioners to recognize alterations and prevent or minimize their effects. Skillful newborn assessment reduces the risks associated with the transition to extrauterine life and pathophysiologic problems of the neonatal period. Yet because assessment skills are such an integral aspect of practice, many individuals take them for granted. To maintain excellence, practitioners must continue to expand, update, and validate their skills. This book provides a resource to do so. As such, it continues to be a significant contribution to neonatal care, for which the editors and authors are to be congratulated.

Susan Tucker Blackburn, RN, PhD, FAAN
Author of Maternal, Fetal, and Neonatal Physiology:
A Clinical Perspective

Introduction

This is the fourth edition of *Physical Assessment of the Newborn.* Our enthusiasm for writing and editing this edition remains as great as it was for the first, nearly 17 years ago. During the years since then, there have been striking changes in our understanding of conditions and diseases of the newborn infant. Despite these changes, the principles of physical assessment have remained the same. Like the three previous editions, this one is intended to be a comprehensive and up-to-date text. The aim was to make the material understandable to a diverse group of individuals ranging from practicing staff nurses, nurse practitioners, and nurse-midwives to medical students and pediatric residents. Our objective is based on the premise that the clinician must be prepared to deal with whatever symptom or sign, common or uncommon, a newborn may present. We believe that clinicians working with newborns need to thoroughly understand and recognize normal findings and conditions before they can identify complications and comprehend their implications in the care of the newborn.

As our neonatal subspecialty continues to emphasize the merit of high-tech diagnostic modalities, physical assessment skills seem to be in danger of becoming a lost art. Diagnosis by physical assessment lacks the glamour of the advanced modalities, but it remains a vital component of our practice. Looking at, listening to, and touching a newborn are critical skills, not only to detect subtleties that may lead to the diagnosis of a serious illness, but also to counsel the family on the common, normal variations. The information contained in the text is only a beginning and, along with other references, is intended to be useful in the clinical decision-making process.

We have retained the features of the previous three editions that were regarded by the readers as most effective and augmented other parts of the text to further enhance the quality of the book. Once again, all chapters are presented in a head-to-toe approach. Each author has written the material in an individual manner, and no attempt has been made to mandate a specific format.

The authors have revised their chapters several times during the months it has taken to complete this edition. We would like to thank each of them for their additional efforts, which result in a more readable and up-to-date text.

In order to retain the quality and vitality seen in the first editions, we have added several new authors. These new voices were sought out for their enthusiasm and expertise, and the additions are healthy for a text in order to ensure its timeliness and freshness.

Because today's students are more visually oriented than in the past, we have expanded our use of illustrations and color photographs to command their interest and add emphasis to the information presented. We offer our thanks to our colleagues who shared their many photographs.

Finally, special words of thanks to the staff at NICU INK for their skill and assistance in the preparation and production of this text.

Ellen P. Tappero, DNP, RN, NNP-BC
Mary Ellen Honeyfield, MS, RN, NNP-BC

ACKNOWLEDGMENTS

Thanks to my husband, Charlie, for his endless patience, guidance, and understanding. Truly, without his willingness to assume many of the day-to-day tasks or to make sacrifices that allowed me the time to pursue my goals, I would not have been able to achieve my successes.

I am grateful to my father, John Paysinger, Jr., for believing in me and encouraging me to pursue my dreams. I wish that he could be here to see another edition in print; he would have been proud of this accomplishment.

I am also grateful to my coworkers at Neonatology Associates, Ltd., and to my many neonatal colleagues in education and clinical practice who have provided their words of encouragement, suggestions, contributions, and, most of all, their commitment to excellence.

Ellen Tappero

As this fourth edition goes to print, I would like to acknowledge all those students I may have touched in the past and those I may yet touch in the future. As our ability to reach out becomes more global, I would also like to recognize the international students of physical assessment. With some 30 years of clinical practice behind me, I realize today more than ever our responsibility as teachers. Our responsibility to the educational process spans our careers. Even when we are students, we are teaching our instructors—that is, if they are paying attention! As we gain in expertise and find our careers winding down, our responsibility is to support the succession of new teachers through mentoring and stepping aside. In this edition, we have provided new authors the opportunity to bring fresh eyes and ideas to a subject that in reality does not change much. They have exceeded our expectations. In the future, one or more of their names may be on the cover of this text!

On a more personal note, I remain most grateful to my family, who continue to support all of my endeavors: Aunt Eleanor, my children, Dave, Mike, and Kathy, their spouses, Carla, Val, and Ty, and my amazing grandchildren, Lincoln, Kylie, Sunny, and Coy. You all make my life blessed.

Mary Ellen Honeyfield

1 Principles of Physical Assessment

Mary Ellen Honeyfield, MS, RN, NNP-BC

The importance of approaching the newborn physical examination with a sense of anticipation cannot be overemphasized. This first exam offers a unique opportunity for early recognition of any problems the infant may have. Seeing each infant as a mystery to be unraveled requires curiosity on the part of the examiner. The inability of the newborn to provide verbal information tests the acuity of the examiner's skills. When the examiner views this responsibility as a diagnostic challenge, newborn physical assessment provides both personal and professional satisfaction, even though most infants examined are normal.

Initially, the inexperienced examiner finds physical assessment time-consuming. Lack of familiarity with the necessary tools and limited practice with the techniques both slow assessment. In fact, the student often views the infant as a series of systems to be examined. Repetition and experience help the practitioner learn to see the newborn as a whole and to process multiple observations while examining individual systems. For example, if the infant begins to cry during palpation of the abdomen, the experienced examiner continues the abdominal exam but also notes the quality of the cry, the infant's color while crying, respiratory effort, facial movements, the tongue, intactness of the palate, and movement of the extremities.

Clinical expertise develops throughout a practitioner's career. With experience, each practitioner develops a unique approach to newborn physical examination. The sequence of how the exam is performed is not as important as that each practitioner develop a consistent and organized approach. Consistency—performing the examination in the same organized manner each time a newborn is examined—maximizes the information gained from each exam performed, thus adding to the practitioner's knowledge base and ensuring that portions of the assessment will not be forgotten.

TECHNIQUES OF PHYSICAL ASSESSMENT

OBSERVATION

Observation, or inspection, is the most important physical assessment technique for the practitioner to master. It is also often the most difficult skill for the fledgling examiner to incorporate into the clinical approach. In 1860, Florence Nightingale wrote these thoughts about the art and skill of observation:

TABLE 1-1 ▲ Observations for Physical Assessment

To Assess	Observe
Distress	Facial expression, respiratory effort, activity, tone
Color	Tongue, mucous membranes (centrally pink vs cyanotic), nail beds, hands, feet (peripherally pink vs cyanotic), skin (jaundice, pallor, ruddiness, mottling), perfusion, meconium staining
Nutrition status	Subcutaneous fat, breast nodule
Hydration status	Skin turgor, anterior fontanel
Gestational age	Skin (smooth vs peeling), ear cartilage, areola and nipple formation, breast nodule, sole creases, descent of testes, rugae, labia
Neurologic status	Posture, tone, activity, response to stimuli, cry, state, state transition, reflexes
Respiratory/chest status	Respiratory rate and effort, retractions, nasal flaring, grunting, audible stridor or wheezing, chest shape, nipples (number and position), skin color
Cardiovascular status	Precordial activity, visible point of maximal intensity, skin perfusion and color
Abdomen	Size (full, distended, taut, shiny), shape (round, concave), distention (generalized or localized), visible peristaltic waves, visible bowel loops, muscular development/tone, umbilical cord, umbilical vessels, drainage from cord, periumbilical erythema (redness)
Head	Size, shape, anterior fontanel, hair distribution, condition of hair
Eyes	Shape, size, position, pupils, blink, extraocular movements, color of sclera, discharge, ability to fix and follow
Ears	Shape, position, external auditory canal, response to sound
Nose	Shape, nares, flaring, nasal bridge
Mouth	Shape, symmetry, movement, philtrum, tongue, palate, natal teeth, gums, jaw size
Neck	Shape, range of motion, webbing
Genitalia (male)	Scrotum, descent of testes, rugae, inguinal canals, foreskin, penile size, urine stream, meatus, perineum, anus
Genitalia (female)	Labia majora, labia minora, clitoris, vagina, perineum, inguinal canals, anus
Skin	Color, texture, firmness, vernix caseosa, masses, lanugo, lesions (pigmentary, vascular, trauma-related, infectious)
Extremities	Posture, range of motion (involuntary movement), digits, palmar creases, soles of feet, nails

In the case of infants, everything must depend upon the accurate observation of the nurse or mother.... For it may safely be said, not that the habit of ready and correct observation will by itself make us useful..., but that without it we shall be useless with all our devotion.... If you cannot get the habit of observation one way or [the] other, you better give up..., for it is not your calling, however kind and anxious you may be.[1]

Using the visual and auditory senses, the practitioner observes the infant and then assesses and makes decisions about what has been seen or heard. A specific observation may alert the examiner to assess a particular system more thoroughly. For example, the observation of an active precordium (visual cardiac pulsations) directs the examiner to careful cardiovascular assessment. Auscultation may reveal a heart murmur. This finding leads the examiner to palpate the precordium and peripheral pulses and to obtain four extremity blood pressures, actions not normally part of the examination of an otherwise healthy-appearing newborn.

The practitioner can collect most of the information needed for a complete physical

FIGURE 1-1 ▲ Bimanual inspection of the kidneys.

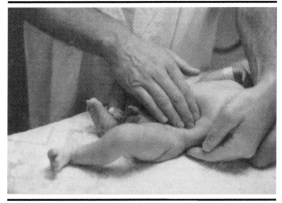

From: Coen RW, and Koffler H. 1987. *Primary Care of the Newborn.* Boston: Little, Brown, 30. Reprinted by permission.

assessment solely through observation (Table 1-1).

AUSCULTATION

Auscultation is the technique of listening to sounds produced by the body (i.e., the lungs, heart, and gastrointestinal tract). Direct auscultation involves application of the examiner's ear to the body surface being assessed. Some sounds, such as stridor, wheezing, and expiratory grunting, may be heard simply by being near the infant. Indirect (mediate) auscultation utilizes a stethoscope to listen to these same sounds.

Accurate indirect auscultation of the newborn requires a stethoscope fitted with a pediatric-sized double-headed chest piece with an open bell and a closed diaphragm. The stethoscope should be placed firmly on bare skin rather than over the infant's clothes. A quiet infant and environment as well as a warm room and warm stethoscope facilitate auscultation.

PALPATION

Palpation is a technique in which the examiner uses the sense of touch to assess both superficial and deeper body characteristics. During palpation, the tips, palmar, and lateral surfaces of the fingers of both hands are used to assess external structures (i.e., skin, hair texture), vibrations (i.e., peripheral pulses, precordial activity, point of maximal impulse of the heart against the chest wall), and internal structures (i.e., liver, spleen, kidneys). One hand can be used, or a bimanual technique may enhance the palpation of deeper organs, such as the kidneys (Figure 1-1).

For accurate palpation, the infant should be quiet and relaxed at the beginning of the abdominal exam. Warm hands, progressing from superficial to deeper palpation, and elevating the infant's hips off the bed keep the abdominal muscles relaxed. The examiner should take care not to palpate too deeply for superficial abdominal organs such as the liver and spleen because the fingertips may be palpating stool-filled intestine or abdominal wall muscle mass rather than the organ itself.

In palpation of the extremities and genitalia, a grasping action of the fingers is used to evaluate such accessible features as skin texture, skin lesions, descent of testes into the scrotum, muscle mass, and muscle strength.

PERCUSSION

Percussion is tapping or striking a part of the body to put the underlying tissue into motion. This movement produces audible sounds and palpable vibrations, which are then assessed for the quality and duration of their tone and notes.

Indirect (mediate) percussion is performed (for a right-handed person) by hyperextending the middle finger of the left hand and placing only the distal interphalangeal joint firmly on the part of the body to be percussed. Contact by any other part of the hand will alter the sounds produced. The right wrist is then hyperextended and the middle right finger partially flexed and "cocked" upward in a position to strike the middle left finger. With a quick wrist motion downward, the tip of the right

FIGURE 1-2 ▲ Transillumination of hydrocele.

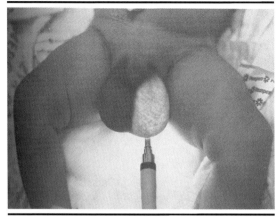

From: Coen RW, and Koffler H. 1987. *Primary Care of the Newborn*. Boston: Little, Brown, 33. Reprinted by permission.

middle finger strikes the left middle finger's distal joint. Vibrations are transmitted through the bones of this joint to the underlying tissue being percussed.

Direct percussion is performed by directly striking the body surface to be assessed with the tip of the middle right finger.

The translation of sounds heard during percussion into descriptive words is difficult at best. It takes practice and multiple examinations of normal infants and those with pathology to develop skill in describing percussed sounds.

Although the technique of percussion is commonly taught to students, in practice it is not a technique universally used on the newborn. When the examiner suspects pathologies, like pleural effusion or air leak, that might be assessed by percussion, the more common approach in the newborn is to confirm the suspected diagnosis by x-ray. A description of the comparative sounds produced during percussion has therefore been omitted.

TRANSILLUMINATION

Transillumination is the technique of applying a high-intensity light directly to a body part, such as the head, chest, or scrotum, and assessing the amount of pink light that can be seen as a corona (halo) around the cuffed flashlight or fiberoptic device.

Transillumination of the enlarged scrotum of an infant with a hydrocele reveals a fluid-filled mass that transmits light rather than a solid mass that does not transmit light, as in the case of an inguinal hernia (Figure 1-2).

As with the other physical assessment techniques described, practice enables the examiner to recognize the difference between normal and abnormal halos of light.

TIMING OF THE EXAM

Timing of newborn physical assessment often depends on circumstance and hospital guidelines. A quick overall exam should be done in the delivery room. It is disconcerting when the parents are the first to discover a problem. A more complete exam is done during the first few hours after birth. Daily and discharge exams are completed thereafter.

BASICS OF PHYSICAL ASSESSMENT

Certain themes recur throughout this text in the discussions of assessments of each system. The repetition is intentional and reflects the importance of these activities. These basic principles of physical assessment include the following:

▶ **Review the perinatal history for clues to potential pathology.** The newborn's history begins with conception and includes events that occurred throughout gestation, labor, and delivery. The newborn is also affected by the genetic histories of both parents and of their families. For example, a maternal history that includes diabetes mellitus directs the experienced practitioner to carefully assess the cardiovascular and neurologic systems and the extremities, because infants of diabetic mothers show an increased incidence of abnormalities in these systems. The labor and delivery history may reveal that the mother received medication for pain relief just before delivery; this could account for the depression of the newborn's respirations and/or muscular tone. With this knowledge, the examiner need not pursue a more serious etiology for the depressed respirations, as long as the respiratory pattern or muscle tone improves over time.

▶ **Assess the infant's color for clues to potential pathology.** The infant's color provides important information about several body systems. For example, the very red or ruddy infant may have polycythemia and may be more prone to complications, such as respiratory distress or hypoglycemia, that are associated with this phenomenon. The infant whose tongue and mucous membranes are pale or blue (central cyanosis) may be anemic or may have a heart lesion or respiratory disease. Proper lighting is essential for accurate assessment of color.

▶ **Auscultate only in a quiet environment.** It is difficult to assess the sounds produced by the body if there are noises, such as people talking or a radio playing, in the room. External interferences inhibit accurate evaluation of heart and breath sounds.

▶ **Keep the infant warm during examination.** After the infant is undressed, preventing heat loss is crucial to the infant's comfort and to maintaining a normal temperature and glucose homeostasis. The undressed infant is examined in a warm environment with an external heat source, such as an overhead radiant warmer. To keep from startling the newborn and to maintain a stable metabolic status, warm the stethoscope and, especially, your hands.

▶ **Have the necessary tools at hand.** A stethoscope, an ophthalmoscope, and a tape measure are used in all newborn examinations. Having them ready saves time.

▶ **Calm the infant before beginning the exam.** A quiet infant provides the best opportunity for data gathering. If a crying infant must be examined, patience—and possibly the aid of a second person to help calm the infant—is required.

▶ **Handle the infant gently.** The newly born infant is amazingly cooperative when the examiner is gentle. A soothing voice and a soft touch often allow the examiner to complete the entire physical assessment without disturbing the infant greatly or at all. Parents enjoy watching their infant interact with the examiner and appreciate the gentleness of touch. Certain portions of the examination cause the infant more distress than others. Examination of the hips is usually the most disturbing part of the exam; it is therefore performed last.

▶ **Complete the exam.** Re-dress the infant to maintain a normal temperature. Notify the primary caregiver that the exam is over and of any abnormalities that were found or observations that need to be made.

A SAMPLE APPROACH

One method of organizing the examination of the newborn is described here as a guide for the inexperienced examiner. As mentioned earlier, with practice, each examiner develops a personal style. It is assumed that the infant is unclothed and supine under a radiant warmer.

OBSERVATION

It can be very difficult for a practitioner to just stand at the crib and observe an infant. The immediate inclination is to touch and talk to the infant. This natural response must be repressed until later in the examination, however, because observation alone produces important information about every organ system. These initial observations allow the practitioner to develop a visual differential diagnosis before employing other assessment techniques (auscultation, palpation). Table 1-1 catalogs the many observations the skilled examiner must process in this initial assessment of the infant's status.

If these multiple observations prove normal, the examiner is less likely to find a significant abnormality upon auscultation and palpation. Each observation of normality serves to reassure the examiner—just as an observation of abnormality should heighten the examiner's suspicion that further inspection is necessary.

Observation is not an isolated technique for use only at the outset of the exam. Although it is important to spend a moment or two observing the infant at the bedside before touching him, observation of the infant's responses takes place throughout the exam. Depending on the infant's state and responses, all the observations listed in Table 1-1 can be made during the hands-on examination. The examiner must learn to take advantage of every opportunity the infant's behavior offers for observation. If, for example, the infant awakens spontaneously during the exam, the examiner should take advantage of that opportunity to examine the eyes.

AUSCULTATION

After observing the infant closely, many examiners next auscultate the lungs, heart, and abdomen. To separate the sounds of the heart from those of the lungs, it is important to concentrate. Listen first to one type of sound, then to the other. For example, listen first to the heart—its rate, rhythm, regularity, and any added sounds. Then listen to breath sounds, ignoring the cardiac sounds.

PALPATION

The exam continues with palpation. Palpating certain parts of the body disturbs the infant more than palpating others. An ordered approach keeps the infant calm through much of the process.

Because femoral pulses are difficult to assess in a crying infant, palpate them first. Then palpate the brachial pulses. Next palpate the abdomen, beginning with the more superficial liver and spleen. (Learning to palpate the liver and spleen with the tips of the fingers as well as with the lateral edges of the index fingers facilitates examination from either side of the bassinet.) Palpate for abdominal masses; then use deeper palpation for the kidneys. At this point, the infant may be disturbed and crying, but this will not impede the remainder of the exam.

HEAD-TO-TOE EXAMINATION

After palpation, the examiner may then assess the infant from head to toe, examining the head and neck, upper extremities, genitalia, lower extremities and back in sequence. This hands-on inspection also includes measurements and tactile examination of the skin. Maneuvers to assess symmetry and reflexes are also done.

THE INTEGRATED EXAM

The skilled examiner integrates examination tasks. For example, after palpating the head, neck, clavicles, arms, and hands, the examiner can perform the pull-to-sit maneuver to assess palmar grasp, arm strength, and tone. At that point, the infant is being held in an appropriate position to elicit the Moro reflex. Genitalia can be examined next, before progressing to the lower extremities. While the infant is positioned prone on the practitioner's hand to assess truncal tone and the truncal incurvation reflex, the back can also be examined. These shortcuts facilitate multiple inspections and save time. The hips should be examined last because this procedure causes the most stress to the infant.

It is usually not necessary to assess reflexes as a separate step. The examiner will likely have observed root and suck by this point. Moro and palmar grasp can be incorporated into the upper-extremity exam, as just explained.

Although an extremely cooperative infant may sleep through the entire exam, the assessment is not complete until the infant has been observed through the various behavioral states. Facial asymmetry, for example, cannot be seen until the infant cries.

Ideally, the parents should observe the first complete examination. Parents appreciate demonstration of their infant's normality and uniqueness as well as early identification of unusual or abnormal findings.

EQUIPMENT

OPHTHALMOSCOPE

In addition to developing hands-on confidence with the newborn and with performing the exam in the parents' presence, the student must become proficient with what may be unfamiliar equipment. Facility with the tools reduces stress to both infant and examiner. Again, practice is the key.

If the ophthalmoscope is not already assembled, attach the head of the device to the handle by pushing the head toward the handle and turning the head clockwise. To turn the ophthalmoscope on, depress the on/off button, usually on the neck of the handle, at the same time turning the button clockwise. To gain familiarity with the various apertures, rotate the aperture selection dial and project the light onto the palm of the hand or a piece of paper. The small and the large round beams are the two apertures used to assess the gemini choroidal light reflex (referred to as the *red reflex)* and pupillary response in newborns. The lens selector compensates for the visual acuity of the individual examiner. Adjust the lens selector dial to bring the structure being examined into focus.[2]

Examination of the undilated eye of the newborn includes assessment of pupillary constriction and the red reflex. The most opportune time to examine a newborn's eyes is when the infant is in the quiet alert state. An infant who is in light sleep will often open the eyes if the room is darkened. To examine the infant's eyes, hold the ophthalmoscope in the right hand, with the viewing aperture as close as possible to the right eye, and use the right index finger to turn the lens selector dial to the appropriate lens for proper focus. While positioning the infant's head with the free hand, align the illuminating light along the infant's visual plane. If both the infant's eyes are open, the Bruckner test, a simultaneous bilateral red reflex test, may be performed. When using the large full spot and holding the ophthalmoscope 18 to 20 inches (45 to 50 cm) from the infant's face, the light circle from the spot will cover both eyes. The examiner assesses symmetry and brightness of the red reflex as well as pupillary constriction.[3,4] The red reflex appears as a homogenous bright red-orange color. Any opacity along the central optical pathway will block all or part of the red reflex. Note that in infants with dark pigmentation, the reflex appears pale or cloudy rather than red.[3] Use the ophthalmoscope to observe pupillary constriction after assessing the red reflex.

STETHOSCOPE

The acoustical stethoscope excludes environmental sounds, making it easier for the examiner to hear sounds coming from the infant; it does not magnify these sounds. The earpieces and connecting binaurals should be angled toward the wearer's nose to project sound onto the examiner's tympanic membrane. To minimize sound distortion, the tubing should be no longer than 12 inches. The chest piece of the stethoscope often has a double head: a flat, closed diaphragm and an open bell. The diaphragm is used to assess high-frequency sounds and the bell, low frequency. Use the diaphragm to assess breath sounds by applying it firmly to the infant's skin so that it moves with the chest wall. Both the diaphragm and the bell are used to assess heart sounds.[4] Do not compress the bell against the chest so firmly that it fills with tissue and acts like a diaphragm (Chapters 6 and 7).

OTOSCOPE

The infant's ears should be assessed for size, shape, and placement. The external auditory canals are examined for patency. Otoscopic examination is not normally done in the newborn period because the ear canals are often filled with vernix. For that reason, use of the otoscope is not described here.

SUMMARY

Each newborn examination is as different as each infant. This text explains basic techniques for examining each body system—to guide examiners with limited experience in performing a thorough newborn physical assessment. It is only through experience, however, that practitioners develop clinical expertise. As their experience and confidence grow, most examiners develop their own unique approach to physical examination, along with the flexibility to adapt their approach to different situations. As long as the necessary equipment is available and basic principles are kept in mind, an infant can be examined in any setting.

REFERENCES

1. Nightingale F. 1969. *Notes on Nursing: What It Is and What It Is Not.* New York: Dover, 112–113.
2. Seidel HM, et al. 2005. *Mosby's Guide to Physical Examination,* 6th ed. Philadelphia: Mosby, 71–72.
3. Wright KW. 1999. *Pediatric Ophthalmology for Pediatricians.* Philadelphia: Lippincott Williams & Wilkins, 36.
4. Fletcher MA. 1998. *Physical Diagnosis in Neonatology.* Philadelphia: Lippincott Williams & Wilkins, 250, 341.

BIBLIOGRAPHY

- Bickley LS, and Szilagyi PG. 2007. *Bates' Guide to Physical Examination and History Taking,* 9th ed. Philadelphia: Lippincott Williams & Wilkins.
- Malasanos L, et al. 1990. *Health Assessment,* 4th ed. Philadelphia: Mosby.
- Orient JM. 2005. *Art and Science of Bedside Diagnosis,* 3rd ed. Philadelphia: Lippincott Williams & Wilkins.
- Scanlon JW, et al. 1979. *System of Newborn Physical Examination.* Philadelphia: Lippincott Williams & Wilkins.
- Vaughan D, Asbury T, and Tabbara KF. 2008. *Vaughn and Asbury's General Ophthalmology,* 17th ed. New York: McGraw-Hill.
- Wong DL, et al. 2005. *Maternal Child Nursing Care,* 3rd ed. Philadelphia: Mosby.

NOTES

2 Recording and Evaluating the Neonatal History

Kimberly Horns LaBronte, PhD, RN, NNP-BC

A comprehensive physical examination of the newborn, performed no later than 18 hours after birth by the physician, nurse practitioner, or physician's assistant, is a standard of perinatal care.[1] This applies to normal newborns; the high-risk newborn, however, requires an early and comprehensive history. Ideally, much of the history can be taken prior to the infant's impending birth. The physical examination must be preceded by a thorough review of the history of the current pregnancy; past obstetric history; intrapartum history; maternal medical, family medical, and social histories; and immediate neonatal adaptation history.[2] It is recommended that admitting nursery personnel evaluate the neonate's status and assess risks through a review of the history documented in the antepartum and intrapartum records no later than 2 hours after birth.[1]

Assessment is the gathering of accurate, detailed data, and it includes four components: (1) reviewing the history, (2) reviewing the results of the physical examination, (3) reviewing available laboratory or other data, and (4) formulating an impression (diagnostic differential). The practitioner then develops a plan of care and evaluates the newborn for actual or potential problems.

IMPORTANCE OF THE HISTORY

A comprehensive history is the prerequisite for adequate assessment. The newly born infant is a unique patient; no thorough history has ever been developed for this patient. When a newborn physical examination is performed without knowledge of the complete history, the information necessary for accurate formulation of an impression may be inadequate or incorrect.

The significance of the initial history and its thorough communication to the neonatal health care providers cannot be overstated. The newly born infant's history originates from the maternal records, but leads up to the individual neonate's transitional experience and plan of care. Commonly, the neonatal health care provider relies on a comprehensive maternal history. However, written, faxed, or electronic information may be incomplete. The salient pertinent negatives and pertinent positives of a neonatal history are extremely important to developing your initial impression (diagnostic differentials).

Knowledge of the history can also be useful in allaying parental anxiety when performing the initial physical examination. A mother whose ultrasound at 20 weeks revealed the possibility of her fetus having a fluid-filled gastrointestinal (GI) mass but whose subsequent ultrasounds appeared to be normal is likely to have an increased level of concern about the status of her neonate's GI tract. Knowledge of this pertinent history allows the examiner to emphasize the normal GI findings, discuss the history of the positive ultrasound findings, and reassure the parents.

The history also alerts the examiner to potential or suspected problems and may indicate the need for more frequent repeat examinations. A cardiac murmur in a neonate with a history of maternal anticonvulsant use throughout pregnancy is of more concern than a murmur in a neonate with a negative history. Embryonic exposure to maternal anticonvulsant therapy increases the risk for structural, congenital cardiac malformations.[3]

The history provides the context in which neonates with identified problems and disorders must be analyzed. Lack of a history or an incomplete history can lead to more extensive testing than would otherwise be necessary or to an incorrect impression or diagnosis. The following case exemplifies the need for obtaining an accurate history.

Baby J, a 36-week gestational age, 3 kg neonate, was admitted to the nursery at 1 AM following vaginal delivery to a 34-year-old, gravida 4, para 3 mother with a history of preeclampsia. His Apgar scores were 7 and 8 at one and five minutes, respectively. His admission was uneventful; his physical examination revealed slightly decreased tone and spontaneous activity. Reevaluation at one and two hours of life revealed continued poor tone and decreased spontaneous activity, with no other abnormal findings on the physical examination. At two and a half hours of life, apnea was noted. After being notified, the on-call health care provider requested that blood for a complete blood count and C-reactive protein level be drawn. On the neonate's next

examination, the findings were consistent with decreased tone and activity. Blood and spinal fluid were obtained for culture and sensitivity, and antibiotic therapy begun. The maternal chart with antepartum and intrapartum history was subsequently delivered to the nursery; it revealed that the mother had received magnesium sulfate. The neonate's magnesium level was obtained and found to be elevated. Review of the history would have given a more accurate context in which to view this infant's poor tone and activity and would have led to an earlier identification of hypermagnesemia, perhaps avoiding unnecessary testing.

THE SUPPLEMENTAL INTERVIEW

Sometimes the mother, or both parents, may need to be interviewed for information not found in the records. Before approaching the parents, review all available medical records and identify the specific information needed. Remember that the first contact with the mother or parents is one of the most important contacts. Introducing yourself and defining the reason for your questions will facilitate your interview. Be sure the parent(s) is comfortable, and maintain a normal conversational distance. Asking what name has been chosen for the baby helps establish a friendly atmosphere.

It is important to make and maintain eye contact and to present questions without reading them. Allow time for the mother to respond to your questions without interrupting her or checking your watch or the clock. Avoid technical language and the tendency to overexplain or lecture as much as possible. If you must take notes, make them brief. Copious note taking detracts from your listening and observing abilities and may be intimidating.[4] Be an active listener: Show that you understand the responses, and request clarification if appropriate. Periodically or at the end of the interview, summarize what you have been told. Evaluate answers to questions for content—what was said—and also for affect or tone—how it was said. A parent who avoids answering a question or answers incompletely may be embarrassed or upset by the question or perceive that the questions are socially or criminally incriminating (such as in a drug history interview).[5] When giving the parents information about the neonate's health status, have them repeat at the end of the interview what they believe the neonate's health status or problems to be so you can clarify any misunderstandings immediately.

ELEMENTS OF A COMPLETE HISTORY

The historic information gathered must then be organized and presented in a systematic format commonly used by other professionals. The history may be hastily presented by health care providers when physical care of the infant is warranted. The physical care of a newly born infant in transition often becomes the priority; however, the comprehensive history is equally important. This is especially true when infants are transported from one institution to another. The comprehensive history is imperative in these situations, and identification of potential problems during and after transport is the common goal. All pertinent information must be included. Elements of a complete history start with the identifying data, followed by the chief complaint, and then the interim history of the neonate or the history of the presenting problem or illness if one exists. This is followed by the antepartum history; obstetric history; intrapartum history; and the maternal medical, family medical, and social histories. In some institutions, these data may be recorded by electronic medical record; in others, a written or dictated history is documented. After the history is compiled, the physical examination data are recorded, followed by any laboratory or radiology studies

obtained. An impression and diagnostic differential of the neonate are then formulated, and a plan for care is outlined.

IDENTIFYING DATA

The identifying data are the patient's name, birth date, and referral source. Both the referring obstetric care provider and the primary care pediatric provider should be listed so that they will receive a copy of the admission history and physical examination. If the patient is admitted to the neonatal intensive care unit, telephone numbers for the primary care providers should be included so that they can receive updates on the neonate's problems and progress. If the patient is transferred in from another facility for care, the name of the referring health care facility should also be included.

CHIEF COMPLAINT

The chief complaint in a neonate is often simply the identification including age, sex, birth and current weights (if greater than one day of age), gestational age by dates and examination, and any presenting clinical signs the infant exhibits. In the normal newborn, the chief complaint might simply be stated as: "3 kg female, 41 weeks gestation by dates, appropriate for gestational age, now 2 hours of age." Or it may include identified problems, as in the following example:

1. 2.5 kg male, 42 weeks gestation by dates, small for gestational age, 3 hours of age
2. Hypoglycemia
3. Tachypnea: Pneumonia versus retained lung fluid
4. Suspected perinatal sepsis

INTERIM HISTORY

The interim history or history of present illness chronologically records the neonate's history from the time of delivery until the present time and, in the well newborn, should include data regarding temperature stabilization, feeding, voiding, stooling, and behavioral adaptation. In the neonate with identified problems, the sequence of the newborn's problem or problems is discussed, as are laboratory or x-ray findings, interventions, and responses to treatment. The age of the mother, type of delivery, neonate's birth weight and current weight, and Apgar scores are sometimes also included to give a more comprehensive picture. Interim histories are often developed and documented when an infant is hospitalized for an extended length of time. A monthly interim history may be helpful in summarizing and developing the final discharge history and physical for a complicated or extremely premature infant.

ANTEPARTUM HISTORY

The antepartum history includes more specific historical data on the pregnancy: maternal age, gravidity, and parity; last menstrual period; and estimated date of confinement or delivery (EDD). The EDD may be revised after serial ultrasound evaluation. The date and gestational age at which prenatal care began, who provided the care, and the number of prenatal visits are recorded. Medical complications and high-risk pregnancy factors (Table 2-1), treatments, and monitoring are recorded. The antepartum history should also include information about exposure of the fetus to radiation; over-the-counter, prescribed, or illicit drugs; and tobacco and alcohol (Table 2-2).

When reviewing the history of the antepartum period, the examiner should note the results of all tests performed on the mother and/or fetus and understand their implications. Usual prenatal screenings may include the following tests: maternal blood type and Rh; antibody screen; serology; VDRL (venereal disease research laboratory) status; rubella immunity testing; cultures for Gonococcus, Chlamydia, and Group B Streptococcus; hepatitis B surface antigen

screening; α-fetoprotein; human immunodeficiency virus (HIV) testing; triple/quadruple screening; and ultrasound. Women with specific high-risk factors for tuberculosis are tested. HIV antibody screening is now universally recommended in prenatal care.[6] Those who acquire HIV infection during pregnancy require more extensive evaluation.[6] Abnormal findings on routine screening tests will prompt follow-up or specialized screenings. A schedule for routine general laboratory examinations during pregnancy appears in Table 2-3. Indications for antepartum fetal assessment are listed in Table 2-4. Appendix A: Antepartum Tests and Intrapartum Monitoring, explains many of the routine and some specialized antepartum screenings and also indicates what the results mean.

OBSTETRIC HISTORY

The mother's obstetric history is reviewed for the number of pregnancies, abortions, stillbirths, living children, types of deliveries, dates of birth or abortion, birth weights, and gestational ages at birth. Particular attention should be paid to serial ultrasound findings, biophysical profiles, and any nonstress or contraction stress tests. Any neonatal problems, previous premature births, or subsequent major medical problems of prior children should be noted. The present age and health status of living children are recorded. If any child is deceased, the cause and date of death are included.

INTRAPARTUM HISTORY

The intrapartum history is evaluated for duration of labor, whether the labor was spontaneous or induced, medications and anesthetics used during labor and delivery, length of the first and second stages of labor, type of delivery, and whether delivery was spontaneous or required forceps or vacuum assistance. The time and duration of rupture of membranes, the use of amnioinfusion, and the status of the

TABLE 2-1 ▲ Categorization of High-Risk Pregnancy Factors

Socioeconomic Factors
1. Inadequate finances
2. Poor housing
3. Severe social problems
4. Unwed, especially adolescent
5. Minority status
6. Nutritional deprivation
7. Parental occupation

Demographic Factors
1. Maternal age under 16 or over 35 years
2. Overweight or underweight prior to pregnancy
3. Height less than 5 feet
4. Maternal education less than 11 years
5. Family history of severe inherited disorders

Medical Factors

A. Obstetric History
1. Infertility
2. Ectopic pregnancy or spontaneous abortion
3. Grand multiparity
4. Stillborn or neonatal death
5. Uterine/cervical abnormality
6. Multiple gestation
7. Premature labor/delivery
8. Prolonged labor
9. Cesarean section
10. Low birth weight infant
11. Macrosomic infant
12. Midforceps delivery
13. Baby with neurologic deficit, birth injury, or malformation
14. Hydatidiform mole or choriocarcinoma

B. Maternal Medical History/Status
1. Cardiac disease
2. Pulmonary disease
3. Metabolic disease—particularly, diabetes mellitus, thyroid disease
4. Chronic renal disease, repeated urinary tract infections, repeated bacteriuria
5. Gastrointestinal disease
6. Endocrine disorders (pituitary, adrenal)
7. Chronic hypertension
8. Hemoglobinopathies
9. Seizure disorder
10. Venereal and other infectious diseases
11. Weight loss greater than 5 pounds
12. Malignancy
13. Surgery during pregnancy
14. Major congenital anomalies of the reproductive tract
15. Mental retardation, major emotional disorders

C. Current Maternal Obstetric Status
1. Late or no prenatal care
2. Rh sensitization
3. Fetus inappropriately large or small for gestational age
4. Premature labor
5. Pregnancy-induced hypertension
6. Multiple gestation
7. Polyhydramnios
8. Premature or prolonged rupture of membranes
9. Antepartum bleeding
   a. Placenta previa
   b. *Abruptio placentae*
10. Abnormal presentation
11. Postmaturity
12. Abnormality in tests for fetal well-being
13. Anemia

D. Habits
1. Smoking during pregnancy
2. Regular alcohol intake
3. Drug use/abuse

From: Aumann GM, and Baird MM. 1993. Risk assessment for pregnant women. In *High-Risk Pregnancy: A Team Approach*, Knuppel RA, and Drukker JE, eds. Philadelphia: Saunders, 23. Reprinted by permission.

amniotic fluid volume and presence or absence of meconium are ascertained. Laboratory and monitoring data obtained during labor are reviewed and noted, as are any maternal complications that occurred during this period (such as fever, bleeding, or hypertension) and the treatment provided. The presentation of the neonate at delivery, the Apgar scores, any resuscitative interventions performed, and the response to resuscitation are documented. If resuscitation is required, the timing of the interventions is equally important.

MATERNAL MEDICAL HISTORY

The maternal medical history is reviewed for chronic health problems and for diseases or

TABLE 2-2 ▲ Maternal Medications and Toxins: Possible Effects on the Fetus and/or Newborn

Medication/Toxin	Possible Effect on Fetus/Newborn
Analgesics and Anti-inflammatories	
Aspirin	Hemorrhage, premature closure of ductus arteriosus, pulmonary artery hypertension
Codeine	Neonatal drug withdrawal reported
Ibuprofen	Reduced amniotic fluid volume when used in tocolysis, theoretic risk for premature ductus arteriosus closure
Indomethacin	Closure of fetal ductus arteriosus, pulmonary artery hypertension
Meperidine	Respiratory depression peaks 2–3 hours after maternal dose
Propoxyphene	Drug withdrawal reported, possible increased risk of anomalies
Anesthetics	
General anesthesia	Respiratory depression of infant at delivery if anesthesia is prolonged before delivery
Lidocaine	High fetal serum levels cause central nervous system depression, accidental direct injection into fetal head causes seizures
Antibiotics	
Aminoglycosides	Ototoxicity reported after first trimester use of kanamycin and streptomycin
Streptomycin	Damage to the eighth cranial nerve, hearing loss
Vancomycin	Potential for ototoxicity
Cephalosporins	Some drugs in this group displace bilirubin from albumin
Isoniazid	Risk for folate deficiency
Metronidazole	Potential teratogen
Sulfonamides	Some drugs in this group displace bilirubin from albumin
Tetracycline	Yellow-brown staining and caries of teeth
Trimethoprim	Folate antagonism
Anticoagulants	
Warfarin (Coumadin)	Warfarin embryopathy
Anticonvulsants	
Carbamazepine	Neural tube defects, midfacial hypoplasia
Phenobarbital	Withdrawal symptoms, hemorrhagic disease
Phenytoin	Hemorrhagic disease, fetal hydantoin syndrome
Trimethadione	Fetal trimethadione syndrome, cleft lip and palate, cardiac and genital anomalies
Valproic acid	Myelomeningocele, facial and cardiac anomalies
Antineoplastics	
Aminopterin	Cleft palate, hydrocephalus, myelomeningocele, growth restriction
Cyclophosphamide	Growth restriction, cardiovascular and digital anomalies
Methotrexate	Absent digits
Antithyroid Drugs	
Iodide-containing drugs	Hypothyroidism
Methimazole	Hypothyroidism, cutis aplasia
Propylthiouracil	Hypothyroidism
Antivirals	
Acyclovir	No known adverse effects reported
Ribavirin	Teratogenic and embryolethal in animals
Zidovudine	Potential fetal bone marrow suppression, reduces perinatal HIV transmission

(continued on next page)

TABLE 2-2 ▲ Maternal Medications and Toxins: Possible Effects on the Fetus and/or Newborn (continued)

Medication/Toxin	Possible Effect on Fetus/Newborn
Cardiovascular Drugs and Antihypertensives	
Angiotensin-converting enzyme inhibitors	Neonatal bradycardia, hypoglycemia
β-blockers (propranolol)	Neonatal bradycardia, hypoglycemia
Calcium channel blockers	If maternal hypotension occurs, could affect placental blood flow
Diazoxide	Hyperglycemia
Digoxin	Fetal toxicity with maternal overdose
Hydralazine	Maternal hypotensive risk with possible effect on placental blood flow
Methyldopa	Mild, clinically insignificant decrease in neonatal blood pressure
Diuretics	
Furosemide	Increases fetal urinary sodium and potassium
Thiazides	Thrombocytopenia
Hormonal Drugs	
Androgenics (danazol)	Masculinization of female fetus
Corticosteroids	Cleft palate reported in animals
Diethylstilbestrol (DES)	DES daughters: genital tract anomalies, increased rate of premature delivery
	DES sons: possible increase in genitourinary anomalies
Estrogens, progestins	Uncertain teratogenic potential, virilization of female fetuses reported with progestins
Tamoxifen	DES-like effect in animal studies
Sedatives, Tranquilizers, and Psychiatric Drugs	
Barbiturates (short-acting)	Theoretic risk for hemorrhage and drug withdrawal
Benzodiazepines	Hypotonia, impaired thermoregulation
Lithium	Cardiac anomalies (Ebstein's), diabetes insipidus, thyroid depression, cardiovascular dysfunction
Thalidomide	Limb reduction and other anomalies
Tricyclic antidepressants	Association with limb reduction defects (causation unproven)
Tocolytics	
Magnesium sulfate	Respiratory depression, hypermagnesemia
Ritodrine	Neonatal hypoglycemia
Terbutaline	Neonatal hypoglycemia
Vitamins and Related Drugs	
A	Excessive doses are teratogenic
D	Megadoses may cause hypercalcemia
Isotretinoin	Ear, cardiac, central nervous system, and thymic anomalies
Menadione (vitamin K_3)	Hyperbilirubinemia and kernicterus at high doses
Miscellaneous	
Antiemetics	Doxylamine succinate and/or dicyclomine hydrochloride with pyridoxine hydrochloride reported to be a teratogen (unproven)
Irradiation	Fetal death, microcephaly, growth restriction
Methyl mercury	Mental retardation, microcephaly
Oral hypoglycemics	Neonatal hypoglycemia

(continued on next page)

TABLE 2-2 ▲ Maternal Medications and Toxins: Possible Effects on the Fetus and/or Newborn (continued)

Medication/Toxin	Possible Effect on Fetus/Newborn
Social and Illicit Drugs	
Alcohol	Fetal alcohol syndrome or effects
Amphetamines	Withdrawal, prematurity, decreased birth weight and head circumference
Cocaine	Decreased birth weight; microcephaly; prematurity; abruptio placentae with possible asphyxia, shock, cerebral hemorrhage, stillbirth
Heroin	Increased incidence of low birth weight and small for gestational age, drug withdrawal, impaired postnatal growth, behavioral disturbances
Marijuana	Decreased fetal growth and increased incidence of acute nonlymphoblastic leukemia in childhood
Methadone	Increased birth weight as compared to heroin, drug withdrawal (worse than with heroin alone)
Phencyclidine (PCP)	Irritability, jitteriness, hypertonia, poor feeding
Tobacco smoking	Decreases birth weight by 175–250 g; increased prematurity rate; increased premature rupture of membranes, placental abruption, and placenta previa; increased fetal death

Adapted from: D'Harlingue AE, and Durand DJ. 2001. Recognition, stabilization, and transport of the high-risk newborn. In *Care of the High-Risk Neonate,* 4th ed., Klaus M, and Fanaroff A., eds. Philadelphia: Saunders, 69–71. Reprinted by permission.

TABLE 2-3 ▲ Recommended Intervals for Routine and Specialized Antepartum Tests

Time (weeks)	Assessment
Initial (as early as possible)	Hemoglobin or hematocrit measurement Urinalysis, including microscope examination and infection screen, measurement of glucose and protein Blood group and Rh type determinations Antibody screen Rubella antibody titer measurement Syphilis screen Cervical cytology—PAP test Hepatitis B surface antigen HIV counseling/testing
Optional labs	Hemoglobin electrophoresis Purified protein derivative (PPD) Chlamydia Gonococcus Tay Sachs/other testing as indicated by history Hepatitis C testing when/if history suggests increased risk
8–20 (depending on test and maternal/fetal history)	Ultrasound Maternal serum α-fetoprotein Amniocentesis Chorionic villus sampling—karyotype, amniotic fluid α-fetoprotein
24–28	Diabetes screening Glucose tolerance testing if diabetes screen abnormal Repeat hemoglobin or hematocrit measurement Repeat antibody test for unsensitized Rh-negative patients
28	Prophylactic administration of Rho(D) immune globulin as indicated
32–36 (when indicated)	Ultrasound Testing for sexually transmitted disease Repeat hemoglobin or hematocrit measurement recommended Group B Streptococcus culture at 35–37 weeks

Adapted from: American Academy of Pediatrics, American College of Obstetricians and Gynecologists. 2007. *Guidelines for Perinatal Care,* 6th ed. Elk Grove Village, Illinois: American Academy of Pediatrics.

disorders treated in the past and/or during the pregnancy. Potential consequences of maternal medical problems for the fetus and/or newborn are listed in Table 2-5. Infections past, present, and during the pregnancy as well as surgical procedures and hospitalizations that occurred before or during the pregnancy are included. Counseling for psychological or social problems should also be noted. Medication use including herbal supplements and over-the-counter preparations for nonpregnancy-related health or medical problems should be explored.

FAMILY MEDICAL HISTORY

The family medical history is reviewed for ages of the infant's mother, father, and siblings; sexes of the other children; and any diagnosed chronic disorders, disabilities, or known hereditary diseases. A genetic history may be required if the neonate is dysmorphic, and further information should be sought regarding other family members affected with a similar disorder. Information about familial disease or disorders can be elicited by asking if anyone else in the immediate or extended family has the same or a related problem or if any relative has a genetic abnormality or an unusual disease or disorder. A finding such as a head circumference several standard deviations above normal with normal weight and length percentiles may raise the possibility of an intracranial abnormality. Review of the family history should include questions regarding any similar finding in the baby's parents when they were children. A grandparent can often provide or confirm this information. The most common cause of a large head in an otherwise normal newborn is benign familial megalencephaly, and one of the parents, usually the father, generally had the same finding in infancy.[7] Preparation of a genetic pedigree chart (Figure 2-1) often helps clarify the relationships of affected family members when the history is positive for similar findings in relatives. The question of

TABLE 2-4 ▲ Maternal and Fetal Indications for Antepartum Fetal Assessment

Chronic hypertension
Pregnancy-induced hypertension
Chronic renal disease
Insulin-dependent diabetes mellitus
Maternal cyanotic congenital heart disease
Rh or other isoimmunization
Homozygous hemoglobinopathies
Maternal abuse of tobacco, alcohol, or drugs
Previous unexplained stillbirth
Hydramnios, oligohydramnios
Decreased fetal movement
Multiple gestation
Premature rupture of membranes
Third-trimester bleeding
Sickle cell anemia
Maternal collagen vascular diseases
Fetal growth restriction
Fetal postmaturity

Adapted from: Gerber SE. 2006. Estimation of fetal well-being. Part 1: Antepartum fetal surveillance. In *Neonatal-Perinatal Medicine: Diseases of the Fetus and Infant,* 8th ed., Martin RJ, Fanaroff AA, and Walsh MC, eds. Philadelphia: Mosby, 167. Reprinted by permission.

consanguinity (mating of individuals related by blood) can be posed by asking the parents if they are related in any way besides by marriage and if there is anyone in the family who was related to both parents before their marriage.

SOCIAL HISTORY

The social history includes the mother's marital status, presence or support of the infant's father, and both parents' occupations and educations. The family's sources of support in the financial, housing, and care areas are noted. The family's religious affiliation and cultural heritage are included. The family unit should be defined, along with the number of people, family and nonfamily, living in the home. The health status of all household members should also be ascertained. Support

TABLE 2-5 ▲ Potential Effects of Maternal Medical Conditions on the Fetus and/or Newborn

Maternal Condition	Potential Fetal/Neonatal Effects
Cardiopulmonary	
Asthma	Increased rates of prematurity, toxemia, and perinatal loss
Congenital heart disease	Effects of cardiovascular drugs (see Table 2-2)
Cystic fibrosis	Prematurity, IUGR, fetal loss
Hypertension, preeclampsia	Premature delivery caused by uncontrolled hypertension or eclampsia; uteroplacental insufficiency, abruptio placentae, fetal loss; IUGR; thrombocytopenia; neutropenia
Endocrine/Metabolic	
Diabetes mellitus	Hypoglycemia, hypocalcemia, macrosomia, polycythemia, hyperbilirubinemia, increased risk for birth defects, birth trauma, small left colon syndrome, cardiomyopathy, RDS
Hypoparathyroidism	Fetal hypocalcemia, neonatal hyperparathyroidism
Hyperparathyroidism	Neonatal hypocalcemia and hypoparathyroidism
Hyperthyroidism (Grave's disease)	Fetal and neonatal hyperthyroidism, IUGR, prematurity, congestive heart failure, tachycardia
Obesity	Macrosomia, birth trauma
Phenylketonuria (untreated pregnancies)	Mental retardation, microcephaly, congenital heart defects
Hematologic	
Fetal platelet antigen sensitization	Thrombocytopenia, CNS hemorrhage
Idiopathic thrombo-cytopenia purpura	Reduced iron stores, lower mental and developmental scores at follow up
Iron deficiency anemia	Potential teratogen
Rh or ABO sensitization	Jaundice, anemia, hydrops fetalis
Severe anemia (hemoglobin <6 mg/dL)	Impaired oxygen delivery, fetal loss
Sickle cell anemia	Increased prematurity, IUGR, fetal distress
Infections	
Chlamydia	Conjunctivitis, pneumonia
Chorioamnionitis	Increased risk for neonatal sepsis, premature labor and delivery
Cytomegalovirus	IUGR, microcephaly, cytomegalovirus inclusion disease, hearing loss
Gonorrhea	Ophthalmia neonatorum
Hepatitis A	Perinatal transmission
Hepatitis B	Perinatal transmission, chronic hepatitis
Hepatitis C	Perinatal transmission, chronic hepatitis
Herpes simplex	Encephalitis, disseminated herpes (risk of neonatal disease is much higher when maternal infection is primary rather than recurrent)
HIV	Risk of infectious transmission
Rubella	Rubella embryopathy, cataracts, cardiac defects
Syphilis	Congenital syphilis, IUGR
Toxoplasmosis	IUGR, microcephaly, hydrocephalus, chorioretinitis, myocarditis
Tuberculosis	Perinatal and postnatal transmission
Varicella	Congenital varicella syndrome, rash, pneumonia, myocarditis, encephalitis

(continued on next page)

TABLE 2-5 ▲ Potential Effects of Maternal Medical Conditions on the Fetus and/or Newborn (continued)

Maternal Condition	Potential Fetal/Neonatal Effects
Inflammatory/Immunologic	
Inflammatory bowel disease	Increase in prematurity, fetal loss, fetal and neonatal growth restriction
Systemic lupus erythematosus	Fetal death, spontaneous abortion, heart block, neonatal lupus, thrombocytopenia, neutropenia, hemolytic anemia, endocardial fibrosis
Neuromuscular	
Maternal seizure disorder requiring anticonvulsants	Teratogenic effects of medications (see Table 2-2)
Myasthenia gravis	Transient neonatal myasthenia, preterm delivery
Myotonic dystrophy	Neonatal myotonic dystrophy
Seizure during pregnancy	Fetal hypoxia
Renal/Urologic	
Chronic renal failure	Prematurity, IUGR, fetal loss
Transplant recipients	Prematurity, IUGR, possible effects of maternal immunosuppressive therapy, and mineral disorders
Urinary tract infection	Prematurity

CNS = Central nervous system

IUGR = Intrauterine growth restriction

RDS = Respiratory distress syndrome

Adapted from: D'Harlingue AE, and Durand D. 2001. Recognition, stabilization, and transport of the high-risk newborn. In *Care of the High-Risk Neonate,* 5th ed., Klaus M, and Fanaroff A., eds. Philadelphia: Saunders, 65. (Compiled from: Creasy RK, and Resnik R. 1999. *Maternal-Fetal Medicine: Principles and Practice,* 4th ed. Philadelphia: Saunders; Barron WM, and Lindheimer MD, eds. 1985. Symposium on medical disorders during pregnancy. *Clinics in Perinatology* 12[3]: 479–713; and Cotton DB, ed. 1986. Critical care in obstetrics. *Clinics in Perinatology* 13[4]: 695–868.) Reprinted by permission.

FIGURE 2-1 ▲ Genetic pedigree chart.

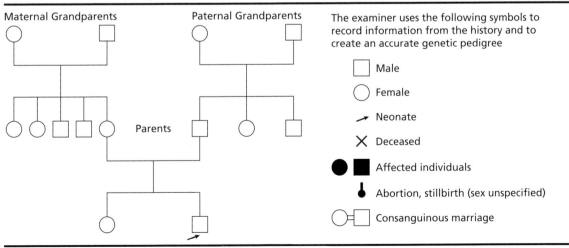

agencies with which the family is now working and the family's current social service contacts are important. Members of the family or others who are planning to help with child care after discharge are included. If and when the mother plans to return to work and what arrangements for infant care are planned should be elicited. Information regarding frequent or recent family moves, deaths in the family, and job changes also gives an idea of the stressors affecting the family. This information will assist the practitioner in planning for necessary services following discharge or can point to the need for referral to social services.

REMAINING ELEMENTS

The physical examination is performed and recorded. Laboratory or radiology data that have been obtained should be noted. An assessment or impression of the infant's status is then made, including a statement of suspected or potential problems. Here is an example for an infant with problems:

1. 3.8 kg preterm female, 35 weeks gestation, born by cesarean section, large for gestational age, infant of a diabetic mother, now 4 hours of age
2. Hypoglycemia
3. Respiratory distress: tachypnea
4. Systolic cardiac murmur at upper left sternal border

An assessment statement for a well newborn with no complications might be similar to this one:

1. 3.5 kg term male, appropriate for gestational age, 4 hours of age
2. Teenage mother with little social support

A plan addressing each of the identified problems should then be written.

SUMMARY

A thorough approach to history exploration, coupled with analysis of antepartum and intrapartum data, provides a comprehensive view of the neonate's present status and potential health problems. Taking the time to review the history facilitates the health care provider identifying problems in context and, in conjunction with the physical examination findings, formulating priorities of care and a deductive plan of care.

REFERENCES

1. American Academy of Pediatrics, American College of Obstetricians and Gynecologists. 2007. *Guidelines for Perinatal Care,* 6th ed. Elk Grove Village, Illinois: American Academy of Pediatrics, 205–249.
2. Narvey M, and Fletcher MA. 2005. Physical assessment and classification. In *Neonatology, Pathophysiology, and Management of the Newborn,* 6th ed., MacDonald MG, Mullett, MD, and Seshia MMK, eds. Philadelphia: Lippincott Williams & Wilkins, 347–350.
3. Thomas SV. 2008. Cardiac malformations are increased in infants of mothers with epilepsy. *Pediatric Cardiology* 29(3): 604–608.
4. Lee RV, et al. 2000. *Medical Care of the Pregnant Patient.* Philadelphia: American College of Physicians, 727.
5. Torrence CR, and Horns KM. 1989. Appraisal and caregiving for the drug addicted infant. *Neonatal Network* 8(3): 49–59.
6. Patterson KB, et al. 2007. Frequent detection of acute HIV infection in pregnant women. *AIDS* 21(17): 2303–2308.
7. Goldbloom RB. 1997. *Pediatric Clinical Skills.* New York: Churchill Livingstone, 51.

BIBLIOGRAPHY

Brodsky D, and Ouellette MA. 2007. *Primary Care of the Premature Infant.* Philadelphia: Saunders.

Johnston PGB, Flood K, and Spinks K. 2002. *The Newborn Child,* 9th ed. New York: Churchill Livingstone.

Knuppell RA, and Drukker JE. 1993. *High-Risk Pregnancy: A Team Approach.* Philadelphia: Saunders.

Seidel HM, et al. 2006. *Primary Care of the Newborn,* 4th ed. Philadelphia: Mosby.

Thureen P, et al. 2005. *Assessment and Care of the Well Newborn,* 2nd ed. Philadelphia: Saunders.

Zaichkin J. 2002. *Newborn Intensive Care: What Every Parent Needs to Know,* 2nd ed. Santa Rosa, California: NICU INK.

3 Gestational Age Assessment

Carol Wiltgen Trotter, PhD, RN, NNP-BC

Gestational age assessment is the process of estimating the age from conception until the time of the evaluation. This is also referred to as the postconceptional age of the neonate. An accurate determination of gestational age is important to the clinician for two reasons. First, knowledge of the neonate's age and the growth patterns appropriate to that age aid in identification of neonatal risks and in development of management plans. This is particularly true for infants born at or near the limit of viability. These infants have numerous medical, social, and ethical issues. Accurate assessment of gestational age is critical for determining morbidity and mortality risks that may be used to counsel families regarding treatment decisions.[1] Based on a review of data from 4,438 infants born at weights between 501 and 1,500 g, Lemons and colleagues have documented large differences in mortality for each week of gestation, particularly for neonates born at less than 30 weeks gestation.[2] These differences are highlighted in Figure 3-1. Pediatrix Medical Group has documented similar outcomes statistics for a larger cohort of neonates (n = 34,475).[3] These data are presented in Figure 3-2. In addition, survival without severe intraventricular hemorrhage or retinopathy of prematurity for 23-week gestational age infants is only 9 percent. This increases to 28 percent for 24-week gestational age infants and to 48 percent for 25-week gestational age infants.[4] The risks associated with the lowest gestational ages are clearly recognized, and identification of those risks requires accurate assessment of gestational age. Second, an accurate determination of gestational age is essential when conducting neonatal research and applying the findings to clinical practice.[5] Gestational maturity is an independent predictor of outcome, so gestational age must be controlled for in clinical trials that evaluate new therapies. Accurate gestational age assessment is also an important factor when comparing outcomes data from different neonatal care facilities.[6]

There are three general methods of determining gestational age in the newborn: (1) calculation of dates based on the mother's last menstrual period, (2) evaluation of obstetric parameters obtained during the prenatal period, and (3) physical examination of the neonate. Although evaluations based on menstrual dates and obstetric methods are discussed briefly, this chapter focuses on determining gestational age through postnatal physical assessment.

The average pregnancy is usually described as lasting 280 days, or 40 weeks from the onset of the last menstrual period.[7] Nägele's

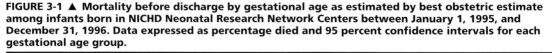

FIGURE 3-1 ▲ Mortality before discharge by gestational age as estimated by best obstetric estimate among infants born in NICHD Neonatal Research Network Centers between January 1, 1995, and December 31, 1996. Data expressed as percentage died and 95 percent confidence intervals for each gestational age group.

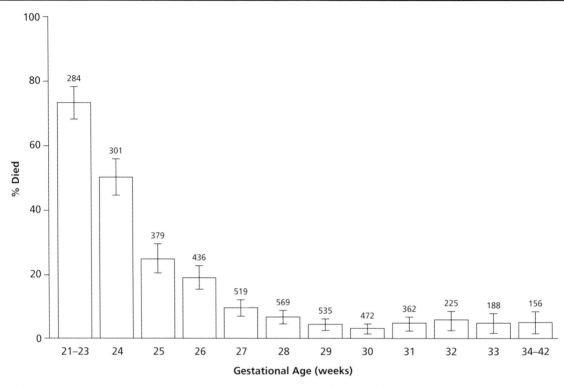

From: Lemons JA, et al. 2001. Very low birth weight outcomes of the National Institute of Child Health and Human Development Neonatal Research Network, January 1995 though December 1996. *Pediatrics* 107(1): e1. Reprinted by permission.

rule, which is based on a 28-day menstrual cycle, can be used to estimate the expected date of confinement (EDC). To calculate the EDC using Nägele's rule, subtract three months from the date of the last menstrual period and add one week and one year.[8] The accuracy with which the EDC can be determined based on the last menstrual period depends on the woman having regular menstrual cycles. If the mother's menstrual cycles are irregular, in pregnancies occurring after cessation of oral contraceptive use and in patients with medically induced ovulation, adjustments need to be made in dating the pregnancy.[9,10] In these cases, ultrasound measurements between the 14th and 20th weeks

of gestation provide an accurate estimate of gestational age.[8]

Obstetric methods for assessing gestational age include maternal physical examination and ultrasound measurements. In the first trimester, crown-rump length is the most sensitive fetal biometric parameter for determining gestational age. During the second and third trimesters, however, the fetus is too large to use the crown-rump length measurement. Instead, measurements of individual structures are used. The four most common measurements are biparietal diameter, head and abdominal circumferences, and femur length.[11] Chervenak and colleagues evaluated 238 pregnancies to determine the accuracy of the four

FIGURE 3-2 ▲ Survival by estimated gestational age and birth weight (%).*

Birth weight (g)	Estimated Gestational Age (weeks)														Total
	23	24	25	26	27	28	29	30	31	32	33	34	35	36	
250 to 500	27	28	53	59											34
501 to 750	33	57	73	82	80	86	84								64
751 to 1,000		64	80	86	93	92	95	99	95	92					88
1,001 to 1,250				91	94	97	97	99	100	99	100	96			97
1,251 to 1,500						97	98	98	98	100	100	100	100		99
1,501 to 1,750							97	99	99	100	100	100	100	100	99
1,751 to 2,000								98	99	100	100	100	100	100	100
2,001 to 2,250									98	100	100	100	100	100	100
2,251 to 2,500										99	100	100	100	100	100
2,501 to 2,750											100	100	100	100	100
2,751 to 3,000												100	100	100	100
≥3,001												100	100	100	100
Total	31	55	75	85	91	95	97	98	99	100	100	100	100	100	97

* The outcomes of 34,475 nonanomalous neonates born at, cared for in, and discharged from 131 hospitals in 28 states from 2003 to 2004. These numbers represent an estimate. The likelihood of a good outcome is influenced by many variables, only two of which are estimated gestational age and birth weight.

From: Data Warehouse 2002–2004. 2005. Sunrise, Florida: Pediatrix Medical Group. Reprinted by permission.

fetal biometric measurements in assigning gestational age. They found head circumference to be the single best predictor, followed by abdominal circumference, biparietal diameter, and then femur length.[12]

Because of the advances that have been made in improving the accuracy of gestational age estimation by obstetric methods, some practitioners believe that formal assessment of gestational age is not required for routine newborn examination. The most accurate guide to gestational age is a combination of menstrual dates and ultrasound measurements.[13] However, when these data are not known, physical examination is appropriate. The physical assessment techniques used in the examination of the neonate for gestational age are inspection and palpation. When rapid assessment of gestational age is necessary, such as in the delivery room, a quick inspection of a few parameters will suffice. A detailed gestational age assessment, however, includes palpation and use of the ophthalmoscope.

HISTORICAL PERSPECTIVE

The gestational age assessment scoring system that provides the basis for many of the tools currently used was published in 1970 by Dubowitz, Dubowitz, and Goldberg.[14] The system is based on assessment of 11 external and 10 neurologic criteria. The external criteria were taken from characteristics defined by Farr and associates.[15] According to Dubowitz, Dubowitz, and Goldberg and Koenigsberger (as well as secondary sources), the development of neurologic criteria to assess gestational age originated in the work of the French schools in the 1950s under Andre Thomas and later Madame Sainte-Anne Dargassies.[14,16] During the 1960s, a number of other investigators helped better define the neurologic criteria. Dubowitz, Dubowitz, and Goldberg selected criteria from the data published by Koenigsberger,

FIGURE 3-3 ▲ Algorithm for the assignment of gestational age.

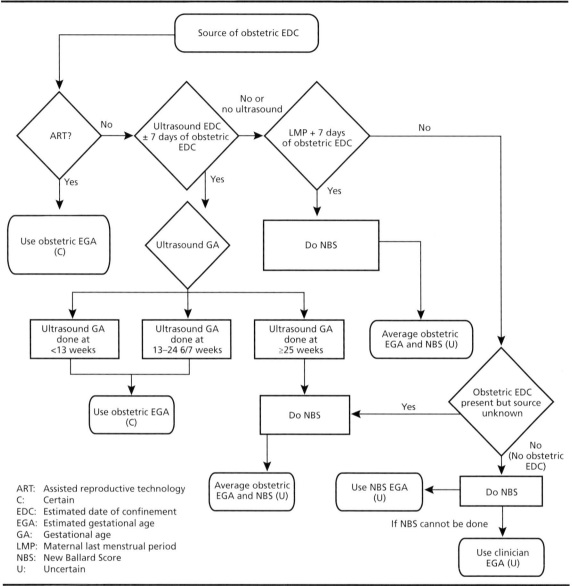

Adapted from: Jacob J, and Hulman S. 2006. A standardized method for assigning gestational age: A tool for measuring gestational age based newborn intensive care outcomes. *American Journal of Perinatology* 23(7): 399. Permission conveyed through Copyright Clearnce center, Inc.

Amiel-Tison, and Robinson to develop the neurologic portion of their scoring system.[14,16,17,18]

Since publication of the system devised by Dubowitz, Dubowitz, and Goldberg, many variations of the tool have been used.[19,20] In 1978, Capurro and coworkers published a simplified method of gestational age assessment using seven of the original variables defined by Dubowitz, Dubowitz, and Goldberg. These investigators identified five physical and two neurologic criteria that most accurately determine gestational age.[21] In 1979, Ballard, Novak, and Driver published a tool

FIGURE 3-4 ▲ The sagittal sections of the eye, showing successive developmental stages of the lens, retina, iris, and cornea.

A. 5 weeks, **B.** 6 weeks, **C.** 20 weeks, **D.** newborn. Note the hyaloid artery and the tunica vasculosa lentis.

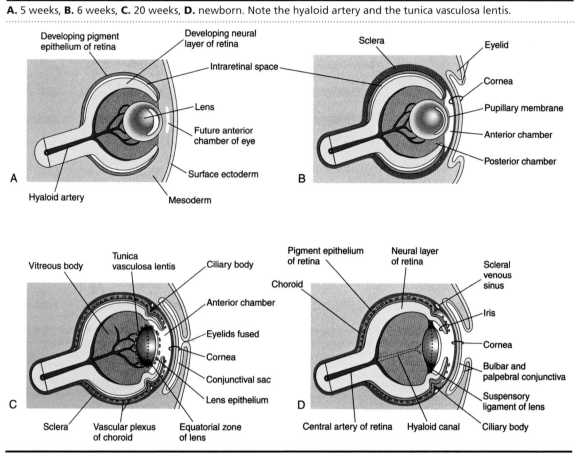

Adapted from: Moore KL, and Persaud TVN. 2008. *The Developing Human: Clinically Oriented Embryology,* 8th ed. Philadelphia: Saunders, 426. Reprinted by permission.

using six neuromuscular criteria and six physical criteria.[22] In addition, other investigators have published reports of determination of gestational age by measuring hand and foot length,[23,24] cerebellar vermis dimensions,[25] postnatal sonographic measuring of femur length,[26] measuring intermamillary distance,[24] and skin reflectance with an optical fiber spectrophotometer.[27]

Both the Ballard and the Dubowitz tools have been criticized for overestimating the actual gestational age by 2 weeks.[28,29] Therefore, Ballard and colleagues expanded their tool to achieve greater accuracy and to include the extremely premature neonate.[30]

According to its authors, this tool, the New Ballard Score (NBS), overestimates gestational age by 0.3 to 0.6 week (two to four days) at gestational ages less than 37 weeks. However, the NBS estimates of gestational age have been shown to exceed actual gestational age by 1.3 to 3.3 weeks in neonates less than 28 weeks.[31] Because of this discrepancy, Sola and Chow state that there is still no absolute "gold standard" for postnatal assessment of gestational age, especially for neonates less than 28 weeks gestation.[32] Practitioners involved in making clinical decisions for extremely premature neonates must be cautious when applying the results of physical examination data. Because

FIGURE 3-5 ▲ Gestational age assessment grading system: Anterior vascular capsule of the lens.

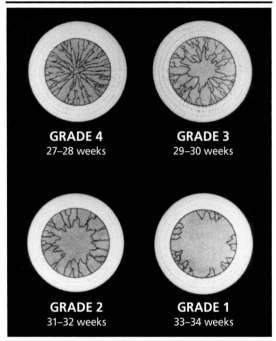

From: Hittner HM, Hirsch NJ, and Rudolph AJ. 1977. Assessment of gestational age by examination of the anterior vascular capsule of the lens. *Journal of Pediatrics* 91(3): 456. Reprinted by permission.

of this variability in accuracy of gestational age assessment, Jacob and Hulman developed an algorithm for gestational age determination (Figure 3-3).[6] They place an emphasis on accurate gestational age assignment for the purpose of comparing outcomes data between institutions. The key component of this algorithm is the obstetrician's assessment of gestational age based on menstrual dates, ultrasound parameters, and maternal physical assessment. The algorithm recommends newborn assessment only if the obstetric parameters are uncertain. The limitations associated with the NBS for gestational age assessment must be kept in mind as it is used throughout this chapter to demonstrate assessment of the neuromuscular and physical criteria associated with various gestational ages.

PHYSICAL ASSESSMENT

There are two methods for determining gestational age by physical examination: (1) assessment of the anterior vascular capsule of the lens (AVCL) using the ophthalmoscope and (2) assessment of neuromuscular and physical criteria by inspection and palpation.

ANTERIOR VASCULAR CAPSULE OF THE LENS

The rationale and technique for examining the AVCL to determine gestational age were described in 1977 by Hittner, Hirsch, and Rudolph.[33] The hyaloid system and the tunica vasculosa lentis are transient embryologic vascular systems that invade the developing eye. The purpose of the vascular system is to nourish the eye during active growth. This system can be seen starting at approximately 27 weeks gestation; it then atrophies progressively until it is gone after week 34. Figure 3-4 depicts the developing eye from 5 weeks to term gestation. Early in fetal life, the lens is invaded by the tunica vasculosa lentis. The hyaloid artery supplies the developing lens and the tunica vasculosa lentis until it disappears late in the fetal period. At that time, the tunica vasculosa lentis atrophies.[34]

To visualize the vessels, the examiner uses a direct ophthalmoscope set between +6 and +12. These settings allow the examiner's eye to focus on the lens rather than on the retina. To the novice practitioner, the image will initially appear blurry. As the ophthalmoscope is moved closer to the infant's eye (within 6 to 10 inches), the vascular system will come into view as the examiner focuses on the more anteriorly placed lens.

Figure 3-5 illustrates the grading system for gestational age assessment based on the pattern and presence of vessels noted. This examination must be performed within the first 24 to 48 hours of life because the vascular system atrophies rapidly after that period.[33] Although

FIGURE 3-6 ▲ Gestational age assessment scoring system: Neurologic and physical criteria (New Ballard score).

Maturational Assessment of Gestational Age (New Ballard Score)

Name_____   Date/time of birth _____   Sex_____

Hospital no._____   Date/time of exam_____   Birth weight _____

Race_____   Age when examined _____   Length _____

Apgar score: 1 minute_____5 minutes _____10 minutes _____   Head circ._____

Neuromuscular Maturity

Examiner _____

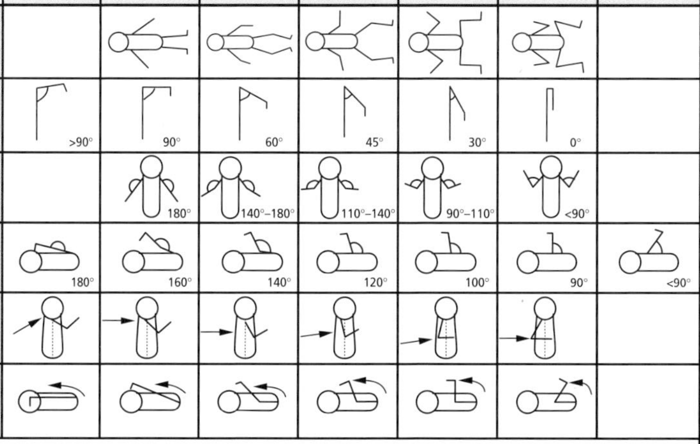

Neuromuscular Maturity Sign	Score							Record Score Here
	−1	0	1	2	3	4	5	
Posture								
Square Window (Wrist)	>90°	90°	60°	45°	30°	0°		
Arm Recoil		180°	140°–180°	110°–140°	90°–110°	<90°		
Popliteal Angle	180°	160°	140°	120°	100°	90°	<90°	
Scarf Sign								
Heel to Ear								

Total Neuromuscular Maturity Score

Physical Maturity

Physical Maturity Sign	Score							Record Score Here
	−1	0	1	2	3	4	5	
Skin	sticky friable transparent	gelatinous red translucent	smooth pink visible veins	superficial peeling and/or rash, few veins	cracking pale areas rare veins	parchment deep cracking no vessels	leathery cracked wrinkled	
Lanugo	none	sparse	abundant	thinning	bald areas	mostly bald		
Plantar Surface	heel-toe 40–50 mm:-1 <40 mm:-2	>50 mm no crease	faint red marks	anterior transverse crease only	creases anterior 2/3	creases over entire sole		
Breast	imperceptible	barely perceptible	flat areola no bud	stippled areola 1–2 mm bud	raised areola 3–4 mm bud	full areola 5–10 mm bud		
Eye/Ear	lids fused loosely: -1 tightly: -2	lids open pinna flat stays folded	sl. curved pinna; soft; slow recoil	well-curved pinna; soft but ready recoil	formed and firm; instant recoil	thick cartilage ear stiff		
Genitals (Male)	scrotum flat, smooth	scrotum empty faint rugae	testes in upper canal rare rugae	testes descending few rugae	testes down good rugae	testes pendulous deep rugae		
Genitals (Female)	clitoris prominent & labia flat	prominent clitoris & small labia minora	prominent clitoris & enlarging minora	majora & minora equally prominent	majora large minora small	majora cover clitoris and minora		

Total Physical Maturity Score

Score

Neuromuscular _____
Physical _____
Total _____

Maturity Rating

Score	Weeks
−10	20
−5	22
0	24
5	26
10	28
15	30
20	32
25	34
30	36
35	38
40	40
45	42
50	44

Gestational Age (weeks)

By dates _____
By ultrasound _____
By exam _____

From: Ballard JL, et al. 1991. New Ballard score, expanded to include extremely premature infants. *Journal of Pediatrics* 119(3): 418. Reprinted by permission.

Dietz, Huppi, and Amato confirmed that the gradual disappearance of the AVCL is not impacted by maternal and neonatal risk factors, Hadi and Hobbs found that maternal chronic hypertension accelerates the atrophy of this system.[35,36] They suggest that chronic intrauterine stress may influence the maturation of this vascular structure.

NEUROMUSCULAR AND PHYSICAL CRITERIA

Ballard and colleagues have defined six neuromuscular and six physical criteria for evaluating gestational age in the newborn.[30,37] The criteria and the scoring tool are depicted in Figure 3-6. A discussion of each criterion follows, and photographs depicting assessment of the criteria accompany the text. Descriptions of the technique for assessment were taken from Dubowitz, Dubowitz, and Goldberg and Ballard unless otherwise noted.[14,30,37]

Neuromuscular Criteria

Posture. The infant is first allowed to assume a baseline position of comfort and is then observed in a supine position. A score is assigned based on the degree of flexion of the arms, knees, and hips. The degree of hip adduction/abduction is also noted. The neonate demonstrates increasing flexion and hip adduction with advancing gestational age, with lower-extremity flexion preceding flexion of the upper extremities (Figures 3-7–3-9).

FIGURE 3-7 ▲ Full-term Infant. Posture score = 4.

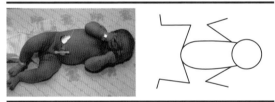

FIGURE 3-8 ▲ Preterm large-for-gestational-age female infant. Posture score = 3.

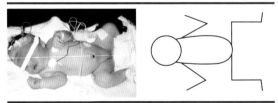

FIGURE 3-9 ▲ Preterm infant with no arm flexion. Posture score = 1.

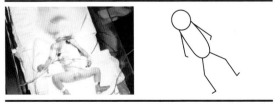

FIGURE 3-10 ▲ Square window in term neonate. Score = 4.

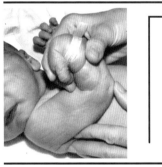

FIGURE 3-11 ▲ Square window in preterm infant. Score = 1.

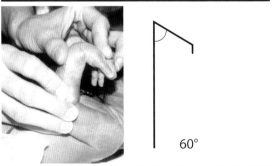

FIGURE 3-12 ▲ Square window in preterm infant. Score = 0.

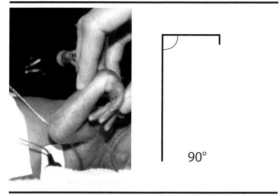

FIGURE 3-14 ▲ Arm recoil maneuver elicited Moro response in this preterm infant. Score = 2.

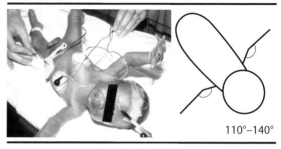

FIGURE 3-13 ▲ Eliciting arm recoil in a term infant.

A. Arms are flexed for five seconds and then extended. **B.** After arms are extended, they are released, and the degree of arm flexion is scored. Score = 4.

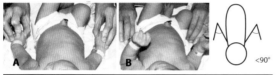

FIGURES 3-15 ▲ Popliteal angle in term infant. Score = 5.

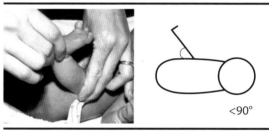

Square window. The infant's fingers are extended and the hand is flexed to the forearm between the examiner's thumb and index finger. Enough pressure is applied to get as full a flexion as possible without rotating the wrist. The angle between the forearm and the palm is measured. The angle decreases with advancing gestational age (Figures 3-10–3-12).

Arm recoil. The neonate's arms are flexed for five seconds while he is in the supine position. The arms are then fully extended by pulling the hands and quickly releasing them. The degree of arm flexion and the strength of the recoil are scored. A sluggish response with little or no flexion receives a low score. A brisk, fully flexed response receives a high score. According to Ballard, a score of 4 requires that the fist

come in contact with the face (Figures 3-13 and 3-14).[37]

Popliteal angle. The neonate should be in a supine position with the pelvis on the mattress. With the thumb and index finger of one hand, the examiner holds the infant's knee and thigh adjacent to the chest/abdomen. At the same time, the examiner grasps the foot and extends the leg gently with the other index finger. The popliteal angle (the angle between the lower leg and thigh, posterior to the knee) is measured. This angle decreases with advancing gestational age (Figures 3-15–3-17).

Scarf sign. With the neonate supine and the head in the midline position, the examiner grasps the infant's hand and pulls the arm across the chest and around the neck. The arm should

FIGURE 3-16 ▲ Popliteal angle in preterm infant. Score = 2.

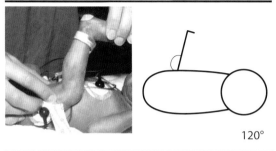

120°

FIGURE 3-17 ▲ Popliteal angle. Score = 1.

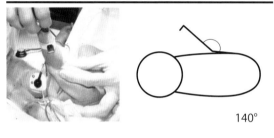

140°

FIGURE 3-18 ▲ Scarf sign in term infant. Elbow drawn to midline of the body. Score = 2.

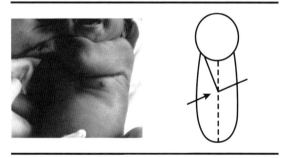

FIGURE 3-19 ▲ Scarf sign in preterm infant with elbow past midline. Score = 1.

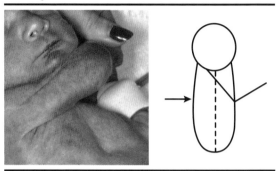

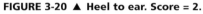

FIGURE 3-20 ▲ Heel to ear. Score = 2.

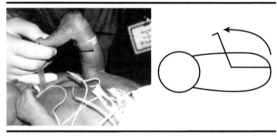

FIGURE 3-21 ▲ Heel to ear maneuver in preterm infant. Score = 1.

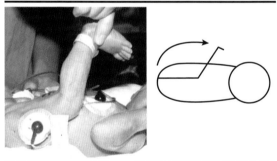

be gently pulled across the chest and posteriorly as far as possible around the opposite shoulder. The examiner scores this item based on the relationship of the elbow to the midline of the body when the arm is pulled across the chest. The neonate demonstrates increasing resistance to this maneuver with advancing gestational age (Figures 3-18 and 3-19).

Heel to ear. With the baby supine and the pelvis flat on the table, the examiner grasps one foot with the thumb and index finger and draws the foot as near to the ear as possible without forcing it.[18] When significant resistance is detected, the examiner notes the distance between the foot and the ear, as well as the degree of knee extension. The neonate demonstrates increasing resistance to this maneuver with advancing gestational age (Figures 3-20 and 3-21).

FIGURE 3-22 ▲ Skin of term infant. Score = 4.

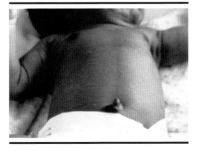

FIGURE 3-23 ▲ Skin of postterm infant. Score = 5.

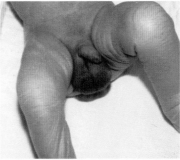

FIGURE 3-24 ▲ Friable, transparent skin of extremely preterm infant. Score = 1.

From: Clark DA. 2000. *Atlas of Neonatology.* Philadelphia: Saunders, 2. Reprinted by permission.

FIGURE 3-25 ▲ Lanugo over shoulders and cheek. Score = 3.

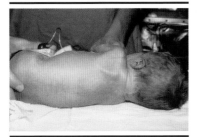

FIGURE 3-26 ▲ Lanugo over back of preterm infant. Score = 2.

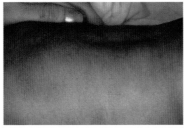

FIGURE 3-27 ▲ Lanugo noted over arm, shoulder, and face of preterm infant. Score 1.

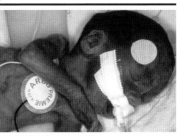

Physical Criteria

Skin. The examiner assesses skin texture, color, and opacity. As the neonate matures, more subcutaneous tissue develops, and there is a gradual loss of the vernix caseosa. Veins become less visible, and the skin becomes more opaque (Figures 3-22–3-24).

Lanugo. Lanugo is the fine downy hair present on the body of the neonate. Lanugo production begins toward the end of the 12th week.[38] Its development peaks at 28 to 30 weeks gestation and then declines as the infant matures.[39] Lanugo acts to retain the vernix caseosa on the surface of the skin.[38] Lanugo is most abundant over the back (particularly between the scapulae), although it will be noted over the face, legs, and arms as well. Thinning of lanugo begins on the back (Figures 3-25–3-27).

Plantar surface. In the extremely premature neonate, the examiner assesses the plantar surface of the foot for length and, as the neonate matures, for creases. Foot length is measured from the tip of the great toe to the back of the heel. Creases should appear between 28 and 30 weeks gestation and should cover the entire plantar surface at or near term (Figures 3-28–3-30).

Breast. The breast is assessed by observing the size of the areola and for stippling, and it is palpated to determine the amount of breast tissue. Breast tissue is measured in millimeters. Breast tissue increases and areola development progresses with advancing gestational age (Figures 3-31–3-33).

Ear/eye. The ear is assessed by observing its form and by palpating for the amount of cartilage present in the pinna and for the recoil

FIGURE 3-28 ▲ Sole creases covering the foot of a term neonate. Score = 4.

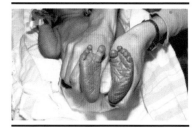

FIGURE 3-29 ▲ Sole creases covering the anterior two-thirds of the foot. Score = 3.

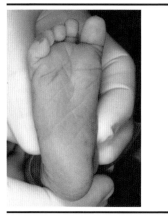

FIGURE 3-30 ▲ Faint red marks over the soles of the feet of a preterm infant. Score = 1.

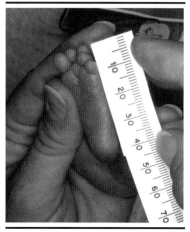

FIGURE 3-31 ▲ Evaluation of breast tissue in postterm infant. Score = 4.

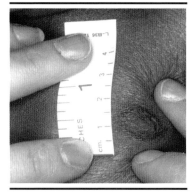

FIGURE 3-32 ▲ Breast tissue in a term neonate. The breast bud is 3–4 mm, and the areola is raised. Score = 3.

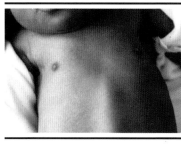

FIGURE 3-33 ▲ Breast tissue in a preterm neonate. There is no breast bud, and the areola is flat. Score = 0.

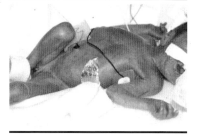

of the pinna when it is folded and released (Figures 3-34–3-36). At the earliest gestations, the eyes are evaluated based on fusion of the eyelids, which occurs at approximately 9 to 10 weeks gestation. The eyelids open during the 26th to the 28th week.[34] Ballard and associates consider loosely fused lids (–1) as closed but able to be separated by gentle manipulation and tightly fused lids (–2) as unable to be separated with gentle manipulation.[30] They collected data on this criterion at gestational weeks 20–28. These data are depicted in Figure 3-37. All eyelids were fused at less than 23 weeks and

open at 28 weeks. Between 23 and 27 weeks gestation, there is variability between the numbers of infants with tightly fused, loosely fused, and open eyelids.

Genitalia. The male genitalia are assessed for the presence of the testes, the degree of descent of the testes into the scrotum, and the development of rugae—creases that appear over the scrotum. Testicular descent begins at approximately 30 weeks gestation, and both testicles should be palpable in the inguinal canal by 34 weeks gestation. Rugae become more prominent as the scrotal sac thickens

FIGURE 3-34 ▲ Fully formed ear of term infant. Score = 4.

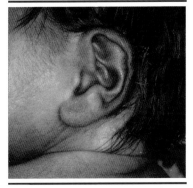

From: Mead Johnson. 1978. *Variations and Minor Departures in Infants.* Evansville, Indiana: Mead Johnson and Company, 32. Reprinted by permission.

FIGURE 3-35 ▲ Ear of preterm infant with a partially curved pinna. Score = 1.

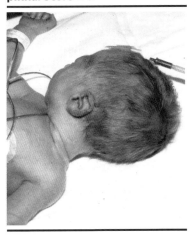

FIGURE 3-36 ▲ Eliciting recoil of pinna.

A. The pinna is folded toward the face and released. Score = 0. **B.** The degree of recoil is scored based on how quickly the folded pinna snaps back when released. The pinna remains folded in this infant. Score = 0.

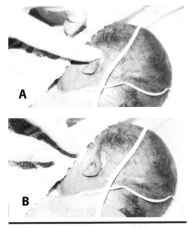

A

B

with advancing gestation (Figures 3-38–3-40). The female genitalia are assessed with the hips abducted to about 45 degrees. Scoring is based on the prominence of the clitoris as well as the development of the labia minora and majora. With advancing gestational age, the labia majora and minora become more developed so that at term they completely cover the clitoris (Figures 3-41 and 3-42).

SCORING THE PHYSICAL EXAMINATION

After the infant has been examined and a score assigned to each criterion, a total score is determined for the neuromuscular category and for the physical category. These two scores are added to obtain the final maturity rating score. As shown in Figure 3-6, the final maturity rating score (in the shaded area) is matched with the corresponding gestational age in weeks (in the unshaded column to the right). If the maturity rating score is 15, for example, the infant is assigned a gestational age of 30 weeks. The NBS authors do not give guidelines for what gestational age to assign

when the maturity score falls between the numbers listed. In my experience, a gestational age that most closely approximates the maturity rating is chosen. For example, if the maturity rating score is 23, a gestational age of 33 weeks is assigned. It is also appropriate

FIGURE 3-37 ▲ Eyelid fusion at gestational weeks 20 through 28 by confirmed-gestational age by last menstrual period (C-GLMP).

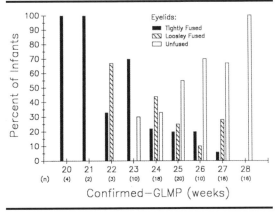

From: Ballard JL, et al. 1991. New Ballard score, expanded to include extremely premature infants. *Journal of Pediatrics* 119(3): 422. Reprinted by permission.

FIGURE 3-38 ▲ Male genitalia in postterm infant. Score = 4.

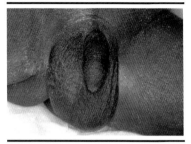

FIGURE 3-39 ▲ Deep rugae of male genitalia. Score = 4.

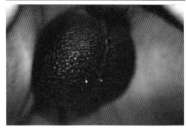

FIGURE 3-40 ▲ Male genitalia in preterm neonate. Score = 0.

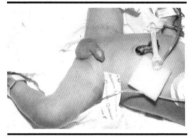

to consider the gestational age determined by dates and obstetric measurements in making a final determination of gestational age.

Infants born before 37 completed weeks of gestation are considered preterm. Infants born between the beginning of week 38 and the completion of week 41 of gestation are considered term. Infants born at 42 weeks gestation or later are considered postterm. These categories are depicted in Figure 3-43.

TIMING OF THE PHYSICAL EXAMINATION

There are no consistent, specific guidelines for optimal timing of the gestational age examination. Ballard and associates state that in extremely premature neonates, prompt examination at a postnatal age of less than 12 hours is essential to ensure validity of the examination.[30] Ballard, Novak, and Driver previously recommended examining all infants between 30 and 42 hours of age.[22] This is to allow for stabilization and adjustment to extrauterine life. Koenigsberger states that the neurologic examination is of little value during the first 48 hours of life because tone and reflexes change rapidly with extrauterine adjustment.[16] Amiel-Tison suggests repeating the examination performed on the first day of age at two to three days of age because tone changes in the days following birth. Amiel-Tison also states that the optimal time for neuromuscular evaluation is one hour before feeding (when the infant is neither too sleepy nor too agitated) because

both sleepiness and agitation affect tone.[18] When conducting their study, Dubowitz, Dubowitz, and Goldberg performed all assessments within five days of delivery. They found that when they did multiple assessments on 70 neonates, the assessments were as reliable during the first 24 hours as during the subsequent four days of life.[14]

Much of the concern regarding gestational age assessment and timing of the exam relates to neuromuscular adjustment following birth. This is further complicated by conditions altering neuromuscular function, such as asphyxia or medications administered during the pre- and postnatal periods. However, Ballard states that the items used to evaluate passive tone on the NBS are not affected by the perinatal events that profoundly affect active tone.[37] This may be the reason that Dubowitz, Dubowitz, and Goldberg did not find differences in their gestational age assessments between examinations performed on the

FIGURE 3-41 ▲ Female genitalia in term infant. Score = 3

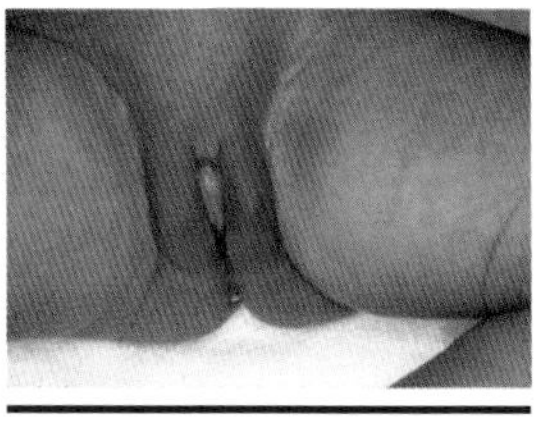

FIGURE 3-42 ▲ Female genitalia in preterm infant. Score = 0.

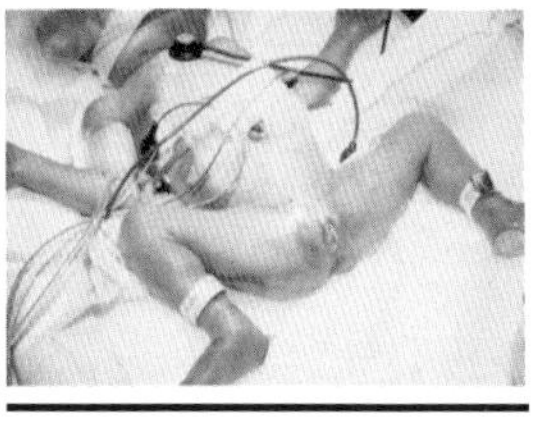

FIGURE 3-43 ▲ Intrauterine growth/gestational age charts.

Classification of Newborns (both sexes) by Intrauterine Growth and Gestational Age

Name_____ Date of exam_____ Length_____

Hospital no._____ Sex_____ Head circ._____

Race_____ Birth weight_____ Gestational age_____

Date of birth_____

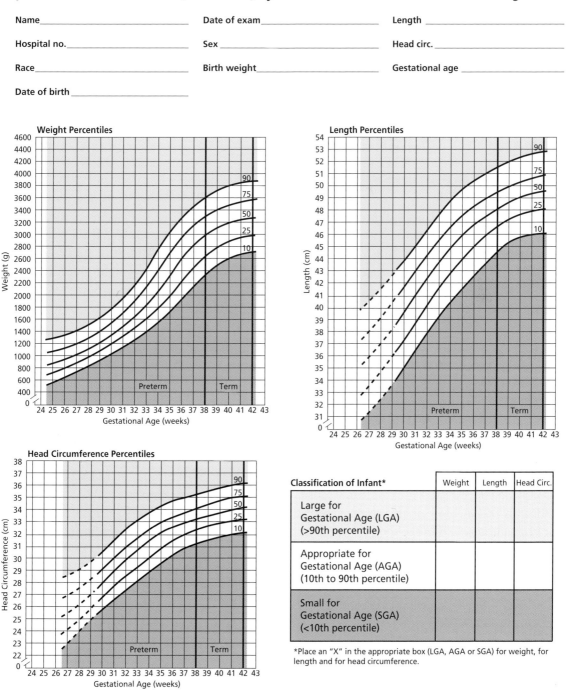

Classification of Infant*	Weight	Length	Head Circ.
Large for Gestational Age (LGA) (>90th percentile)			
Appropriate for Gestational Age (AGA) (10th to 90th percentile)			
Small for Gestational Age (SGA) (<10th percentile)			

*Place an "X" in the appropriate box (LGA, AGA or SGA) for weight, for length and for head circumference.

From: Ross Laboratories publication 10–91; (0.05) A-58560. Constructed from Battaglia FC, and Lubchenco LO. 1967. A practical classification of newborn infants by weight and gestational age. _Journal of Pediatrics_ 71(2): 159–163; and Lubchenco LO, Hansman C, and Boyd E. 1966. Intrauterine growth in length and head circumference as estimated from live births at gestational ages from 26 to 42 weeks. _Pediatrics_ 37(3): 404. Reprinted by permission.

TABLE 3-1 ▲ Clinical Features of Intrauterine Growth Restriction

Relatively large head compared with whole body
Shrunken abdomen with "scaphoid" appearance (must be distinguished from diaphragmatic hernia)
Loose skin, sometimes dry, peeling, with the appearance of "hanging," occasionally meconium stained
Long fingernails, especially in term and postterm infants with severe IUGR, occasionally meconium stained
Face with shrunken appearance or wizened
Widened or overriding cranial sutures, anterior fontanel larger than usual
Thin umbilical cord, sometimes meconium stained

From: Subhani M. 2005. Intrauterine growth restriction. In *Intensive Care of the Fetus and Neonate,* 2nd ed., Spitzer AR, ed. Philadelphia: Mosby, 139. Reprinted by permission.

first day of life and those done at four days of life.[14]

Still, it is clear that controversy exists as to the optimal timing for the gestational age examination. In general, it is advisable that the initial examination be performed within the first 48 hours of life. Follow-up examinations may be indicated if the findings from the first examination disagree with gestational age assessments based on menstrual dates or obstetric methods. However, most clinicians will assign the gestational age based on dates and obstetric measurements. When using the NBS tool, if the neuromuscular condition of the neonate is unreliable at birth, the examiner may assess the physical criteria, multiply the score by a factor of two, and then assign a gestational age based on this total score. Although the validity of this approach has not been addressed, it is based on the fact that Dubowitz, Dubowitz, and Goldberg, when analyzing their data, found that external characteristics scored collectively gave a better age index than did the neurologic criteria scored collectively.[14] However, the total score using both parameters was the most accurate.

EVALUATION OF GROWTH INDICES

When the gestational age of the neonate has been determined, the examiner plots the gestational age by the neonate's weight, length, and occipital-frontal head circumference (OFC)

on growth charts like those in Figure 3-43. For example, an examiner using the weight chart would define a neonate as being appropriate for gestational age (AGA) if his weight falls between the 10th and 90th percentiles (the unshaded area of the weight graph in Figure 3-43). A small-for-gestational-age (SGA) neonate is one whose weight falls below the 10th percentile for gestational age (heavily shaded area). A large-for-gestational-age (LGA) neonate is one whose weight falls above the 90th percentile for his gestational age (lightly shaded area). On the basis of the relationship between weight and gestational age, each neonate will fall into one of nine categories: preterm SGA, AGA, or LGA; term SGA, AGA, or LGA; or postterm SGA, AGA, or LGA. These classifications are important because neonatal risk factors are identified based on intrauterine growth patterns and the gestational age of the neonate.

A low birth weight infant is defined as one with a birth weight of less than 2,500 g. A very low birth weight infant is one weighing less than 1,500 g.[2] An intrauterine growth restricted (IUGR) neonate is one who has not grown at the expected *in utero* rate for weight, length, or OFC. Generally, an IUGR infant demonstrates restricted fetal growth subsequent to a pathophysiologic process occurring during the perinatal period. Table 3-1 summarizes the clinical features of the IUGR infant.

TABLE 3-2 ▲ Symmetric and Asymmetric Intrauterine Growth Restriction

	Symmetric	Asymmetric
Etiology	Usually intrinsic to the infant	Usually extrinsic to the infant
Affected gestation	Quite early, in first trimester	Most in third trimester, some in late second trimester onward
Body affected	Yes	Yes
Bone growth affected	Yes	No
Biparietal diameter	Low profile type	Low flattening type
Brain affected	Yes, symmetrically to body size	No (known as "brain sparing")
Ponderal index	Normal	Low
Genetic disorders	Yes	No
Risk for hypoglycemia	Low	High
Risk for perinatal asphyxia	Low	High
Blood flow in internal carotid artery	Normal	Redistribution
Maternal and fetal arterial waveform velocity	Normal	Decreased
Glycogen and fat content	Relative	Decreased
Fetal distress	No	Yes
Examples	Chromosomal disorders, genetic disorders, infections (e.g., TORCH)	Chronic fetal distress, preeclampsia, chronic hypertension

TORCH = toxoplasmosis, rubella, cytomegalovirus, herpes simplex

From: Subhani M. 2005. Intrauterine growth restriction. In *Intensive Care of the Fetus and Neonate,* 2nd ed., Spitzer AR, ed. Philadelphia: Mosby, 139. Reprinted by permission.

Intrauterine growth retardation and intrauterine growth restriction have been used to refer to the same phenomenon. However, intrauterine growth restriction is the preferred nomenclature to avoid the use of the term "retardation," which may indicate mental retardation.[10] The term IUGR has also been used interchangeably with SGA, which is not appropriate. Practically speaking, IUGR infants are often SGA, but this is not always the case. Some neonates may be growth restricted, yet not fall below the tenth percentile. For example, a 36-week gestational age infant with a birth weight of 2,000 g is well below the 50th percentile for weight on the graph depicted in Figure 3-43 which indicates a significant restriction of growth. However, this infant does not fall below the 10th percentile for weight so cannot be identified as SGA. Additionally, not all infants identified as SGA have experienced a pathologic process. They may simply be infants who are constitutionally small and represent one of the normal outliers for the newborn population.[10]

There are two types of IUGR patterns: symmetric and asymmetric. Generally, symmetric growth restriction involves both the head and the infant's weight. Asymmetric growth restriction involves just the infant's weight. Table 3-2 summarizes the characteristics of these two types of infants. Generally, symmetric IUGR is caused by factors that produce a diminished overall growth rate and typically exert their effects early in gestation. Examples include congenital viral infections, single-gene defects, and chromosomal disorders. These conditions have a significant impact on cell replication and overall growth potential.[40] Infants with asymmetric IUGR are typically those with normal OFC and length measurements, but who have a relatively low weight. These infants appear thin and wasted, with a head that is disproportionately large when compared with body size. This pattern of growth restriction is associated with poor placental perfusion or nutritional deficits to the fetus during the third trimester. Conditions predisposing the neonate to asymmetric growth restriction include maternal preeclampsia, poor caloric intake during pregnancy, and chronic fetal distress.

LGA infants are frequently born to diabetic mothers with poor glucose control. Maternal hyperglycemia results in fetal hyperglycemia and hyperinsulinemia. The high insulin levels act as a fetal growth hormone, causing macrosomia and resulting in hypoglycemia postnatally. The term "macrosomia" is frequently used interchangeably with LGA. A macrosomic infant is one who weighs more than 4,000 g at birth. Risks associated with macrosomic or LGA infants are typically related to difficult deliveries and the postnatal hyperinsulinemia that occurs after prolonged maternal hyperglycemia.

Summary

Assessment of the neonate's gestational age is an essential component of the neonatal physical examination. Knowledge of gestational age and appropriate growth patterns assists the practitioner in identifying potential risks to the neonate. With experience and a cooperative neonate, the examiner should be able to perform the gestational age examination in five minutes. Infants born with altered neuromuscular states may require an additional gestational age examination at a later date.

References

1. MacDonald H, American Academy of Pediatrics, Committee on Fetus and Newborn. 2002. Perinatal care at the threshold of viability. *Pediatrics* 110(5), 1024–1027.

2. Lemons JA, et al. 2001. Very low birth weight outcomes of the National Institute of Child Health and Human Development Research Network, January 1995 through December 1996. *Pediatrics* 107(1):1–8.

3. Pediatrix Medical Group. 2005. Survival by estimated gestational age and birth weight. Pediatrix Medical Group database. Available at www.pediatrix.com/body–university.cfm?id=596.

4. Pediatrix Medical Group. 2005. Survival without severe IVH or ROP, by estimated gestational age and birthweight. Pediatrix Medical Group database. Available at www.pediatrix.com/body–university.cfm?id=596.

5. DiPietro JA, and Allen MC. 1991. Estimation of gestational age: Implications for developmental research. *Child Development* 62(5): 1184–1199.

6. Jacob J, and Hulman S. 2006. A standardized method for assigning gestational age: A tool for measuring gestational age based newborn intensive care outcomes. *American Journal of Perinatology* 23(7): 397–402.

7. Savitz DA, et al. 2002. Comparison of pregnancy dating by last menstrual period, ultrasound scanning, and their combination. *American Journal of Obstetrics and Gynecology* 187(6): 1660–1666.

8. Katz VL. 2003. Prenatal care. In *Danforth's Obstetrics and Gynecology*, 9th ed., Scott JR, et al., eds. Philadelphia: Lippincott Williams & Wilkins, 1–33.

9. Attico NB, et al. 1990. Gestational age assessment. *American Family Physician* 41(2): 553–560.

10. Subhani M. 2005. Intrauterine growth restriction. In *Intensive Care of the Fetus and Neonate,* 2nd ed., Spitzer AR, ed. Philadelphia: Mosby, 135–148.

11. American Institute of Ultrasound in Medicine. 2007. *AIUM Practice Guideline for the Performance of Obstetric Ultrasound Examinations.* Laurel, Maryland: AIUM, 1–11. Retrieved October 18, 2007, from http://www.aium.org/publications/clinical/obstetric.pdf.

12. Chervenak FA, et al. 1998. How accurate is fetal biometry in assessment of fetal age? *American Journal of Obstetrics and Gynecology* 178(4): 678–686.

13. Lissauer T. 2006. Physical examination of the newborn. In *Neonatal-Perinatal Medicine: Diseases of the Fetus and Infant,* 8th ed., vol. 1, Martin RJ, Fanaroff AA, and Walsh MC, eds. Philadelphia: Mosby, 513–528.

14. Dubowitz LMS, Dubowitz V, and Goldberg C. 1970. Clinical assessment of gestational age in the newborn infant. *Journal of Pediatrics* 77(1): 1–10.

15. Farr V, et al. 1966. The definition of some external characteristics used in the assessment of gestational age in the newborn infant. *Developmental Medicine and Child Neurology* 8(5): 507–511.

16. Koenigsberger MR. 1966. Judgment of fetal age. Part 1: Neurologic evaluation. *Pediatric Clinics of North America* 13(3): 823–832.

17. Robinson RJ. 1966. Assessment of gestational age by neurological examination. *Archives of Disease in Childhood* 41: 437–447.

18 Amiel-Tison C. 1968. Neurological evaluation of the maturity of newborn infants. *Archives of Disease in Childhood* 43(227): 89–93.

19. Bhagwat VA, Dahat HB, and Bapat NG. 1990. Determination of gestational age of newborns: A comparative study. *Indian Pediatrics* 27(3): 272–275.

20. Eregie CO. 1991. Assessment of gestational age: Modification of a simplified method. *Developmental Medicine and Child Neurology* 33(7): 596–600.

21. Capurro H, et al. 1978. A simplified method for diagnosis of gestational age in the newborn infant. *Journal of Pediatrics* 93(1): 120–122.

22. Ballard JL, Novak KK, and Driver M. 1979. A simplified score for assessment of fetal maturation of newly born infants. *Journal of Pediatrics* 95(5): 769–774.

23. Kumar GP, and Kumar UK. 1993. Estimation of gestational age from hand and foot length. *Medicine, Science, and the Law* 34(1): 48–50.

24. Amato M, Huppi P, and Claus R. 1991. Rapid biometric assessment of gestational age in very low birth weight infants. *Journal of Perinatal Medicine* 19(5): 367–371.

25. Anderson N, et al. 1996. Cerebellar vermis measurement at cranial sonography for assessing gestational age in the newborn weighing less than 2,000 grams. *Early Human Development* 44(1): 59–70.

26. Mackanjee HR, Iliescu BM, and Dawson WB. 1996. Assessment of postnatal gestational age using sonographic measurements of femur length. *Journal of Ultrasound in Medicine* 15(2): 115–120.

27. Lynn C, et al. 1993. Gestational age correlates with skin reflectance in newborn infants of 24–42 weeks gestation. *Biology of the Neonate* 64(2-3): 69–75.

28. Sanders M, et al. 1991. Gestational age assessment in preterm neonates weighing less than 1,500 grams. *Pediatrics* 88(3): 542–546.

29. Alexander GR, et al. 1992. Validity of postnatal assessments of gestational age: A comparison of the method of Ballard JL, et al., and early ultrasonography. *American Journal of Obstetrics and Gynecology* 166(3): 891–895.

30. Ballard JL, et al. 1991. New Ballard score, expanded to include extremely premature infants. *Journal of Pediatrics* 119(3): 417–423.

31. Donovan EF, et al. 1999. Inaccuracy of Ballard scores before 28 weeks' gestation. *Journal of Pediatrics* 135(2 part 1): 147–152.

32. Sola A, and Chow, L. 1999. The coming of (gestational) age for preterm infants. *Journal of Pediatrics* 135(2 part 1): 137–139.

33. Hittner HM, Hirsch NJ, and Rudolph AJ. 1977. Assessment of gestational age by examination of the anterior vascular capsule of the lens. *Journal of Pediatrics* 91(3): 455–458.

34. Moore KL, and Persaud TVN. 2003. The eye and ear. In *The Developing Human: Clinically Oriented Embryology,* 7th ed. Philadelphia: Saunders, 466–483.

35. Dietz U, Huppi P, and Amato M. 1993. Influence of perinatal risk factors on the involution of the irido-pupillary membrane. *Journal of Perinatal Medicine* 21(1): 53–57.

36. Hadi HA, and Hobbs CL. 1990. Effect of chronic intrauterine stress on the disappearance of the tunica vasculosa lentis of the fetal eye: A neonatal observation. *American Journal of Perinatology* 7(1): 23–25.

37. Ballard JL. 1993. *New Ballard Score: A Maturational Assessment of Gestational Age.* Bethesda Hospitals, Clinical Staff Development, 619 Oak Street, Cincinnati, Ohio 45206.

38. Moore KL, and Persaud TVN. 2003. The integumentary system. In *The Developing Human: Clinically Oriented Embryology,* 7th ed. Philadelphia: Saunders, 489–501.

39. Robertson A. 1979. Commentary: Gestational age. *Journal of Pediatrics* 95(5): 732–734.

40. Kliegman RM. 2006. Intrauterine growth restriction. In *Neonatal-Perinatal Medicine: Diseases of the Fetus and Infant,* 8th ed., vol. 1, Martin RJ, Fanaroff AA, and Walsh MC, eds. Philadelphia: Mosby 271–306.

Notes

NOTES

4 Skin Assessment

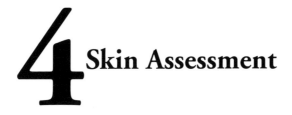

Catherine Witt, RN, MS, NNP-BC

Assessment of the skin is an important element of the newborn physical exam. Valuable information regarding the neonate's health and well-being can be obtained by observing the color, integrity, and characteristics of the skin. Close examination can aid the practitioner in determining gestational age, nutritional status, functioning of organ systems, and the presence of cutaneous or systemic disease.

Newborn rashes, birthmarks, and lesions can be a source of questions and anxiety for parents. Those caring for newborns must be well versed in normal and abnormal variations, for both educational and diagnostic purposes.

A complete examination of the skin involves both inspection and palpation. Most skin variations can be noted by inspection alone, but palpation is essential to avoid missing less obvious problems. Palpation is also important for determining the thickness, turgor, and consistency of the skin.

ANATOMY AND PHYSIOLOGY

The skin serves a number of basic functions in the neonate. These include physical and immunologic protection, thermoregulation, sense perception, and self-cleaning. An understanding of the skin's structure is essential to careful examination and to recognition of irregularities in appearance or function.

The skin consists of three layers: the epidermis, the dermis, and the subcutaneous layer (Figure 4-1). The epidermis, or outermost

FIGURE 4-1 ▲ Cross-section of human skin and the anatomic relationships among the various structures.

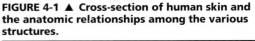

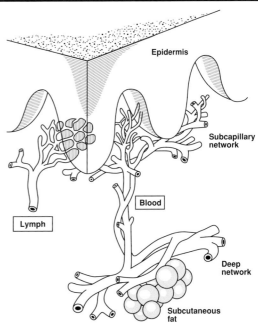

From: Nasemann T, Sauerbrey W, and Burgdorf W. 1983. *Fundamentals of Dermatology.* New York: Springer-Verlag, 11. Reprinted by permission.

layer, is subdivided into five layers. The top layer is the stratum corneum, consisting of dead cells that are constantly being brushed off and replaced. This constant replacement of the epidermis prevents bacterial colonization of the skin and is well developed in the term newborn[1,2] The epidermis is only about 0.01 to 0.05 mm thick, but the close adherence of the stratum corneum cells to one another prevents chemicals and microorganisms from entering the body and prevents significant insensible water loss through the skin in the term infant and the adult.[1]

The lower layers of the epidermis contain keratin-forming cells and melanocytes. Melanocytes are pigment-producing cells and provide for protection from ultraviolet radiation. Different numbers of melanocytes are found in various regions of the skin, with more in the facial area than on the trunk.[1] The amount of pigmentation in the skin depends on the development of the melanocytes, with more advanced melanocytes producing and dispersing more pigment.

The dermis lies directly under the epidermis. The epidermis and dermis are attached by means of a basement membrane referred to as the dermal-epidermal junction. This junction consists of various structures that anchor and attach the epidermis to the dermis. This membrane is well established in the fetus in the third trimester, although the anchoring is less secure than in the adult.

The dermis consists of fibrous and elastic tissues, sweat glands, sebaceous glands, and hair shafts, as well as blood vessels and cutaneous nerves. The fibrous, elastic tissues are what give the dermis its strength and elasticity. Sweat glands and blood vessels help maintain body temperature, and cutaneous nerves protect the skin from injury and provide the sensations of touch, temperature, and pain.

The third layer of the skin consists of subcutaneous fat. This fat layer serves as insulation, protection for internal organs, and calorie storage.

The skin of the newborn is similar to that of the adult in its basic structure. As with any other organ, however, the less mature the infant, the less mature the function of the skin.

The more immature the skin, the thinner and more permeable it is. Fibrils that connect the dermis and the epidermis are more fragile in term and preterm skin than in adult skin, and the stratum corneum is thinner.[1] Sweat glands, although present at birth, do not reach full adult functioning until the second or third year of life.

Fetal skin is covered *in utero* with vernix caseosa, a greasy white or yellow material composed of sebaceous gland secretions and exfoliated skin cells. Vernix becomes thicker during the third trimester and provides protection for the skin *in utero.* It gradually decreases as the infant approaches 40 weeks gestation.[3]

In utero the fetus is covered also with a fine, soft, downy type of hair called lanugo. Lanugo first appears at approximately 20 weeks gestation and covers most of the body, including the face. Most of it disappears by 40 weeks gestation.

BEGINNING THE EXAMINATION

Several factors influence the appearance of the newborn's skin and affect the examiner's ability to note normal and abnormal variations. A consistent, systematic approach to examining the skin increases the likelihood of gathering all the information.

A family and maternal history and an account of the labor and delivery are useful to the examiner because they may highlight items that should be inspected with extra care. For example, a forceps- or vacuum-assisted delivery may lead to disruption of skin integrity. A family history of neurofibromatosis would alert the examiner to search for café au lait spots.

Before beginning the exam, consider the infant's environment. The amount and type of light and the temperature of the room will affect the appearance of the skin. Adequate lighting, preferably bright natural light, is important. Ideally, the infant should be examined under a radiant heat source so that he can be completely undressed. This allows the examiner to observe vascular changes.

To begin the exam, undress the infant, and inspect the general color, consistency (smooth, peeling), thickness, and opacity of the skin. Note distribution of hair and any obvious markings or anomalies. Then begin a closer inspection of the infant. It is important to follow the same pattern every time to avoid missing subtle deviations. Many examiners find it easiest to begin at the head and progress downward toward the feet. While looking closely at the skin, note the size, color, and placement of any discolorations, markings, or variations. The infant should be turned over for a complete examination of the back. Inspect all skin crevices, including the axillae and the groin.

Palpation is an equally important aspect of the exam. It permits the examiner to assess the underlying dermis, thickness of the skin and subcutaneous fat, presence of edema, and any irregularities in texture or consistency. Palpation is also necessary to determine the size or configuration of certain lesions or variations that may be observed during the exam. Blanching of lesions should be assessed by pressing the pad of the thumb or finger against the lesion for a few seconds and observing for color changes.

Hydration and nutrition can also be assessed by examination of the skin. Poor skin turgor or loose, hanging skin indicates dehydration or poor nutritional status. Excessive fluid, or edema, can be noted by pressing the pad of the thumb into the skin and looking for pitting. Edema may be especially noted in dependent areas or on the scalp if the delivery was difficult. Most newborns will have some edema around the face and eyes as a result of excess fluid volume after delivery.

To determine the amount of subcutaneous fat, pinch a skin fold between thumb and forefinger. Loose skin folds will be present in the term baby who has a decreased amount of fat—for example, the infant who has intrauterine growth restriction or the postterm infant who has lost some weight in the week or two before delivery.

USING CORRECT TERMINOLOGY

When reporting skin irregularities, correct terminology facilitates accurate description of observations. The following terms are commonly used to define skin irregularities.

Bulla: A vesicle greater than 1 cm in diameter containing serous or seropurulent fluid

Crust: A lesion consisting of dried serous exudate, blood, or pus on the surface of the skin

Cyst: A raised, palpable lesion with a fluid or semisolid filled sac

Ecchymosis: A large area of subepidermal hemorrhage, initially bluish black in color, then changing to greenish brown or yellow, that does not blanch with pressure

Lesion: An area of altered or abnormal tissue

Macule: A discolored, flat spot less than 1 cm in diameter that is not palpable

Nodule: An elevated, palpable lesion with indistinct borders; some of the lesion is palpable below the skin outside the elevated area

Papule: An elevated, palpable lesion, solid and circumscribed, less than 1 cm in diameter

Patch: A macule greater than 1 cm in diameter

FIGURE 4-2 ▲ Harlequin color change.

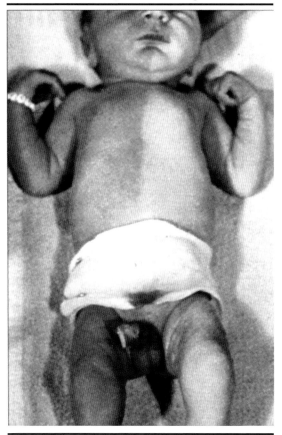

From: Solomon LM, and Esterly NB. 1973. *Neonatal Dermatology.* Philadelphia: Saunders. Reprinted by permission.

Petechia: A small, purplish, hemorrhagic spot on the skin, pinpoint in size

Plaque: An elevated, palpable lesion with circumscribed borders greater than 1 cm or a fusion or coalescence of several papules

Purpura: A small hemorrhagic spot larger than a petechia, 1 to 3 mm in size

Pustule: An elevation of the skin filled with cloudy or purulent fluid

Scale: An exfoliation of dead or dying bits of skin; can also result from excess keratin

Vesicle (blister): An elevation of the skin filled with serous fluid and less than 1 cm in diameter

Wheal: A collection of fluid in the dermis that appears as a reddened, solid elevation of the skin

It is important to describe the color of the lesion and the distribution. Lesions may be arranged in distinct patterns, such as linear, circular, or distinct separated lesions.

RECOGNIZING COMMON VARIATIONS IN NEWBORN SKIN

A number of changes occur in the newborn skin during the first few days and weeks after birth. Most are benign, transient lesions that do not require therapeutic intervention. It is important to be familiar with these normal changes and to be able to distinguish them from signs of serious disease.

COLOR VARIATIONS

Acrocyanosis

Acrocyanosis refers to bluish discoloration of the palms of the hands and the soles of the feet. Most infants present with acrocyanosis at birth. It may persist for up to 48 hours after delivery and is exacerbated by low environmental temperatures. It is benign in the otherwise normal infant. Circumoral (around the mouth) cyanosis may also be present during the first 12 to 24 hours after birth. Acrocyanosis that persists beyond the first few days after birth or circumoral cyanosis lasting longer than 24 hours should be investigated.

Plethora

Plethora describes the ruddy or red appearance present in some newborns. It may be indicative of a high hemoglobin level. The infant who is ruddy, or plethoric at birth and demonstrates clinical signs such as jitteriness, hypoglycemia, or respiratory distress should have hemoglobin and hematocrit checked by heelstick or central venipuncture. Newborns with central hematocrits greater than 65 percent are considered polycythemic and should be watched closely for symptoms such as hypoglycemia, cyanosis, respiratory distress, and jaundice.[4]

Jaundice

Jaundice is the term used to describe a yellow coloring of the skin and the sclera. The color is caused by the deposition of bile pigment resulting from hyperbilirubinemia, or excess bilirubin in the blood. The presence of jaundice in a newborn should be noted, with particular attention paid to the age of the infant and the degree of jaundice present. As a general rule, jaundice first appears in the head or face, and then progresses head to toe as the bilirubin level rises. Because it is difficult, if not impossible, to estimate serum bilirubin levels on the basis of clinical appearance, transcutaneous or serum bilirubin levels must be obtained to determine the presence of hyperbilirubinemia.

Cutis Marmorata

The bluish mottling or marbling of the skin seen in response to chilling, stress, or overstimulation is called cutis marmorata. It is caused by the constriction of capillaries and venules and usually disappears when the infant is warmed. Persistent cutis marmorata may be seen in infants with trisomy 21, trisomy 18, and Cornelia de Lange syndrome.[5]

Harlequin Color Change

Seen only in the newborn period, harlequin color change appears to be more common in the low birth weight infant.[6] When the infant is lying on one side, a sharply demarcated red color is seen in the dependent half of the body, with the superior half appearing pale (Figure 4-2). If the infant is rotated to the other side, the color reverses.

The color change may last anywhere from 1 to 30 minutes and disappears slowly if the infant is returned to the back or abdomen. This phenomenon occurs in both healthy and ill infants and is of no pathologic significance.[6,7]

FIGURE 4-3 ▲ Erythema toxicum.

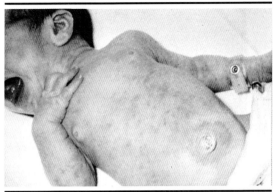

Courtesy of Barbara Quissell, MD, Presbyterian/St. Luke's Medical Center, Denver, Colorado.

It has been attributed to a "temporary imbalance of [the] autonomic regulatory mechanism of the cutaneous vessels."[7] This phenomenon can be observed for up to three weeks of age.

COMMON NEWBORN SKIN LESIONS

Erythema Toxicum

A benign rash, erythema toxicum is found in up to 70 percent of term newborns.[1] The rash consists of small white or yellow papules or vesicles with erythematous bases. It may be found on any part of the body, but it is most commonly seen on the face, trunk, and extremities (Figure 4-3). This rash often disappears and then reappears moments or hours later on a different part of the body. It may last anywhere from a few hours to several days. The peak incidence is from 24 to 48 hours of life, but it can continue to occur until the infant is three months of age. The cause is unknown; however, it may be exacerbated by handling or chafing of linen. No treatment is necessary. In fact, use of lotions or creams may make the rash worse.

Diagnosis is generally made by visual recognition of the eruption. A definitive diagnosis can be made by observation of the presence of numerous eosinophils in a smear of an aspirated papule.

FIGURE 4-4 ▲ Milia.

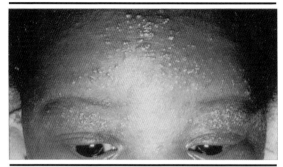

From: Cohen BA. 2005. *Pediatric Dermatology,* 3rd ed.
Philadelphia: Mosby, 22. Reprinted by permission.

Milia

Milia are multiple yellow or pearly white
papules about 1 mm in size (Figure 4-4). They
are usually found on the brow, cheeks, and
nose of up to 40 percent of newborns.[1] When
found in the mouth, they are called Epstein
pearls. Milia are epidermal cysts caused by
accumulation of sebaceous gland secretions.
They resolve spontaneously during the first
few weeks of life.

Sebaceous Gland Hyperplasia

Sebaceous gland hyperplasia is characterized
by numerous tiny (less than 0.5 mm) white or
yellow papules found on the nose, cheeks, and
upper lips. These enlarged sebaceous glands
are caused by maternal androgenic stimulation and occur in approximately 50 percent of
newborns.[1] They will spontaneously decrease
in size after birth and require no treatment.

Miliaria (Heat Rash)

Miliaria is caused by obstruction of the sweat
ducts as a result of an excessively warm, humid
environment. It is seen primarily over the forehead, on the scalp, in creases, or in the groin
area. Miliaria is classified as one of four types
depending on its severity. *Miliaria crystallina*
consists of clear, thin vesicles, 1–2 mm in
diameter, that develop in the epidermal portion of the sweat glands. The vesicles rupture
at about 24 to 48 hours, leaving a white scale.

FIGURE 4-5 ▲ Hyperpigmented macule.

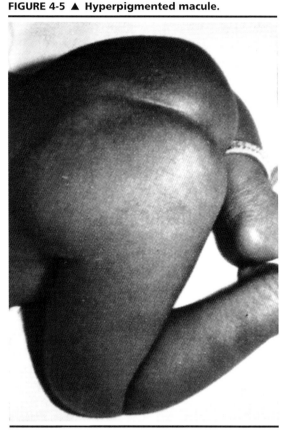

Courtesy of Barbara Quissell, MD, Presbyterian/St.
Luke's Medical Center, Denver, Colorado.

Prolonged obstruction of the ducts of the sweat
glands, leading to release of sweat into adjacent
tissue, is termed *miliaria rubra* and is accompanied by a prickly sensation (prickly heat).
Miliaria rubra appears as small erythematous
papules about 2–4 mm in diameter. They are
found most often in the neck, axilla, and groin
areas, where sweat is likely to accumulate.

Continued occlusion results in progression
to *miliaria pustulosa,* caused by leukocyte infiltration of the papule. If the condition is not
resolved, it can lead to a secondary staphylococcal infection of the deeper dermal portions
of the sweat glands. This condition, termed
miliaria profunda, is extremely rare.

Treatment of miliaria consists of eliminating
precipitating factors, such as excessive heat and

humidity. Eliminating overheating and keeping the infant dry often cause the lesions to resolve within a few hours.

Sebaceous Nevus

The sebaceous nevus is a small yellow or yellowish-orange papule or plaque. It is most often found on the scalp or face, but it may be seen on other parts of the body. It consists of immature hair follicles and sebaceous glands. The sebaceous nevus is devoid of hair when found on the scalp because of the rudimentary hair follicles found in the lesion. It may remain unchanged until puberty, when it enlarges and becomes raised. Approximately 7 to 14 percent of these lesions become basal cell epitheliomas; therefore, surgical removal is recommended.[1,3,6,8]

COMMON PIGMENTED LESIONS

Hyperpigmented Macule (Mongolian Spot)

The most common pigmented lesion in the newborn, the hyperpigmented macule is seen in up to 90 percent of African American, Asian, and Hispanic infants and up to 10 percent of Caucasian infants.[1,3] These large macules or patches are seen most commonly over the buttocks, flanks, or shoulders (Figure 4-5). They are gray or blue-green in color. Hyperpigmented macules may be mistaken for bruising because of their color and location, so it is important to document the size and distribution of the lesion to avoid later suspicion of nonaccidental trauma.

Hyperpigmented macules are caused by melanocytes that infiltrate the dermis. The macules tend to fade gradually over the first three years of life and will become less apparent as the infant's skin darkens. Some may persist into adulthood.

Transient Neonatal Pustular Melanosis

Transient neonatal pustular melanosis begins with superficial, vesiculopustular lesions

FIGURE 4-6 ▲ **Multiple papules present in neonatal pustular melanosis.**

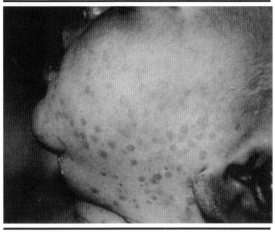

From: Clark DA. 2000. *Atlas of Neonatology.* Philadelphia: Saunders, 261. Reprinted by permission.

(Figure 4-6), often causing some alarm when present at birth. These vesicles rupture within 12 to 48 hours, leaving small pigmented macules. The macules are often surrounded by a ring of very fine white scales. Any stage or combination of stages (vesicles, pustules, or scaling of ruptured vesicles) may be present at birth. These small hyperpigmented macules may remain for up to three months after birth. Transient neonatal pustular melanosis is benign, requiring no treatment. Aspiration of the vesicles reveals numerous neutrophils and almost no eosinophils. This skin lesion is found in up to 5 percent of African American infants and about 0.2 percent of Caucasian infants.[1,9]

Congenital Melanocytic Nevi (Pigmented Nevi)

Dark brown or black macules, congenital melanocytic nevi are caused by proliferation of melanocytes within the epithelial structures and sometimes extend into the subcutaneous fat. Pigmented nevi are most commonly seen on the lower back or buttocks, but may occur anywhere on the body. The skin may be smooth over the lesion or may be nodular or

FIGURE 4-7 ▲ Congenital melanocytic nevi.

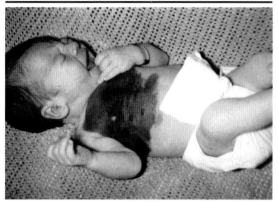

Courtesy of Peter Honeyfield, MD, Presbyterian/St. Luke's Medical Center, Denver, Colorado.

FIGURE 4-8 ▲ Café au lait spots.

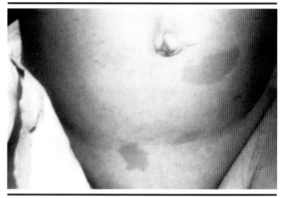

Courtesy of Eva Sujansky, MD, associate professor of pediatrics, University of Colorado Health Sciences Center.

irregular. Lesions range in size from less than 1 cm to more than 20 cm in diameter (Figure 4-7). Lesions may be with or without tufts of hair. Small to moderate sized lesions (less than 20 cm in diameter) are generally benign, but may pose a small risk of developing malignant melanoma and should be either excised or watched closely.[3] Six to eight percent of larger lesions (greater than 20 cm in diameter) can demonstrate malignant changes.[10,11] These larger lesions then should be observed closely for changes in size or shape. Treatment with a Q-switched ruby laser may be useful in reducing the size of some lesions, but surgical excision may be required.[10–13]

Café au Lait Patches

Café au lait patches are tan or light brown, oval-shaped macules or patches with well-defined borders (Figure 4-8). When less than 3 cm in length and less than three to five in number, they are of no pathologic significance. Up to 40 percent of normal children have one or more café au lait spots. They are more common in African American infants. The presence of six or more spots greater than 0.5 cm in length may indicate cutaneous neurofibromatosis.[3,6,14]

Neurofibromatosis (von Recklinghausen disease) is an autosomal dominant disorder in which tumors of various sizes form on peripheral nerves. Cranial nerves may also be affected. Ninety percent of patients with neurofibromatosis have café au lait patches.[14] Neurofibromas, small skin-colored nodules, may be present at birth or may not appear until adolescence in children with neurofibromatosis.

Tuberous Sclerosis

Tuberous sclerosis is a hereditary disorder characterized by cutaneous and central nervous system tumors resulting in seizures, developmental delays, and behavioral problems.[15–17] It presents with hypopigmented, white macules that may be thumb- or leaf-shaped. They are sometimes referred to as ash leaf macules. They may number up to 100 and are found anywhere on the newborn's skin, most often on the trunk and buttocks. Infants who present with unexplained seizures should be examined closely for these lesions. Most patients with tuberous sclerosis will have these macules at birth or soon afterward. Because of their light color, the lesions may not be readily apparent in fair-skinned infants. A Wood (ultraviolet) light may be helpful in illuminating white or hypopigmented lesions. Up to 5 percent of the

FIGURE 4-9 ▲ Forcep mark.

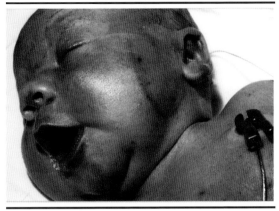

Courtesy of Peter Honeyfield, MD, Presbyterian/St.
Luke's Medical Center, Denver, Colorado.

FIGURE 4-10 ▲ Subcutaneous fat necrosis.

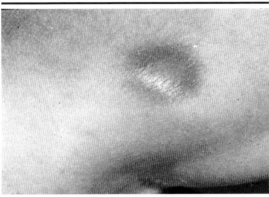

Courtesy of Barbara Quissell, MD, Presbyterian/St.
Luke's Medical Center, Denver, Colorado.

population has one hypopigmented lesion.[1,15] If more than three are present, further evaluation is indicated.[15–17]

SKIN LESIONS SECONDARY TO TRAUMA

Forcep Marks

Forcep marks may be seen on the cheeks, scalp, and face of infants born following the use of forceps (Figure 4-9). The marks are generally red or bruised areas where the forceps were applied. The skin may also be abraded. The infant should be examined for other complications of birth trauma, such as facial palsy, fractured clavicles, or skull fractures.

Subcutaneous Fat Necrosis

Subcutaneous fat necrosis is a subcutaneous nodule that is hard, nonpitting, and sharply circumscribed (Figure 4-10). It may have a red or purplish color. It is thought to be caused by trauma, cold, or asphyxia.[18,19] The nodule appears during the first weeks of life, grows larger over several days, and then resolves on its own over several weeks. There may be more than one lesion present. Occasionally, hypercalcemia may occur in infants with more than one nodule. Serum calcium levels should be monitored, and intervention may be necessary.[18]

Subcutaneous fat necrosis usually requires no treatment, with the exception of correcting any underlying cause, such as hypoglycemia or asphyxia, or the resulting hypercalcemia.

Sucking Blisters

Vesicles or bullae may appear on the lips, fingers, or hands of newborns as a result of vigorous sucking, either *in utero* or after birth. These sucking blisters (Figure 4-11) may be intact or ruptured and require no treatment.

Scalp Lesions

Scalp abrasions or lacerations may occur as a result of trauma during delivery or the insertion of a scalp electrode. Application of a suction cup for vacuum-assisted delivery may result in bruising or abrasions. Scalp pH measurements are used less often than in the past, but may result in lacerations to the fetal scalp. Treatment of lacerations or abrasions consists of keeping the area clean and dry and observing for secondary infections. Facial bruising may also be significant following delivery.

VASCULAR SKIN LESIONS

Nevus Simplex

The nevus simplex, also called salmon patch or stork bite, is the most common of the vascular birthmarks. It is seen in over 40 percent of newborns.[1] The nevus simplex is an irregularly

FIGURE 4-11 ▲ Sucking blister.

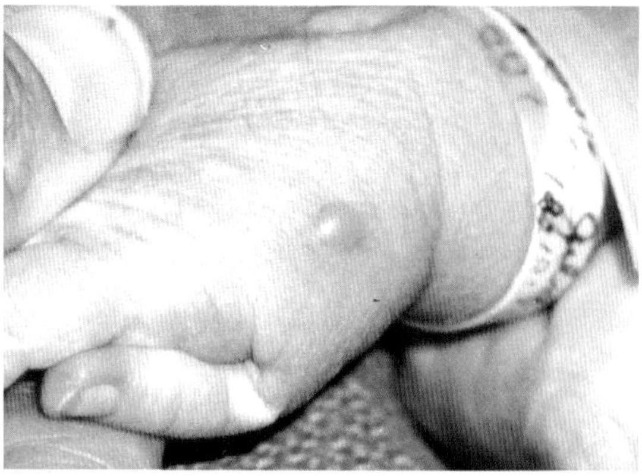

Courtesy of Peter Honeyfield, MD, Presbyterian/St.
   Luke's Medical Center, Denver, Colorado.

FIGURE 4-12 ▲ Nevus simplex.

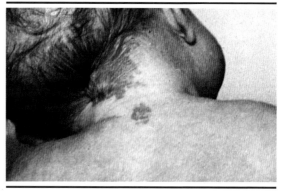

Courtesy of Barbara Quissell, MD, Presbyterian/St.
   Luke's Medical Center, Denver, Colorado.

bordered pink macule composed of dilated, distended capillaries (Figure 4-12). The lesion is most often found on the nape of the neck, the upper eyelid, the bridge of the nose, or the upper lip. Nevi simplex blanch with pressure and frequently become more prominent with crying. They generally fade by the second year of life, although those on the nape of the neck may persist.

Port Wine Nevus (Nevus Flammeus)

The port wine nevus is a flat pink or reddish purple lesion consisting of dilated, congested capillaries directly beneath the epidermis. (In African American infants, it is a jet black color.) It has sharply delineated edges and does not blanch with pressure (Figure 4-13). The port wine nevus does not grow in size or spontaneously resolve. It may be small or may cover almost half of the body. It is usually unilateral, but may occasionally cross the midline. Unfortunately, the lesion most often occurs on the face, but it may appear on other parts of the body.[1,3]

Initially, the best treatment is to cover the lesion with a water-repellent cosmetic cream. Flashlamp-pulsed dye laser therapy can be successful in eliminating or reducing port wine nevi. Pulsed dye laser works

by photocoagulation and destruction of the blood vessels in the lesion without damaging surrounding healthy skin. The treatment is more effective in infants and young children because the lesion tends to become darker and thicker with time.[20,21] Despite report of good results in the newborn period, up to 10 percent of port wine stains have been noted to reoccur seven months to 15 years after treatment.[22,23]

Most port wine nevi are isolated, but those that follow a pattern similar to the branches of the trigeminal nerve (the forehead and upper eyelid) may be associated with Sturge-Weber syndrome. This disorder causes a proliferation of endothelial cells, particularly in the small blood vessels. Intracerebral calcifications and atrophic changes may be present.

Children with Sturge-Weber syndrome may present with seizures, mental retardation, hemiparesis, and glaucoma. The cause of this syndrome is unknown. It does not appear to be hereditary.

Strawberry Hemangioma

A strawberry hemangioma is a bright red, raised, lobulated tumor that occurs on the head, neck, trunk, or extremities. It is soft and compressible, with sharply demarcated margins (Figure 4-14). The tumor may also occur in the throat, causing airway obstruction. Strawberry

FIGURE 4-13 ▲ Port wine nevus.

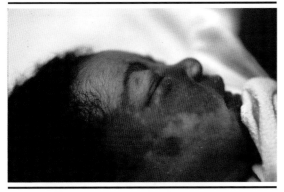

From: Clark DA. 2000. *Atlas of Neonatology.*
Philadelphia: Saunders, 267. Reprinted by
permission.

FIGURE 4-14 ▲ Strawberry hemangioma.

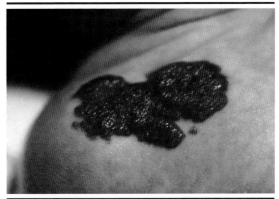

From: Clark DA. 2000. *Atlas of Neonatology.*
Philadelphia: Saunders, 265. Reprinted by
permission.

hemangiomas occur in up to 10 percent of newborns and are more common in female and premature infants.[1,3]

The lesion is caused by dilated capillaries, with associated endothelial proliferation in the dermal and subdermal layers. Twenty to 50 percent are present at birth; the others are usually apparent by six months of age.[1,3,24] It is not uncommon for an infant to have more than one of these lesions.

The strawberry hemangioma grows rapidly for approximately six months and then gradually begins to regress spontaneously. Complete regression may take several years.

Complications of strawberry hemangiomas include bleeding, ulceration, infection, or compression of vital organs or orifices. The preferred treatment is to allow natural spontaneous regression. If the lesion is interfering with vital functions (such as the airway or vision), systemic corticosteroids may be helpful. Interferon has also been used with some success. Yellow flashlamp-pulsed dye lasers may reduce the extent of vascular proliferation and may increase healing in ulcerated hemangiomas or those likely to cause disfigurement.[24] Laser therapy is not generally recommended for small nonulcerated lesions.[25]

Cavernous Hemangioma

The cavernous hemangioma is similar to the strawberry hemangioma, but consists of larger, more mature vascular elements lined with endothelial cells and involving the dermis and subcutaneous tissues. The overlying skin is bluish red in color. On palpation, the cavernous hemangioma is soft and compressible, with poorly defined borders (Figure 4-15).

The cavernous hemangioma usually increases in size during the first 6 to 12 months, then involutes spontaneously. Treatment is unnecessary unless the lesion is interfering with vital functions. In those cases, treatment with systemic corticosteroid therapy has been shown to cause some shrinkage.[6,26]

Two syndromes are related to cavernous hemangiomas. The first, Kasabach-Merritt syndrome, is a cavernous hemangioma associated with sequestration of platelets, thrombocytopenia, and consumption of fibrinogen and coagulation factors. Mortality can be as high as 20 to 30 percent, usually resulting from infection, severe hemorrhage, or iatrogenic complications.[26] It has been suggested that these tumors are not hemangiomas, but rather lymphatic malformations that have an underlying venous connection.[26] Treatment

FIGURE 4-15 ▲ Cavernous hemangioma.

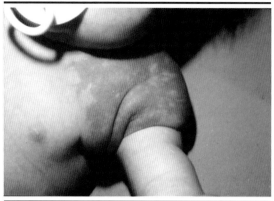

Courtesy of Barbara Quissell, MD, Presbyterian/St. Luke's Medical Center, Denver, Colorado.

FIGURE 4-16 ▲ Klippel-Trenaunay-Weber syndrome.

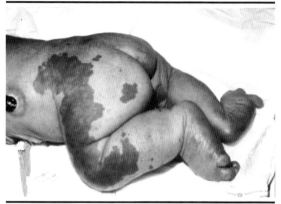

Courtesy of Peter Honeyfield, MD, Presbyterian/St. Luke's Medical Center, Denver, Colorado.

consists of supportive therapy, such as platelet transfusions and administration of corticosteroids. Angiogenesis inhibitors may restrain the growth of these tumors by inhibiting the growth of new blood vessels surrounding them.[24,26]

The second, Klippel-Trenaunay-Weber syndrome, consists of a vascular nevus with hypertrophy of the bone and soft structures of an extremity or other organs (Figure 4-16). The hypertrophy is probably the result of excess blood flow and malformed vessels.[24] This is a rare congenital anomaly, seen more frequently in males.[24] Prognosis depends on the severity of limb hypertrophy and other organ involvement.[27]

INFECTIOUS LESIONS

Thrush

A common infection in the newborn, thrush is an oral fungal infection caused by the organism *Candida albicans*. It appears as patches of white material scattered over the tongue and mucous membranes. The material is adherent and cannot be scraped off with a tongue blade. Thrush is treated with an oral antifungal solution.[6]

Candida Diaper Dermatitis

Diaper dermatitis is common in newborns and generally needs no treatment other than frequent diaper changes and the diaper area kept clean and dry. Barrier ointments such as petroleum or zinc oxide help keep urine and feces away from the skin. Diaper dermatitis can be caused by *C. albicans*. This rash is a moist erythematous eruption with small white or yellow pustules. Small areas of skin erosion may also be seen. It is found primarily over the buttocks and perianal region, occasionally spreading to the thighs. Treatment consists of keeping the area clean and dry and applying an antifungal cream several times a day. If the rash is persistent or severe, an oral antifungal solution may be recommended to prevent reinfection resulting from Candida passing through the gastrointestinal tract.[6] Infants may present with both an oral Candida infection (thrush) and Candida diaper dermatitis.

Herpes

Neonatal herpes is one of the most serious viral infections in the newborn, with a mortality rate of up to 40 percent in those infants with disseminated disease.[28,29] The rash appears as vesicles or pustules on an erythematous base (Figure 4-17). Clusters of

FIGURE 4-17 ▲ Blisters on trunk seen with neonatal herpes.

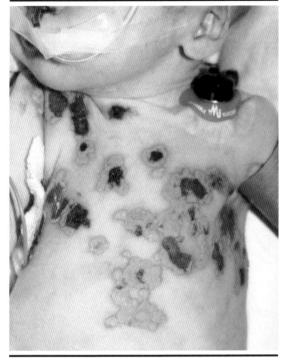

From: Weston WL, Lane AT, and Morelli JG. 2007. *Color Textbook of Pediatric Dermatology*, 4th ed. Philadelphia: Mosby, 130. Reprinted by permission.

FIGURE 4-18 ▲ Scalded skin syndrome secondary to staphylococcal infection.

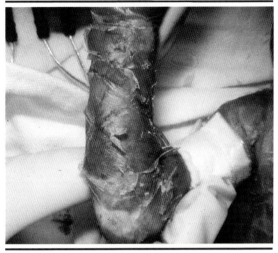

Courtesy of Dr. David A. Clark, Albany Medical Center and Wyeth-Ayerst Laboratories. Philadelphia, Pennsylvania. Reprinted by permission.

lesions are common. The lesions ulcerate and crust over rapidly. Fifty to 70 percent of infants with neonatal herpes eventually develop this characteristic rash, but not always before they exhibit other clinical signs.[28,29] Absence of vesicles does not rule out the presence of the disease.[28,29] Treatment includes use of an intravenous antiviral agent such as acyclovir. Topical ophthalmic antiviral therapy should be used if there is ocular involvement.[29] Other signs such as seizures should be treated as they occur. Precautions for blood and body secretions must be observed.

Staphylococcal Scalded Skin Syndrome

Staphylococcal scalded skin syndrome begins with a generalized, tender erythema, followed by bullous eruption and peeling of the epidermis, often in large sheets (Figure 4-18). The eruption is caused by a *Staphylococcus aureus* infection, which produces a toxin damaging to epidermal cell walls. Treatment includes systemic antistaphylococcal antibiotics and isolation to prevent spread of the infection. There may be extensive insensible water loss, so fluids and electrolytes should be closely monitored.

Other Congenital Viral Infections

Infections caused by viruses such as cytomegalovirus, rubella virus, or enterovirus may present with dermatologic findings. Most frequently, these consist of jaundice and petechiae or purpura seen on the head, trunk, and extremities. Often described as "blueberry muffin" spots, these lesions are caused by thrombocytopenia and dermal erythropoiesis. One associated finding is hepatosplenomegaly. Treatment depends on the specific viral agent present.

Miscellaneous Skin Lesions

Aplasia Cutis Congenita

Aplasia cutis congenita (ACC) is a congenital abnormality characterized by the absence of some or all layers of the skin (Figure 4-19). It most often appears as an ulceration or scarred

FIGURE 4-19 ▲ Aplasia cutis congenita.

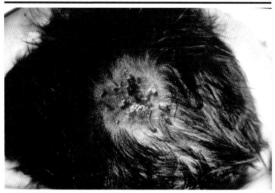

Courtesy of Peter Honeyfield, MD, Presbyterian/St. Luke's Medical Center, Denver, Colorado.

area on the scalp (on the parietal bones or near the sagittal suture), but it can occur on other parts of the body.

ACC may be an isolated defect, or it can be associated with other anomalies, such as midline defects and chromosomal disorders (trisomy 13).[5,6] The cause is unclear, but ACC may result from vascular disruptions, midline developmental disruptions, trauma, or uterine or amnionic abnormalities (amniotic disruption sequence). Treatment consists of keeping the area clean and dry. Use of antibacterial dressings may be helpful. Large defects may require surgery.

INSPECTING THE NAILS

The examination of the skin is not complete without close attention to the nails on the hands and feet. The nail consists of hard keratin. Damage to the nail matrix can be caused by trauma, inflammation, or genetic abnormalities. This damage can appear as pits, ridges, aplasia, or hypertrophy.[1,6] Most defects in the neonatal period are congenital rather than traumatic in origin.

ABSENCE OR ATROPHY OF NAILS

Absence or atrophy of nails is seen in a number of congenital syndromes, including trisomy 13, trisomy 18, and Turner syndrome.[5]

Inherited ectodermal dysplasias and skeletal anomalies may also be seen with absent or dystrophic nails.[30]

HYPERTROPHY OF NAILS

Hypertrophic nails are rarely seen in the newborn period. They may occur in diseases such as congenital hemihypertrophy or familial onychogryposis.

ABNORMALLY SHAPED NAILS

Spoon- or racquet-shaped nails may occur as a result of a congenital or hereditary anomaly. They may be associated with anomalies of the hair or skin. Spoon-shaped nails may also be a temporary finding in an otherwise healthy infant.[30]

SUMMARY

Careful assessment of the skin gives the examiner insight into the overall health of the newborn as well as any underlying pathology. Although numerous other anomalies may occur in newborn skin, this overview of the most common variations should aid the practitioner in performing a complete and thorough newborn skin examination.

REFERENCES

1. Weston W, Lane A, and Morelli JC. 2007. *Color Textbook of Pediatric Dermatology,* 4th ed. Philadelphia: Mosby, 1–9, 195–212, 309–333, 381–411.
2. Behne JM, et al. 2003. Neonatal development of the stratum corneum pH gradient: Localization and mechanisms leading to emergence of optimal barrier function. *Journal of Investigative Dermatology* 120(6): 998–1006.
3. Conlon JD, and Drolet BA. 2004. Skin lesions in the neonate. *Pediatric Clinics of North America* 51(4): 863–888, vii–viii.
4. Diehl-Jones W, and Askin DF. 2004. Hematologic disorders. In *Core Curriculum for Neonatal Intensive Care Nursing,* 3rd ed., Verklan MT, and Walden M, eds. Philadelphia: Saunders, 728–758.
5. Jones KL. 2005. *Smith's Recognizable Patterns of Human Malformation,* 6th ed. Philadelphia: Saunders, 7–12, 13–17, 18–21, 76–81.
6. Dinulos JGH, and Darmstadt GL. 2005. Dermatologic conditions. In *Neonatology: Pathophysiology and Management of the Newborn,* 6th ed., MacDonald MG, Mullett MD, and Seshia MMK, eds. Philadelphia: Lippincott Williams & Wilkins, 1485–1505.

7. Solomon LM, and Esterly NB. 1973. *Neonatal Dermatology.* Philadelphia: Saunders, 43–48, 60–80.

8. Wyatt AJ, and Hansen RC. 2000. Pediatric skin tumors. *Pediatric Clinics of North America* 47(4): 937–962.

9. Ramamurthy RS, et al. 1976. Transient neonatal pustular melanosis. *Journal of Pediatrics* 88(5): 831–835.

10. Sahin S, et al. 1998. Risk of melanoma in medium-sized congenital melanocytic nevi: A follow-up study. *Journal of the American Academy of Dermatology* 39(3): 428–433.

11. Marghoob AA, et al. 1996. Large congenital melanocytic nevi and the risk for development of malignant melanoma: A prospective study. *Archives of Dermatology* 132(2): 170–175.

12. Marghoob AA, et al. 2000. Large congenital melanocytic nevi. *Current Problems in Pediatrics* 30(9): 286–292.

13. Arneja JS, and Gosain AK. 2007. Giant congenital melanocytic nevi. *Plastic and Reconstructive Surgery* 120(2): 26e–40e.

14. Landau M, and Krafchik BR. 1999. The diagnostic value of café-au-lait macules. *Journal of the American Academy of Dermatology* 40(6 part 1): 877–890.

15. Vanderhooft SL, et al. 1996. Prevalence of hypopigmented macules in a healthy population. *Journal of Pediatrics* 129(3): 355–361.

16. Sidbury R, and Pallar AS. 2000. Dermatologic clues to inherited diseases. *Pediatric Clinics of North America* 47(4): 825–839.

17. Schwartz RA, et al. 2007. Tuberous sclerosis complex: Advances in diagnosis, genetics, and management. *Journal of the American Academy of Dermatology* 57(2): 189–202.

18. Karochristou K, et al. 2006. Subcutaneous fat necrosis associated with severe hypercalcemia in a neonate. *Journal of Perinatology* 26(1): 64–66.

19. Burden AD, and Krafchik BR. 1999. Subcutaneous fat necrosis of the newborn: A review of 11 cases. *Pediatric Dermatology* 16(5): 384–387.

20. Morelli JG. 1998. Use of lasers in pediatric dermatology. *Dermatology Clinics* 16(3): 489–495.

21. Alster TS, and Railan D. 2006. Laser treatment of vascular birthmarks. *Journal of Craniofacial Surgery* 17(4): 720–723.

22. Soueid A, and Waters R. 2006. Re-emergence of port wine stains following treatment with flashlamp-pumped dye laser 585 nm. *Annals of Plastic Surgery* 57(3): 260–263.

23. Huikeshoven M, et al. 2007. Redarkening of port-wine stains 10 years after pulsed-dye-laser treatment. *New England Journal of Medicine* 356(12): 1235-1240. (Comment in *New England Journal of Medicine,* 2007, 356[26]: 2745–2746.)

24. Young AZ, Cohen BA, and Siegfried EC. 2004. Cutaneous congenital defects. In *Avery's Diseases of the Newborn,* 8th ed., Taeusch WH, Ballard RA, and Gleason CA, eds. Philadelphia: Saunders, 1521–1538.

25. Batta K, et al. 2002. Randomised controlled study of early pulsed dye laser treatment of uncomplicated childhood haemangiomas: Results of a 1-year analysis. *Lancet* 360(9332): 521–527. (Comment in *Lancet,* 2002, 360[9332]: 502–503; Author reply, 2003, 361[9354]: 349.)

26. Enjolraso O, et al. 1997. Infants with Kasabach-Merritt syndrome may not have "true" hemangiomas. *Journal of Pediatrics* 130(4): 631–640.

27. Dhamecha RD, and Edwards-Brown MK. 2001. Klippel-Trenaunay-Weber syndrome with hemimegalencephaly. *Journal of Craniofacial Surgery* 12(2): 194–196.

28. Enright AM, and Prober CG. 2004. Herpesviridae infections in newborns: Varicella zoster virus, herpes simplex virus, and cytomegalovirus. *Pediatric Clinics of North America* 51(4): 889–908, viii.

29. Freoj BJ, and Sever JL. 2005. Viral and protozoal infections. In *Avery's Neonatalogy: Pathophysiology and Management of the Newborn,* 6th ed., MacDonald MG, Mullett MD, and Seshia MMK, eds. Philadelphia: Lippincott Williams & Wilkins, 1274–1356.

30. Pappert AS, Scher RK, and Cohen JL. 1991. Nail disorders in children. *Pediatric Clinics of North America* 38(4): 921–940.

NOTES

NOTES

5 Head, Eyes, Ears, Nose, Mouth, and Neck Assessment

Patricia J. Johnson, DNP, MPH, RN, NNP

Examination of the infant's head and neck requires visual inspection, obtaining measurements, palpation, use of an ophthalmoscope, brief auscultation, and, in rare cases, transillumination. After initial close surveillance, the exam should proceed from the top of the head down to the neck. Attention should be given to the infant's state to facilitate optimal assessment with minimal discomfort. Portions of the exam may need to be delayed until the infant is in a more relaxed state. Examination of the eyes is easier when the infant is in the quiet alert state, and examination of the oropharynx is easier when the infant is crying.

General initial observations should include the infant's state; color of the skin and mucous membranes; size and symmetry of the head and face; and obvious deformations, malformations, or evidence of birth trauma. Minor anomalies of the head and neck are common. Up to 90 percent of all anomalies seen at birth occur in this region.[1] Furthermore, the initial inspection will provide important clues to possible birth trauma and will often reveal important race-specific variations.

CRANIUM

HEAD SIZE

Measurement of the occipital-frontal circumference (OFC) is the first step in assessing head size. This measurement may be unsettling for the infant and can be deferred to the end of the exam. A nonstretchable paper tape measure should be used to obtain three measurements of the OFC; the largest of these should be recorded. Accuracy of this measurement depends on encircling the head at the widest occiput prominence and anteriorly 1–2 cm above the glabella space at the largest frontal prominence. The average OFC at 40 weeks is 35 cm, ranging from 33 to 37 cm between the 10th and 90th percentile.[2] Before closure of the fontanels, the measurement of the OFC is an indirect measure of intracranial contents including the brain, cerebrospinal fluid, cerebral blood volume, and bone.[3] The OFC is often misleading immediately after birth due to cranial molding, scalp edema, or hemorrhage under the periosteum. Subsequent measurement(s) should be obtained several

FIGURE 5-1 ▲ Transillumination.

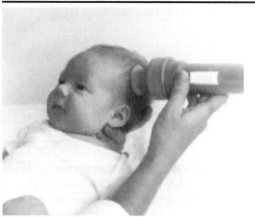

From: Jarvis C. 1992. *Physical Examination and Health Assessment.* Philadelphia: Saunders, 297. Reprinted by permission.

FIGURE 5-2 ▲ Head molding in the newborn infant.

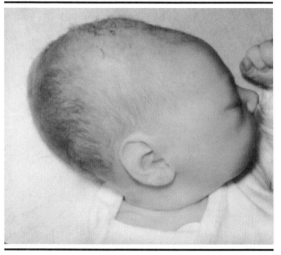

Courtesy of Dr. David A. Clark, Albany Medical Center.

days after birth once the initial distortions resulting from the birth process resolve. The OFC should be plotted on a standard growth chart and the gestation specific percentile in which the measurement falls noted. The percentile of the OFC, along with those for weight and length for gestational age, are necessary to diagnose symmetric vs asymmetric growth restriction and micro- or macrocephaly.[4]

Microcephaly (OFC below the tenth percentile for gestational age) is caused by poor brain growth. The sutures often become prematurely fused because the expansive force of brain growth that enlarges the cranial vault is lacking. Microcephaly can be an isolated finding, or it may be associated with a genetic syndrome or congenital infection.[4–7] As with the other growth parameters, OFC in the infant born prematurely tends to be lower than expected for gestational age. Discrepancies may be due to inaccurate dating and/or pathologic restriction of growth, which occurs more frequently than growth acceleration.[8] In addition, many non-Caucasian infants born in the U.S. have at birth a smaller head circumference that is reported to be merely a characteristic racial variation. This common variation illustrates

the need for race-specific population growth references, which are currently not available.[9]

Macrocephaly is diagnosed when the OFC is above the 90th percentile despite appropriate weight and length for gestational age. Macrocephaly may be familial, caused by hydrocephalus, or associated with dwarfism or osteogenesis imperfecta.[4,10] Familial macrocephaly is more often macrencephaly or large brain volume without hydrocephalus. Confirmation requires obtaining measurements of the parent's heads and plotting on a Weaver curve.[11]

Transillumination of the skull is not part of the routine newborn physical exam, but it may be helpful when the infant's head has an unusual shape or size or the neurologic examination is abnormal. A transilluminator or a flashlight with a rubber cuff may be placed flat against the infant's head in a dark room (Figure 5-1). A ring of light more than 2 cm larger than the light source implies increased fluid or decreased brain tissue in the cranium. A false positive transillumination may occur with a large caput because the scalp edema will transmit a halo of light. More definitive

FIGURE 5-3 ▲ Sutures, fontanels, and bones of the neonatal skull.

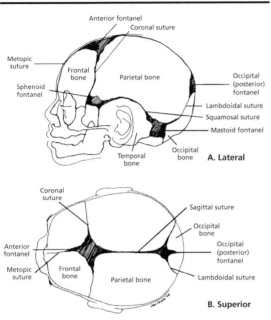

A. Lateral

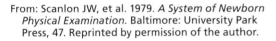

B. Superior

From: Scanlon JW, et al. 1979. *A System of Newborn Physical Examination*. Baltimore: University Park Press, 47. Reprinted by permission of the author.

FIGURE 5-4 ▲ Measurement of the anterior fontanel: bone to bone.

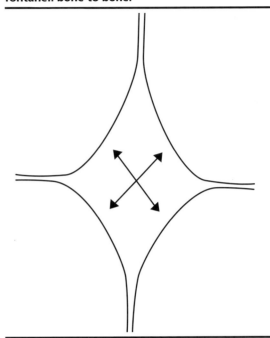

studies are necessary for diagnosis.[1,4,5] In the infant presenting with a high level of suspicion for hydrocephalus, transillumination is often replaced by one of the more definitive studies, i.e. cranial ultrasound, computed tomography scan, or magnetic resonance imaging scan.

HEAD SHAPE

The shape of the infant's head usually relates to molding of the skull during delivery (Figure 5-2). An infant delivered by cesarean section will usually have a well-rounded head. The breech position may cause the head to be molded posteriorly into an egg shape, with a prominent occiput. Prolonged diagonal pressure may cause the head to appear "out of round," or asynclitic, when viewed from above. Distortion of the skull due to positional, external pressures *in utero* or during labor can be expected to self-correct. Parents can be reassured that molding usually resolves within a few weeks after birth.[4,5,7,12]

SKULL

Inspection and careful palpation of the infant's skull are necessary to identify bones, sutures, and fontanels (Figure 5-3). Sutures separate bones, and fontanels occur where two sutures meet. The metopic suture extends midline down the forehead between the two frontal bones and intersects with the coronal suture, which separates the frontal and parietal bones. The anterior fontanel (AF) is formed at the intersection of the metopic, coronal, and sagittal sutures. The size of the AF varies from 0.6 to 3.6 cm across, and in African American infants, it is commonly larger—from 1.4 to 4.7 cm.[13] Fontanels are measured diagonally from bone to bone rather than from suture to suture (Figure 5-4). Because there is a wide variation in fontanel size at birth, the measurement may serve only as a baseline for serial comparison. Individual measurements have no

FIGURE 5-5 ▲ Bulging anterior fontanel.

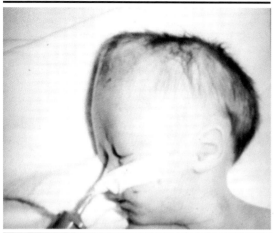

Courtesy of Dr. David A. Clark, Albany Medical Center and Wyeth-Ayerst Laboratories, Philadelphia, Pennsylvania. Reprinted by permission.

FIGURE 5-6 ▲ Cross-section of sutures.

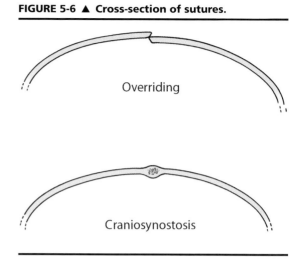

clinical significance, have limited reproducibility, and are not useful as a single examination finding. The AF is normally described as flat and soft if assessed with the infant in a quiet state and held in the sitting position. A tense or bulging fontanel may be a sign of increased intracranial pressure or may occur when the infant is crying (Figure 5-5).[1,14] If the examiner is uncertain whether the fontanel is flat or bulging, it should be palpated with the infant in an upright, sitting position. A sunken fontanel is a sign of severe dehydration and is rarely seen in the newborn nursery. However, it may indicate excessive or acute decompression in an infant with a newly inserted external ventricular drain for treatment of hydrocephalus. A very large AF can be associated with hypothyroidism.[15] The AF normally closes by 6 to 24 months of age.[4,5,16]

Auscultation over the fontanels and lateral skull bones is performed during examination of the head and neck. Auscultation of the fontanels is specifically indicated in infants with multiple hemangiomas or heart failure.[13] In the normal infant, auscultation of a bruit (murmurlike sound) over the fontanels or the lateral skull can be a normal finding. Evidence of a bruit over the fontanel in an infant with suspected cardiac failure is associated with an intracranial arteriovenous malformation, which may be the cause of the congestive heart failure.[4,17–19]

The sagittal suture extends midline between the two parietal bones to the posterior fontanel (PF). This fontanel is formed where the sagittal suture meets the lambdoidal suture, which extends posterolaterally to separate the occipital from the parietal bones. The PF is usually small, 0.5 cm in diameter in Caucasian newborns and 0.7 cm in African American newborns, and closes by approximately two to three months of age.[4,5,13] If palpable, the PF should be soft and flat. A third "fontanel" may occur along the sagittal suture between the anterior and posterior fontanels. This is really a defect of the parietal bone and not a true fontanel. It can be a normal variant or may be associated with Down syndrome or congenital hypothyroidism.[20]

The squamosal suture extends above the ear to separate the temporal bone from the parietal bone. This suture and the sphenoid and mastoid fontanels are usually apparent only when there is increased intracranial pressure, as with severe hydrocephalus, but may be palpable in the premature infant with rapid brain growth.[4]

Mobility of sutures is assessed by placing the thumbs on the bones on either side of the suture and gently pressing down alternately with one thumb and then the other. Normal sutures may be described as approximated and mobile. Sutures may be split (separated) up to 1 cm. More widely split sutures may indicate increased intracranial pressure and require further investigation. With molding, the edge of the bone on one side of the suture will feel as if it is on top of the edge of the opposing bone; these sutures are described as overriding. It is common for the lambdoidal sutures to be overriding, with the parietal bone on top of the occipital due to molding after birth or with minor decrease in hydration. It is important to differentiate an overriding suture from one that feels ridged and immobile. This apparent overriding suture actually presents as a peaking of the approximated bones that can be mistaken as overriding where the involved boney edges overlap. The suture that peaks and is immobile implies premature fusion of the suture, or craniosynostosis (Figure 5-6).[1,4,6]

Premature closure of a suture stops bone growth perpendicular to the suture, but allows continued parallel growth and compensatory expansion at the functional sutures, leading to abnormal head shape.[1,4–7,16,21] Abnormal head shape resulting from craniosynostosis may be noted at birth, or the premature fusion may not be suspected until later in infancy (Figure 5-7). Fused coronal sutures limit forward growth of the skull and lead to a broad skull (brachycephaly). Early closure of the sagittal suture limits lateral growth and results in a long, narrow head (scaphocephaly). Plagiocephaly is an asymmetric skull resulting from closure of the sutures on one side. The premature infant's head may develop the shape termed dolichocephaly, which is flattened side to side

FIGURE 5-7 ▲ Normal skull and shapes that result from craniosynostosis.

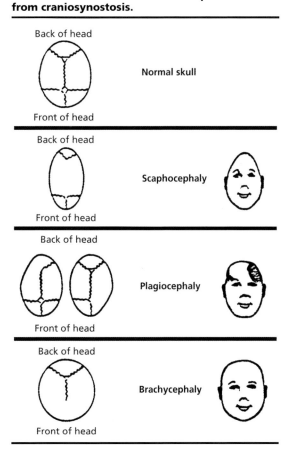

From: Disabato J, and Wulf J. 1989. Nursing strategies: Altered neurologic function. In *Family-Centered Nursing Care of Children,* Foster RL, Hunsberger MM, and Tackett JJ, eds. Philadelphia: Saunders, 1731. Reprinted by permission.

without craniosynostosis. Viewing the head from above may facilitate assessment of skull shape. Craniosynostosis may be primary (isolated), associated with a genetic syndrome such as Apert or Crouzon, or the result of a metabolic disorder such as hyperthyroidism.[6,7,16,21] The incidence of isolated craniosynostosis in the U.S. is reported to be 0.4 to 1 per 1,000 live births.[6,21]

Palpation of the skull may reveal areas of soft or thinning bone, called craniotabes. Pressing on the bone elicits collapse with recoil of the underlying bone and a snapping sensation similar to pressing on a Ping-Pong ball, known

FIGURE 5-8 ▲ Hemorrhages of the scalp.

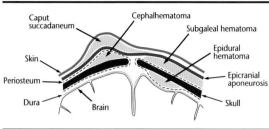

From: Sheikh AMH. Public domain with credit.

FIGURE 5-9 ▲ Cephalhematoma.

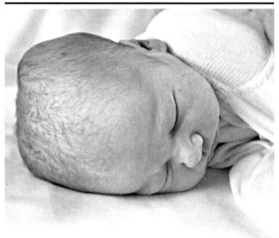

From: Mead Johnson. 1978. *Variations and Minor Departures in Infants.* Evansville, Indiana: Mead Johnson and Company, 10. Reprinted by permission.

as Macewen sign. Craniotabes, an incidental finding evident upon palpation of parietal bones near the sagittal suture, are most often due to external pressure from prolonged vertex engagement or pressure of the fetal head on the uterine fundus with breech position.[1] They may also be due to internal pressure on the fetal head from hydrocephalus. When due to external pressures, craniotabes can be expected to resolve in a few weeks. If they are due to hydrocephalus, resolution will depend on the degree and persistence of internal pressure causing the characteristic bone thinning.[1,4,5]

While palpating the skull, the examiner also inspects the scalp and head for evidence of birth trauma and other abnormalities. The most common form of trauma to the head is caput succedaneum (caput). This is edema of the presenting part of the scalp caused by pressure that restricts the return of venous and lymph flow during labor and delivery. It can be accentuated by vacuum-assisted delivery. The edema pits on pressure, usually crosses suture lines, and has edges that are poorly defined. Caput is noted immediately after birth and resolves within a few days, which can help differentiate it from a cephalhematoma (Figure 5-8).[4,5,12]

A cephalhematoma results from the collection of blood between the periosteum and the skull. It may not be evident at birth because of an associated caput. A cephalhematoma has clearly demarcated edges confined by suture lines (Figure 5-9). With time, it may liquefy and become fluctuant on palpation; it may take weeks or months to resolve completely. The most common locations for a cephalhematoma are the parietal and occipital bones. Associated depressed skull fractures are very rare.[1,4,5,12,14]

A subgaleal hemorrhage is the third and potentially most serious lesion resulting from birth trauma. It is most common with instrumented vaginal delivery, especially vacuum-assisted delivery. However, it has been reported with cesarean births or any maneuver during delivery that produces a shearing force to the scalp resulting in tearing of the large emissary veins. With a subgaleal hemorrhage, there is bleeding into the Galen aponeurotica or sub-aponeurotic space, which extends from the orbital ridges to the nape of the neck and laterally to the ears (Figure 5-10). This potential space produces a large compartment capable of containing the total blood volume of an infant and therefore has a 5 to 22 percent mortality rate if blood loss is extensive and undiagnosed.[22] It presents with generalized scalp edema, usually with ecchymosis, and

FIGURE 5-10 ▲ Subgaleal hemorrhage, sagittal view.

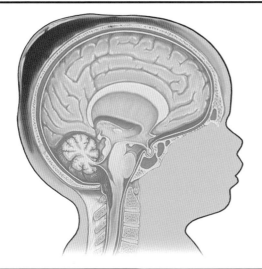

FIGURE 5-11 ▲ Aplasia cutis congenita.

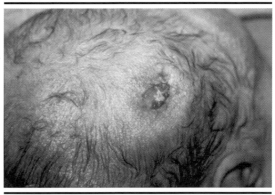

From: Blunt K, et al. 1992. Aplasia cutis congenita: A clinical review and associated defects. *Neonatal Network* 11(7): 18. Reprinted by permission.

often with bilateral or unilateral periorbital and periauricular edema. The ballotable fluid mass crosses the sutures and can be manually repositioned from the eyebrows to the nape of the neck, differentiating it from a large caput. If progressive, it can result in severe anemia, hypotension, and death unless diagnosed early. Effective treatment may involve volume resuscitation, blood replacement, and treatment of presenting clotting abnormalities.

Trauma to the scalp may include puncture from a scalp electrode; lacerations from fetal blood sampling or uterine incision; and bruises, abrasions, or subcutaneous fat necrosis from an instrument (forcep or vacuum) delivery.[5,14,23] The trauma should be described by its appearance, size, and location near sutures, fontanel, or underlying bones. Open scalp defects, known as aplasia cutis congenita (Figure 5-11), are associated with trisomy 13, but they may also be seen as a normal variant.[1,15] Other skin lesions are described in Chapter 4.

Malformation of the skull associated with incomplete neural tube closure results in an encephalocele. Central nervous tissue can protrude from a defect anywhere on the skull, most commonly midline and in the occipital area.[5]

SCALP HAIR

Examination of the scalp should include assessment of the hair for quantity, texture, distribution, and hair whorls. Low hairline, increased quantity of hair, and brittleness may be associated with congenital anomalies. The slope of each hair follicle appears to be associated with the stretch of the skin during brain growth. The most rapid brain growth occurs at 16 to 19 weeks gestation and results in the formation of a hair whorl in the posterior parietal region. One or two hair whorls can be normal. An abnormally placed whorl, absence of hair whorl, or unusual hair growth may be associated with aberrant brain growth and mental retardation.[15] Scalp hair in the newborn has variable coarseness, and the thickness of scalp hair growth patterns correlates with central nervous system development. There are racial variations in color, consistency, and growth patterns, and parental concordance is expected.[15]

Alopecia is an abnormal deficiency of hair that is diffuse or focal. Diffuse alopecia is more

FIGURE 5-12 ▲ Facial asymmetry.

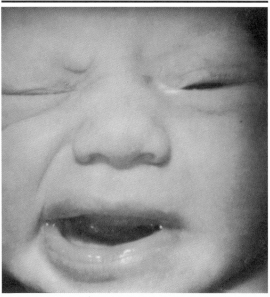

Courtesy of Dr. David A. Clark, Albany Medical Center and Wyeth-Ayerst Laboratories. Philadelphia, Pennsylvania. Reprinted by permission.

commonly due to a genetic anomaly in the hair follicles or is syndromic. Focal alopecia is often traumatic or associated with underlying scalp lesions. Hirsutism or excess hair growth may be genetic, syndromic, metabolic, drug-induced, or an isolated finding. Hair consistency and growth patterns commonly reflect developmental, familial, and racial variations of no clinical significance.[24]

Aplasia cutis congenita is an uncommon scalp lesion found primarily at the vertex just in front of the lambda. This lesion is a hairless, circumscribed area of 1 cm or more, and its surface is often shiny, cicatricial, and flat or keloid in appearance. Occasional blistering or ulceration is evident with serosanguinous exudate or fresh granulation. There is a risk of underlying defect and associated major defects in some infants with this lesion necessitating careful evaluation of the infant for major abnormalities. In most infants with aplasia cutis congenita, the defect is an isolated find-

ing that resolves with residual scar formation and absence of hair growth.[25]

FACE

Examination of the face should begin with observation of the relationships between all the facial components: eyes, ears, nose, and mouth. The forehead of a newborn takes up the upper half of the face, reflecting the large cranial volume needed for rapid brain growth. In childhood, the growth of the mid- and lower face exceeds that of the upper face, eventually resulting in the face and skull shape of the adult.[7,16]

The shape and symmetry of the face, as well as evidence of trauma, should be noted. Face or brow presentation or the presence of a nuchal cord (cord around the neck) may cause facial bruising, petechiae, and progressive edema. Unusual flattening of facial features may occur as a result of prolonged intrauterine compression from oligohydramnios. Forceps application can cause bruises, abrasions, or subcutaneous fat necrosis.[5] The location and extent of any trauma should be carefully described. Other skin lesions that may be seen on the face are described in Chapter 4.

Many malformation syndromes have very distinctive facial features. These minor anomalies may serve as aids in the diagnosis of a particular syndrome.[1,15] The examiner should also remember that unusual facial characteristics might be familial.

Facial movements during crying are assessed for symmetry. Damage to the facial nerve (seventh cranial nerve) prior to or during delivery can result in paralysis of the affected side of the face. Extensive damage can involve the entire side of the face innervated by the damaged nerve and cause drooping of the muscles on the affected side of the face. More commonly, the damage involves only the lower branch (mandibular branch) of the facial nerve, which controls the muscles around the lips. This presents with the characteristic decreased movement on the affected side of the face when the infant cries because the weakened facial muscles of the affected side allow the mouth to be pulled to the unaffected side ("drooping mouth" appearance). These infants often have loss of forehead wrinkling and nasolabial fold and partial closing of the eye on the affected side, differentiating them from congenital asymmetric crying facies (ACF) (Figure 5-12). If the nerve damage is caused by pressure, then the facial effects resolve within hours to weeks after birth. Congenital facial palsy is often spontaneous, but is also associated with difficult or instrumented delivery requiring forceps. A persistent palsy may be an indication of an underlying, more central abnormality. ACF, for example, is a congenital absence or hypoplasia of the depressor anguli oris muscle (DAOM) on one side. The DAOM controls frowning, with resulting asymmetry of the face with crying. There is an association with other anomalies, and further evaluation, especially for cardiovascular abnormalities, is warranted.[26] (Chapter 11 provides guidelines for a complete neurologic assessment.)

EARS

Abnormal formation or placement of the ears can be associated with chromosomal anomalies and syndromes; however, a wide variety of minor structural variations falls within the normal range. Ear anomalies are usually nonspecific and supportive of a diagnosis rather than presence of the anomaly being diagnostic in and of itself.[4,5,12,15] To describe abnormalities, the examiner should be familiar with the normal anatomy and descriptive nomenclature of the ear (Figure 5-13). In a term infant, the pinna should be well formed, with cartilage that recoils easily after folding (Chapter 3). Temporary asymmetry of the

FIGURE 5-13 ▲ Normal external newborn ear (pinna).

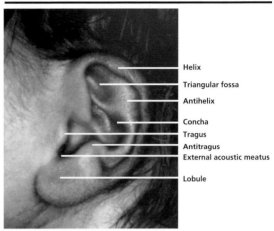

From: Mead Johnson. 1978. *Variations and Minor Departures in Infants.* Evansville, Indiana: Mead Johnson and Company, 32. Reprinted by permission.

ears from unequal intrauterine pressure on the sides of the head is common.[4] Especially hairy ears, involving both the pinna and lobes, are familial, syndromic, or associated with infants of mothers with poorly controlled diabetes mellitus.

Minor malformations, such as pits and skin tags, may be familial or associated with other anomalies (Figure 5-14).[4,5,12,15,27] These minor malformations are usually located anterior to the tragus and are thought to be embryologic remnants of the first branchial cleft or arch. A preauricular sinus may be blind, or it may communicate with the internal ear or brain. Chronic infection could necessitate surgical removal of the entire sinus tract. Darwinian tubercle is a normal variant, appearing as a small nodule on the upper helix. A very poorly formed external ear should alert the examiner to a possible chromosomal anomaly or syndrome.[12,15]

The position of the external ear on the head can be assessed by extending a line from the inner to the outer canthus of the eye toward the ear (Figure 5-15). If the insertion of the ear falls below this line, it is low set. It is

FIGURE 5-14 ▲ Variations and minor malformations of the ear.

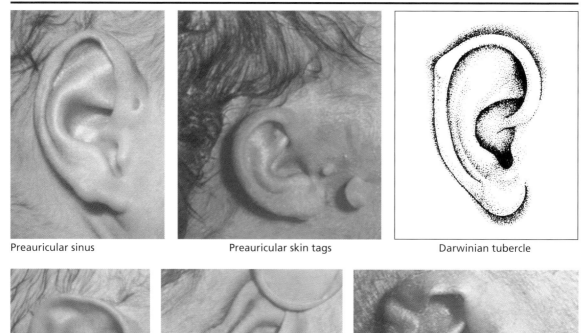

Preauricular sinus   Preauricular skin tags   Darwinian tubercle

Poorly formed helix   Abnormal ear attachment (Trisomy 17, 18)   Malformed ear (Trisomy 17, 18)

From: Mead Johnson. 1978. *Variations and Minor Departures in Infants*. Evansville, Indiana: Mead Johnson and
   Company, 34, 36. Reprinted by permission.

important to assess both ears because one may be posteriorly rotated and give the appearance of being low set.[12,14,15]

The newborn infant's external auditory canal is short and may contain vernix, interpartum blood, or meconium debris, making otoscopic examination difficult. This is not part of the routine newborn exam; it can be done later at the first well-baby visit. The ear should be inspected visually to assess presence and patency of the auditory canal.[4,5,14]

Significant hearing loss is one of the most common major abnormalities present at birth.[28] However, assessment of an infant's hearing during an examination can be difficult. The infant should startle, cry, or stiffen at the sound of a loud noise or alert to the sound of a voice, but may be responding to air movement rather than noise and can quickly habituate to a repeated stimulus.[4,5] Any infant with a small or abnormally developed ear is at increased risk for hearing loss in that ear. Current recommendations endorse universal hearing screening of all newborns, with a goal of appropriate intervention by six months of age.[28]

FIGURE 5-15 ▲ The normal ear position.

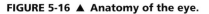

FIGURE 5-16 ▲ Anatomy of the eye.

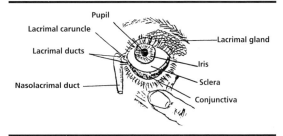

EYES

Eyes are usually a major area of interest when parents are viewing their newborn infant. Parents will need reassurance about common eye trauma, such as bruises or edema of the eyelids and hemorrhages seen around the iris that can occur with a normal vaginal delivery. Conjunctival or subconjunctival hemorrhage results from rupture of a capillary of the mucous membrane that lines the eyelids and is reflected onto the eyeball (conjunctiva) (Figure 5-16). It is seen as a bright red area on the white part of the eye (sclera) near the iris and usually resolves within a week to ten days without residual effects. Inflammation of the conjunctiva can be caused by prophylaxis of the eyes with silver nitrate drops and less often with erythromycin ointment.[1,5,10,12,14,29] Malformation of the eyelids is uncommon, but coloboma (an absence or defect of some ocular tissue, including the eyelid) may be seen. Ptosis, a paralytic drooping of an eyelid when the lids are fully open, may also be seen. Nevus simplex is a common vascular birthmark seen on the eyelids and glabella (area above the nose and between the eyebrows) (Chapter 4).[1,12,30]

Tear formation does not usually begin until two to three months of age. The nasolacrimal duct is not fully patent until five to seven months, and purulent or mucoid eye drainage is common. Unless accompanied by

FIGURE 5-17 ▲ Eye measurements.

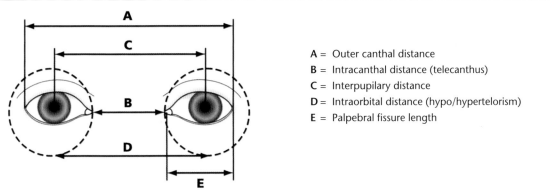

A = Outer canthal distance
B = Intracanthal distance (telecanthus)
C = Interpupilary distance
D = Intraorbital distance (hypo/hypertelorism)
E = Palpebral fissure length

Adapted from: Cheng KP, and Biglan AW. 2007. Ophthalmology. In *Atlas of Pediatric Physical Diagnosis,* 5th ed., Zitelli BJ, and Davis HW, eds. Philadelphia: Mosby, 727. Reprinted by permission.

FIGURE 5-18 ▲ Congenital cataracts.

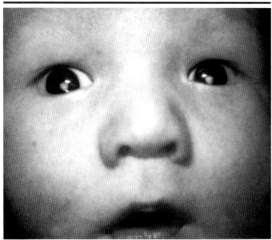

From: Clark DA. 2000. *Atlas of Neonatology.*
   Philadelphia: Saunders, 280. Reprinted by
   permission.

conjunctival inflammation with redness or swelling, this drainage can generally be treated by lacrimal massage and gentle cleansing with water and a cotton ball.[4,5,14]

Abnormal placement of the eyes or small palpebral fissures (eye openings) can alert the examiner to the presence of a syndrome or chromosomal anomaly. The distance between the outer canthi can be divided into equal thirds, with one normal palpebral fissure length fitting into the inner canthal distance (Figure 5-17). Hypertelorism exists if the eyes are more widely spaced; hypotelorism is present if the eyes are more closely spaced. Small palpebral fissures can give the appearance of hypertelorism.[4,5,15,31]

If the outer canthus of the eye is higher than the inner canthus, the eye is said to be upslanting; if the outer canthus is lower than the inner canthus, the eye is downslanting. The epicanthal fold is a vertical fold of skin on either side of the nose that covers the lacrimal caruncle and, although a characteristic finding in Asians, occurs in 20 percent of non-Asians, usually disappearing by ten years of age as the growth of the nasal bridge catches up to that of the medial canthal skin.[32] Epicanthal folds with upslanting palpebral fissures are common in infants of Asian descent. They may suggest Down syndrome in other ethnic groups, especially if associated with hypertelorism.[1,5,15]

The eyebrows normally extend above the eye in a curve approximately the length of the palpebral fissure. Eyebrows that meet at the glabella and abnormally long or tangled eyelashes are associated with some syndromes, such as Cornelia de Lange.[1,15]

Examination of the eyes is much easier if they are opened spontaneously by the infant. This may be accomplished at the beginning of the exam by giving an auditory stimulus, changing the infant's position from supine to upright, gently swinging the infant in an arc on the examiner's arm, or dimming the lights. If the eyes are forcefully opened, the eyelids will often evert, making visualization impossible. The eye exam will be more difficult if attempted within several hours after eye prophylaxis.

A full ophthalmoscopic exam is not practical, so the examiner must be alert to obtain the information needed in a limited time.[1,5,14,30] The ophthalmoscope should first be adjusted for focus and then for supply of a small round white beam of light. The examiner directs the light into the infant's pupils from a distance of about 6 inches to assess equality of size, pupillary reflex (constriction with bright light), and red retinal reflex. The notation "PERL" can be used if pupils are noted to be equal and reactive to light. When a bright light is directed at the newborn's lens, a clear red color is reflected from the retina back to the examiner. Opacity of the lens or cornea interrupts the reflection; lack of the red reflex could imply congenital cataract, retinoblastoma, or glaucoma (Figure 5-18).[1,4,5,30,33] In dark-skinned infants, the red reflex pales from orange toward gray in the most pigmented infants. The lens vessels of the premature infant can be examined to help determine gestational age (Chapter 3). A keyhole-shaped pupil, also known as coloboma of the iris, may be associated with other anomalies.[4,5,14,30]

The iris of a newborn infant is generally dark gray, blue, or brown at birth and will acquire final pigment color at about six months of age. Brushfield spots are white specks scattered linearly around the entire circumference of the iris. They are associated with Down syndrome, but may be seen as a normal variant.[15] The sclera of a term infant is generally white to bluish white. A blue sclera is associated with osteogenesis imperfecta. The sclera may become jaundiced with hyperbilirubinemia. In a normal gaze, no sclera should be visible above the iris. The "sunset sign" is often seen in infants with hydrocephalus, where there is lid retraction and a downward gaze.[4,5,12,14,30]

Observation of eyeball movements during neurologic assessment is discussed in detail in Chapter 11. Nystagmus is a rapid, searching movement of the eyeballs. Limited horizontal nystagmus may be elicited with rotational eye movement, but disappears by three to four months of age. Spontaneous horizontal, vertical, or torsional nystagmus and persistent nystagmus are always aberrant and likely associated with visual and/or neurologic abnormalities. Strabismus results from muscular incoordination and gives the appearance of crossed eyes (Figure 5-19). Pseudostrabismus from a flat nasal bridge or epicanthal folds usually resolves by one year of age and is differentiated from strabismus by the presence of symmetric corneal light reflex. Unusual protrusion (proptosis) or enlargement of the eyeball is associated with hyperthyroidism and congenital glaucoma and can be associated with damage to the eye with hemorrhage into its orbit.[5,12,30,33,34]

FIGURE 5-19 ▲ Strabismus.

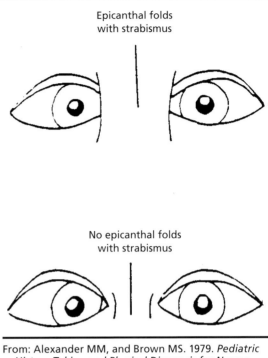

Epicanthal folds with strabismus

No epicanthal folds with strabismus

From: Alexander MM, and Brown MS. 1979. *Pediatric History Taking and Physical Diagnosis for Nurses,* 2nd ed. Philadelphia: Mosby, 97. Reprinted by permission of the authors.

NOSE

The size and shape of the nose may be racially characteristic and familial, but the infant's nose is generally smaller and flatter than an adult's. The nose should be symmetric and placed vertically in the midline. Nasal flaring is abnormal and is a sign of respiratory distress. Sneezing is common and normal unless excessive or continuous. Nasal stuffiness can be normal in the newborn period; however, chronic breathing difficulty or chronic nasal discharge is abnormal.[4,5,14,35]

A very low nasal bridge with a broad base may be associated with Down syndrome.[5,15] Deviation of the nasal septum to one side may be a deformation from position *in utero,* or it may be caused by a dislocated septum. If the septum will not easily straighten and the nares remain asymmetric when the tip of the nose

FIGURE 5-20 ▲ Nasal deformity.

This infant incurred dislocation of the triangular cartilage of the nasal septum during delivery. Inspection of the nose reveals deviation of the septum to the right and asymmetry of the nares (left). When the septum is manually moved toward the midline, the asymmetry persists, confirming the dislocation (right).

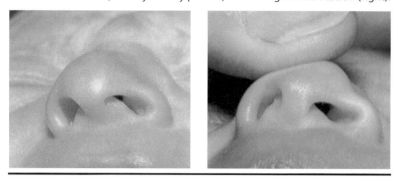

From: Brozanski BS, and Bogen DL. 2007. Neonatology. In *Atlas of Pediatric Physical Diagnosis*, 5th ed., Zitelli BJ, and Davis HW, eds. Philadelphia: Mosby, 44. Reprinted by permission.

is pushed to midline, the septum is dislocated and will require treatment (Figure 5-20).[4,6]

The examiner can elevate the tip of the nose slightly to view the nasal septum, the floor of the nose, and the turbinates.[29] Patency can be assessed by watching the infant breathe in a quiet state. Because infants are obligate nose breathers, bilateral choanal atresia (obstruction of the posterior nasal passages) will cause them to be cyanotic at rest and pink when crying and breathing through the mouth. If obstruction is suspected, a soft #5 French catheter can be gently passed through both nostrils to assess patency. If an infant has noisy nasal respirations, a piece of cold metal can be held under the nose to observe for mist formation under both nares. If the turbinates are swollen from previous suctioning, passing a catheter to assess patency may only make the edema worse.[4,5] Nasal occlusion can also be acquired from accumulation of secretions resulting in noisy respirations, feeding difficulties, respiratory distress, or apnea. Excessive bulb suctioning may aggravate the occlusive tendency, and normal saline irrigation or intermittent installation of normal saline drops may facilitate resolution of obstruction from secretions.

With increased use of nasal continuous airway pressure in premature infants, erosive trauma to the nasal labia, nasi columella, and nares is more common. Preventative and protective skin coverings can help, but monitoring the area for ulceration will minimize long-term disfiguring and scarring.

Major abnormalities of the nose, including clefts, single nares, masses, and partial or complete hypoplasia, are usually syndromic or associated with major central nervous system anomalies.

MOUTH

The lips and mucous membranes of a healthy term infant should be pink. Mild circumoral cyanosis is normal during transition and with crying during the first few days.

Abnormal shape and size of the oral opening, lips, philtrum (midline groove between the nose and upper lip), and mandible may be associated with a syndrome. A small oral opening, known as microstomia, may be seen in some syndromes. Macrostomia is seen with storage diseases such as the mucopolysaccharidoses. Lip thickness is related to racial and familial characteristics, and many infants have calluses on the lips from sucking. Unusually thick or thin lips are abnormal and require further evaluation for trauma or underlying mass. A thin upper lip with a smooth philtrum and short palpebral fissures may be seen in fetal alcohol syndrome. Cleft lip may be unilateral or bilateral and may be small or extend to the floor of the nose. Micrognathia, or abnormally small lower jaw, is seen in Robin sequence and other syndromes (Figure 5-21).[4,5,15,21]

During the examination, assess the cry for quality, strength, pitch, and hoarseness or stridor. Inspect the symmetry of facial movements during the cry, and assess rooting and sucking reflexes (Chapter 11).

Visual examination inside the mouth is easiest when the infant is crying. Use of a tongue depressor may stimulate a strong protrusion reflex, making assessment difficult. The mouth may be opened by gently pressing down on the chin. Abnormalities of the oropharynx are unusual, but a quick look is necessary to ensure absence of a structural anomaly or tumor. If possible, the uvula should be visualized at the back of the soft palate. A bifid uvula may be associated with other congenital anomalies.[5,15]

The tongue should fit well into the floor of the mouth and appear symmetric. A large tongue (macroglossia) impedes closure of the mouth and is associated with Beckwith-Wiedemann syndrome, hypothyroidism, and mucopolysaccharidosis. The tongue may *appear* large when the lower jaw is small, micrognathia with cleft palate, as is found with Robin sequence.

The frenulum attaches the underside of the tongue to the floor of the mouth, usually midway between the tongue's ventral surface and tip. A very thick or prominent frenulum, or "tongue tie," is rare, but if the frenulum limits movement of the tongue or pulls the tongue to a "V" at the tip, it is abnormal and may limit suck effectiveness. White patches on the tongue and mucous membranes may be from residual milk, and leukoplakia is normal in darkly pigmented infants. If the white coating cannot be easily removed with a tongue blade or cotton swab, it may be lesions of a Candida (oral thrush). A translucent or bluish swelling under the tongue is a mucocele or ranula.

FIGURE 5-21 ▲ Robin sequence (micrognathia).

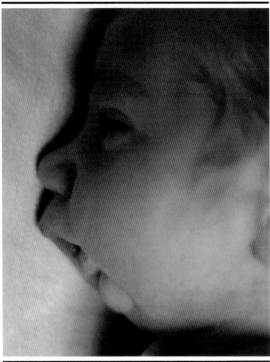

From: Clark DA. 2000. *Atlas of Neonatology.* Philadelphia: Saunders, 144. Reprinted by permission.

These mucous or salivary gland retention cysts usually resolve spontaneously.[5,12]

A gloved finger inserted into the infant's mouth with the finger pad up may be used to assess for continuity of the hard and soft palates, strength and coordination of suck, and for a gag reflex. A finger can also be used to run along the gum line to assess for lumps or masses. Small whitish-yellow clusters of Epstein pearls may be seen at the junction of the hard and soft palates and on the gums. Epstein's pearls are epithelial inclusion cells and usually disappear by a few weeks of age. They are histologically the same as Bohn's nodules found on the gums and milia seen on the skin.[4,5,12]

The gums should be pink and smooth. Natal teeth are rarely seen in Caucasian infants, but are a common variant in Native American infants.[36] Natal teeth or eruption

FIGURE 5-22 ▲ Cystic hygroma, with extension to the axilla.

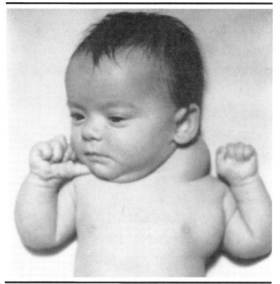

From: Koop CE. 1976. *Visible and Palpable Lesions in Children.* New York: Grune & Stratton, 35. Reprinted by permission of the author.

cysts with teeth appearing after birth (neonatal teeth) are usually seen in the lower incisor region. These are usually immature caps of enamel and dentine with poor root formation and may be very mobile. They may cause ulceration of the infant's tongue and pain with feeding, and there is a presumed risk of aspiration. For these reasons, removal is generally recommended, after consultation with a dentist and the family. If the tooth is firmly implanted, removal may impact future dentition, and the dentist may choose to leave it in place and do follow-up examinations to assess for any complications.[5,12,37,38]

Excessive oral secretions requiring frequent suctioning are abnormal in the newborn infant. The etiology could be esophageal atresia or poor swallow from a neurologic abnormality. Strength and coordination of swallow should be assessed at every feeding. If there is concern, patency of the esophagus is assessed by passage of a large bore (usually #10 French) orogastric tube with confirmation x-ray.[5]

FIGURE 5-23 ▲ Webbed neck—Turner syndrome.

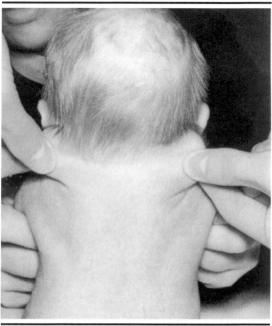

From: Milner RDG, and Herber SM. 1984. *Color Atlas of the Newborn.* Oradell, New Jersey: Medical Economics, 102. Reprinted by permission of Blackwell Scientific Publications.

NECK

The infant's neck is normally short, but severe shortness may be syndromic. To observe the shape and symmetry of the neck, elevate the shoulders, allowing the head to fall back slightly. Asymmetry is most likely the result of *in utero* positioning.

The neck must be visualized and palpated anteriorly, laterally, and posteriorly. The thyroid gland is difficult to palpate unless it is enlarged. Goiter, caused by intrauterine deprivation of thyroid hormone, is very unusual.[5]

Cystic hygroma is the most commonly seen neck mass (Figure 5-22). It is caused by development of sequestered lymph channels, which dilate into large cysts. Cystic hygroma is soft and fluctuant, transilluminates well, and is usually seen laterally or over the clavicle. Its size can range from only a few centimeters to massive, and it may cause severe feeding difficulties or airway compromise. Very small lesions may regress spontaneously, but surgical resection is usually required.[1,4]

A mass high in the neck may be a thyroglossal duct cyst or a branchial cleft cyst. A branchial sinus may also be seen anywhere along the sternocleidomastoid muscle. It may communicate with deeper structures, and infection may necessitate surgical removal of the entire sinus tract.[1,27]

During palpation of the neck, redundant skin or webbed neck may be noted. This is associated with Turner (Figure 5-23), Noonan, and Down syndromes.[1,4,14,15]

The clavicles should be palpated to assess for fracture, especially if there is a history of shoulder dystocia or macrosomia. Some infants present with nonrespiratory tachypnea due to discomfort from the fracture. Movement of the bone ends and crepitus may be felt soon after birth, or a fracture may not be evident for weeks, until callus has formed and can be palpated as a mass over the clavicle.

Assessment of neck reflexes, range of motion, and tone is described in Chapters 10 and 11.

Summary

Careful examination of the head and neck is important because abnormalities presenting at birth in this region are often indicative of other anomalies or a specific syndrome. Examination of the eyes and mouth requires the infant's cooperation, and the examiner needs to be alert for opportune times. States are now adopting the current recommendation for universal hearing screening for all newborns.

References

1. Fletcher MA. 1998. *Physical Diagnosis in Neonatology.* Philadelphia: Lippincott Williams & Wilkins, 173–299.
2. Lissauert T. 2006. Physical examination of the newborn. In *Neonatal-Perinatal Medicine: Diseases of the Fetus and Infant,* 8th ed., Martin RJ, Fanaroff AA, and Walsh MC, eds. Philadelphia: Mosby, 513–528.
3. Boom JA. Head growth: Evaluating macrocephaly and microcephaly. *UptoDate.* Retrieved from www.uptodate.com/patients/content/topic.do?topicKey=~NN6sGu1OzJ7QzLN.
4. Scanlon JW, et al. 1979. *A System of Newborn Physical Examination.* Baltimore: University Park Press, 45–60.
5. Seidel HM, et al. 2006. *Mosby's Guide to Physical Examination,* 6th ed. Philadelphia: Mosby, 254–359.
6. Disabato J, and Wulf J. 1994. Nursing strategies: Altered neurologic function. In *Family-Centered Nursing Care of Children,* 2nd ed., Betz CL, Hunsberger MM, and Wright S, eds. Philadelphia: Saunders, 1717–1790.
7. Dirks PB, and Rutka JT. 2007. The neurogenetic basis of pediatric neurosurgical conditions. In *Principles and Practice of Pediatric Neurosurgery,* 2nd ed., Albright AL, Pollack IF, and Adelson PB, eds. New York: Thieme Medical, 23–45.
8. Blair EM, et al. 2005. Optimal fetal growth for the Caucasian singleton and assessment of appropriateness of fetal growth: An analysis of a total population perinatal database. *BMC Pediatrics* 5(13): 1–12.
9. Goldenberg RL, et al. 1991. Black-white differences in newborn anthropometric measurements. *Obstetrics and Gynecology* 78(5 part 1): 782–788.
10. Cole TR, and Hughes HE. 1991. Autosomal dominant macrocephaly: Benign familial macrocephaly or a new syndrome? *American Journal of Medical Genetics* 41(1): 115–124.
11. Weaver DD, and Christain JC. 1980. Familial variation of head size and adjustment for parental head circumference. *Journal of Pediatrics* 96(6): 990–994.
12. Mead Johnson. 1978. *Variations and Minor Departures in Infants.* Evansville, Indiana: Mead Johnson and Company.
13. Kiesler J, and Ricer R. 2003. The abnormal fontanel. *American Family Physician* 67(12): 2547–2552.
14. Rennie JM. 2005. Examination of the newborn. In *Robertson's Textbook of Neonatology,* 4th ed., Rennie JM, and Robertson NRC, eds. Philadelphia: Churchill Livingstone, 249–266.
15. Jones KL. 2006. *Smith's Recognizable Patterns of Human Malformation,* 6th ed. Philadelphia: Saunders.
16. Gleeson JG, et al. 2006. Congenital structural defects. In *Pediatric Neurology: Principles and Practice,* 4th ed., Swaiman KF, Ashwal S, and Ferriero DM, eds. Philadelphia: Mosby, 363–490.
17. McMahon WS. 1998. Arteriovenous fistulae. In *The Science and Practice of Pediatric Cardiology,* 2nd ed., vol. 2, Garson A, et al., eds. Philadelphia: Lippincott Williams & Wilkins, 1677–1688.
18. Musewe NN, et al. 1992. Arteriovenous fistulae: A consideration of extracardiac causes of congestive heart failure. In *Neonatal Heart Disease,* Freedom RM, Benson LN, and Smallhorn JF, eds. New York: Springer-Verlag, 759–761.
19. Pellegrino PA, et al. 1987. Congestive heart failure secondary to cerebral arterio-venous fistula. *Child's Nervous System* 3(3): 141–144.
20. Taeusch HW, and Sniderman S. 2007. Initial evaluation: History and physical examination of the newborn. In *Avery's Diseases of the Newborn,* 8th ed., Taeusch HW, and Ballard RA, eds. Philadelphia: Saunders, 334–353.

21. Snively SL. 1987. Craniofacial anomalies. Part 2: Congenital syndromes and surgical treatment. *Selected Readings in Plastic Surgery* 4(25): 1–25.

22. Reid J. 2007. Neonatal subgaleal hemorrhage. *Neonatal Network* 26(4): 219–227.

23. Brozanski BS, and Bogen DL. 2007. Neonatology. In *Atlas of Pediatric Physical Diagnosis,* 5th ed., Zitelli BJ, and Davis HW, eds. St. Louis: Mosby, 29–57.

24. Furdon SA, and Clark DA. 2003. Scalp hair characteristics in the newborn infant. *Advances in Neonatal Care* 3(6): 286–296.

25. Currarino G. 1976. Normal variants and congenital anomalies in the region of the obelion. *American Journal of Roentgenology* 127(3): 487–494.

26. McKee-Garrett TM. Examination of the newborn. *UptoDate.* Retrieved from www.utdol.com.

27. Nicklaus PJ, and Kelley PE. 1996. Management of deep neck infection. *Pediatric Clinics of North America* 43(6): 1277–1296.

28. American Academy of Pediatrics, Joint Committee on Infant Hearing. 2007. Year 2007 position statement: Principles and guidelines for early hearing detection and intervention programs. *Pediatrics* 120(4): 898–921.

29. Swartz MH. 2006. *Textbook of Physical Diagnosis: History and Examination,* 5th ed. Philadelphia: Saunders, 762–785.

30. O'Doherty N. 1985. *Atlas of the Newborn,* 2nd ed. Lancaster, England: MTP Press, 45–53.

31. Aase JM. 1990. *Diagnostic Dysmorphology.* New York: Plenum, 34–118.

32. Jarvis C. 2007. *Physical Examination and Health Assessment,* 5th ed. Philadelphia: Saunders, 325.

33. Yanoff M. 1998. *Ophthalmic Diagnosis and Treatment.* Philadelphia: Current Medicine.

34. Gnanaraj L, and Rao VJ. 2000. Corneal birth trauma: A cause for sensory exotropia. *Eye* 14(part 5): 791–792.

35. Perry S. 1991. Normal newborn. In *Essentials of Maternity Nursing,* 3rd ed., Bobak IM, and Jensen MD, eds. Philadelphia: Mosby, 441–481.

36. Adam M, and Hudgins L. 2003. The importance of minor anomalies in the evaluation of the newborn. *NeoReviews* 4(4): e99–e103.

37. Mathewson RJ, and Primosch RE. 1995. *Fundamentals of Pediatric Dentistry,* 3rd ed. Chicago: Quintessence Publishing, 101–102.

38. Nik-Hussein NN. 1990. Natal and neonatal teeth. *Journal of Pedodontics* 14(2): 110–111.

NOTES

6 Chest and Lungs Assessment

Debbie Fraser Askin, MN, RNC-NIC

Physical assessment of the lungs should begin with a thorough review of the infant's history. Physical findings will vary greatly with the infant's gestational age and the time elapsed since delivery. Other important factors from the infant's prenatal, intrapartum, and postnatal history are outlined in Table 6-1.

Physical examination of the chest generally begins with observation so as not to disturb the infant before assessing breath sounds. Auscultation and palpation follow. Depending on the infant's physical condition, it may be necessary to allow him to rest between parts of the examination. Provisions should also be made to ensure that the infant does not become cold during the examination; cold stress will precipitate or further aggravate respiratory distress.

LANDMARKS AND STRUCTURE

The chest cavity is bounded by the sternum, 12 thoracic vertebrae, and 12 pairs of ribs (7 true vertebrocostal pairs and 5 false, or vertebrochondral, dyads). The ribs in the neonate are much more cartilaginous than in the adult, accounting in part for increased chest wall compliance and for the retractions seen in the infant with respiratory distress. The lower boundary of the thorax is formed

TABLE 6-1 ▲ Historic Factors the Examiner Should Note

Prenatal/Intrapartum History
Gestational age
Maternal drug ingestion
Fetal distress
Maternal health (i.e., diabetes, fever)
Prolonged rupture of membranes
Meconium-stained fluid
Delivery mode
Apgar scores

Postnatal History
Corrected age
Duration of mechanical ventilation
History of respiratory distress syndrome or bronchopulmonary dysplasia
History of pneumonia
Difficulty feeding
Apnea

by the diaphragm, normally a convex muscular sheath. The diaphragm inserts on the sternum, the first 3 lumbar vertebrae, and the lower 6 ribs.[1]

Other palpable thoracic landmarks include the suprasternal notch, found on the upper aspect of the sternum, and the xiphoid process,

FIGURE 6-1 ▲ Bony structure of the chest.

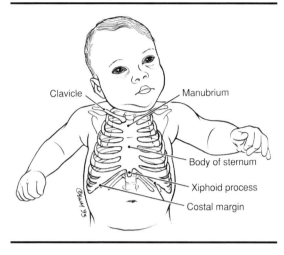

FIGURE 6-3 ▲ Reference lines.

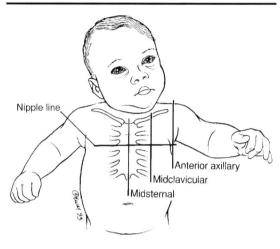

which protrudes below the sternum. The clavicles and scapulae complete the bony structure of the chest (Figure 6-1).

The chest cavity consists of three potential spaces: the mediastinum and the right and left pleural cavities. The mediastinum contains the heart, esophagus, trachea, mainstem bronchi, thymus, and major blood vessels. The three lobes of the right lung and the two lobes of the left lung are encased in serous membranes,

FIGURE 6-2 ▲ Internal structure of the chest.

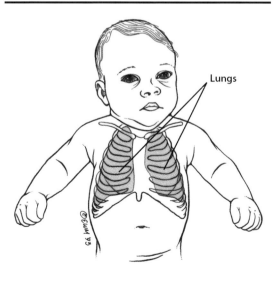

which make up the visceral and parietal pleura (Figure 6-2).

Reference Lines

When describing the location of a physical finding during the examination of chest and lungs, use the following reference lines to aid accuracy (Figure 6-3):

▶ **Anterior axillary line:** extends from the anterior axillary fold

▶ **Midclavicular line:** vertical line drawn through the middle of the clavicle

▶ **Midsternal line:** bisects the suprasternal notch

▶ **Nipple line:** horizontal line drawn through the nipples

Inspection

General

Inspection should begin with an overall assessment of the infant's color, tone, and activity. These findings provide clues to oxygenation and respiratory status.

Color

Observe the color of the infant's skin and mucous membranes. In the normal neonate, the lips and mucous membranes are pink and well perfused. Acrocyanosis (bluish coloration of the hands and feet) after birth is common and may persist during transition (up to 24 hours) following delivery.[2]

Color deviations might include cyanosis (either generalized or central [lips, tongue, and mucous membranes]) and acrocyanosis or mottling in the infant beyond transition. Other abnormalities in color—such as ruddiness and paleness—are discussed in Chapter 7.

Tone and Activity

Observe the infant's muscle tone and level and type of activity. Normal findings include flexed posture and active movement of all four limbs when awake. (Please note that the ability to attain and maintain flexion is decreased with prematurity.) Deviations include hypotonia and inactivity.

RESPIRATIONS

Rate

Count the infant's respirations for one full minute. Normal findings are 30 to 60 breaths per minute, with wide variations. If the room is very warm or cool, the infant's respiratory rate may vary. Most infants experiencing temperature stress will be tachypneic, but occasionally, they may demonstrate bradypnea (respirations less than 40 breaths per minute). Because of the increased likelihood of retained fetal lung fluid, babies delivered by cesarean section generally have a more rapid respiratory rate in the first 12 to 24 hours than do those delivered vaginally.[3]

Although respiratory rates vary, tachypnea (respirations greater than 60 breaths per minute) that persists beyond two hours of age may indicate underlying lung pathology (transient tachypnea of the newborn, respiratory distress syndrome, meconium aspiration, pneumonia), hyperthermia, or pain.

Bradypnea or shallow respirations are associated with central nervous system depression secondary to factors such as maternal drug ingestion, asphyxia, or birth injury.

Quality

Observe the general appearance of the infant. Relaxed, symmetric diaphragmatic respirations are normal. The newborn infant uses the diaphragm as the primary muscle of respiration. For the diaphragm to work efficiently, the rib cage must be stabilized by the intercostal muscles and the abdomen by the abdominal muscles. Coordination of this activity is still developing in term infants; it is less well developed in preterm infants, especially during rapid eye movement sleep, when respiratory instability may be seen.[1] To compensate for chest wall instability, the diaphragm is situated higher in the chest and is more concave in shape than the adult diaphragm, allowing for more efficient contractions.[1]

During normal respiratory efforts in the neonate, the lower thorax pulls in, and the abdomen bulges with each respiration. Deviations include asymmetric chest movement and excessive thoracic expansion. Paradoxical or seesaw respirations where the chest wall collapses and the abdomen bulges on inspiration suggest poor lung compliance and loss of lung volume.[4]

Babies are generally nose breathers, although most term infants will breathe through their mouth if the nares are occluded.[5] Nasal flaring and grunting may be noted immediately following birth. Mild nasal flaring, grunting, and substernal or intercostal retractions may be seen immediately after birth as the infant attempts to clear fetal lung fluid from the lungs. Beyond this period, flaring, grunting, and retractions suggest respiratory problems (transient tachypnea of the newborn, respiratory distress syndrome, atelectasis, pneumonia). Suprasternal retraction, especially if accompanied by gasping or stridor, may indicate upper airway obstruction (laryngeal webs or cysts,

FIGURE 6-4 ▲ Retraction sites.

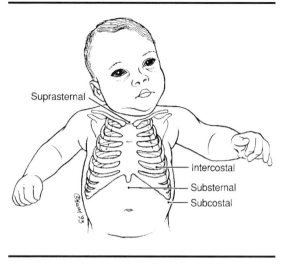

tumors, or vascular rings). Figure 6-4 shows the most common sites for retractions.

In 1956, Silverman and Andersen developed a scoring system (upon which many of today's scoring systems are based) to measure respiratory distress objectively.[6] This scoring system, shown in Table 6-2, can be used to quantify the extent of respiratory distress experienced by the infant at the time of examination.

Asymmetric chest movement may result from conditions such as diaphragmatic hernia, cardiac lesions inducing failure, pneumothorax, or phrenic nerve damage. Sneezing is a common finding because it helps to clear the nasal passages. Coughing in the newborn is considered abnormal.

Pattern

While counting respirations, note the pattern (regularity) of inspiration. Normal newborns have an irregular pattern of respirations, one that varies with environmental temperature, sleep, and state following a feeding. The less mature the infant, the more likely the breathing pattern is to be irregular. Periodic breathing (vigorous breaths followed by up to a 20-second pause) is common in preterm infants and may persist for up to several days

after birth in term infants. Periodic breathing persists in premature infants until they approach term.

A lapse of 15 seconds or more between respiratory cycles (one inspiration and one expiration) accompanied by bradycardia or color changes indicates apnea.[7] This condition, associated with prematurity, is gradually outgrown as the infant approaches term. Apnea in the term or close-to-term infant should be considered abnormal and may indicate underlying illness (sepsis, hypoglycemia, central nervous system injury or abnormality, seizures) or factors such as maternal drug ingestion.

COMPONENTS OF THE RESPIRATORY SYSTEM

Airways

The nasal portion of the airway is supported by bony and cartilaginous structures. Resistance to airflow in the nasal passages comprises about one-third of the total pulmonary resistance.[8] The pharyngeal component of the airway system is shorter than in adults and very compliant. In the absence of good muscle tone, the tongue can fall back against the soft palate and obstruct the airway, a process accentuated by neck flexion.[9] Observe for the presence of nasal flaring or obvious signs of obstruction. In particular, infants with poor tone, a large tongue (macroglossia), or a small jaw (micrognathia) may experience upper airway obstruction.

Larynx and Trachea

In the newborn, the tracheal cartilages (hyoid, thyroid, and cricoid) are supported by superficial fascia. In premature infants, this fascia is less well developed which increases the risk for airway obstruction.[8,10] The trachea and bronchi are supported by cartilaginous rings; however, in newborns, the cartilage is less well developed which can lead to an increased risk of airway collapse and air trapping.

TABLE 6-2 ▲ Assessment of Respiratory Distress

Criterion	Score		
	0	1	2
Chest movement	Chest moves with abdomen	Chest sinks minimally as abdomen rises	Seesaw respirations; chest sinks as abdomen rises
Intercostal retractions	None	Minimal	Marked
Xiphoid retractions	None	Just visible	Marked
Expiratory grunting	None	Heard only with stethoscope	Audible with naked ear
Nasal flaring	None	Minimal	Marked

Note: The distress score is calculated by adding the values (0, 1, 2) assigned to each category. A score of 10 indicates maximum distress.

Adapted from: Silverman WA, and Andersen DH. 1956. A controlled clinical trial of water mist on obstructive respiratory signs, death rate, and necropsy findings among premature infants. *Pediatrics* 17(1): 4. Reprinted by permission.

Chemoreceptors in the larynx trigger reflex apnea to prevent entry of foreign substances. Infants have the ability to alter laryngeal airway diameter by active movement of the vocal cords with breathing. Expiratory grunting in an infant with respiratory distress illustrates the infant's attempt to increase laryngeal airway resistance and ultimately to increase functional residual capacity in the lungs.

On x-ray, the trachea is normally midline. Deviation suggests pneumothorax, a space-occupying lesion, or significant atelectasis. Rotation of the infant on the x-ray cassette may result in the false appearance of tracheal deviation.

Thorax

Observe the infant's chest and measure its circumference. The average chest circumference in term infants is 30 to 36 cm or 2 cm less than the normal occipital-frontal head circumference.[11,12] The difference between head and chest circumference is more exaggerated in premature infants and in those with intrauterine growth restriction, where the chest circumference will be small in comparison to that of the head.

In infants, the thorax is normally rounded rather than dorsoventrally flattened, as in older children. The ribs are oriented more horizontally, limiting the potential for expansion of the rib cage.[13] The soft cartilaginous structure of the newborn's chest results in a tendency for the chest wall to collapse inward in the presence of decreased lung compliance. To preserve end-expiratory lung volume, the infant compensates by increasing the respiratory rate, shortening the inspiratory time, and closing the larynx.[9]

The anterior-posterior (AP) diameter of the thorax is approximately equal to the transverse diameter. A small thorax is seen in pulmonary hypoplasia, and a bell-shaped thorax may be an indication of neurologic abnormalities or dwarfing syndromes.[14] A barrel chest characterized by an increased AP diameter is a finding characteristic of the air trapping seen in conditions such as transient tachypnea of the newborn, meconium aspiration, and overzealous mechanical ventilation. Other deviations include protrusion of the sternum outward (pectus carinatum) or indented sternum (pectus excavatum), which are rarely clinically significant, but may be seen with rickets or Marfan syndrome.[14] Flaring of the lower ribs, known as Harrison's groove, is another finding that may be normal or associated with rickets (Figure 6-5).[11] Abdominal distention may accompany hyperinflation as

FIGURE 6-5 ▲ Different chest shapes.

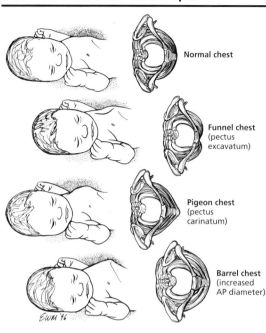

Normal chest

Funnel chest
(pectus
excavatum)

Pigeon chest
(pectus
carinatum)

Barrel chest
(increased
AP diameter)

the diaphragm is pushed downward by air trapped in the lungs.[4]

Muscle

Observe the chest for development, symmetry, and bulges or masses. The normal chest wall is symmetric and relatively smooth. Deviations include bulges or masses, atrophy, agenesis, and hypertrophy. Unilateral hypoplasia or absence of the pectoralis major muscle is a feature of Poland syndrome; other features of this syndrome include rib defects and upper limb hypoplasia.[14]

Nipples

Look at the number, placement, shape, and pigmentation of the nipples. Also inspect the nipples for fissures and secretions.

In the term infant, the areolae normally are raised and stippled, with 0.75 to 1 cm of palpable breast tissue. The distance from the outside of one areola to the outside of the other should be less than one-quarter of the chest circumference.[12] Size is also a useful indicator in gestational age assessment (Chapter 3).

In some infants, the influence of maternal estrogen results in breasts that are enlarged and engorged with a milky secretion known as "witch's milk." Secretion of this liquid may last one to two weeks and the enlargement, several months. Rarely, newborn infants may develop mastitis, characterized by redness, tenderness, breast enlargement, and discharge of pus.

Wide-spaced nipples are a feature of Turner syndrome; associated findings include lymphedema and redundant skin at the nape of the neck.[14] Supernumerary (accessory) nipples are most commonly seen as raised or pigmented areas 5 to 6 cm below the normal nipple but can be located anywhere on a vertical line drawn through the true nipple. Accessory nipples are commonly seen in African American infants.[11] In Caucasian infants, the association between supernumerary nipples and congenital renal anomalies has been disproven.[15]

ORAL AND NASAL SECRETIONS

Observe the quantity and quality of the infant's oral and nasal secretions. During transition, the appearance of oral and nasal secretions reflect the lungs' attempt to clear fetal fluid. Normal secretions are usually clear to white frothy mucus. Oral secretions will also reflect the stomach contents swallowed during delivery and therefore may be yellow or green in the presence of meconium or blood tinged if maternal blood was swallowed.

Deviations include excessive frothy oral secretions, which may indicate the presence of an esophageal atresia. Nasal stuffiness is associated with maternal drug use.[16] Snuffles (rhinitis) may be found with congenital syphilis.[17] Thick yellow secretions may be seen in the presence of a respiratory infection, and copious white nasal secretions are associated with respiratory syncytial virus infection.

FIGURE 6-6 ▲ **Sequence for breath sound auscultation: anterior and posterior chest.**

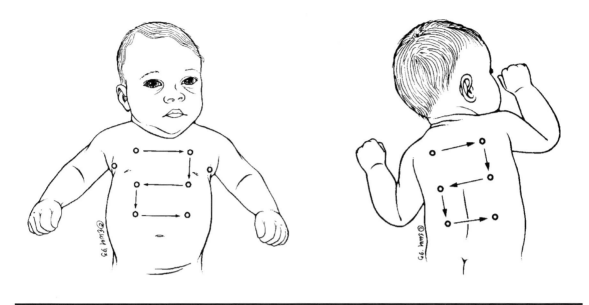

AUSCULTATION

Breath sounds are louder and coarser in the neonate than in the adult because the infant has less subcutaneous tissue to muffle transmission. Sounds are very readily referred in the neonate's chest because of its small size; therefore, localization of adventitious sounds is difficult. In addition, breath sounds may be decreased but are seldom absent, even over areas of atelectasis or pneumothorax. Breath sounds are less readily transmitted if (1) the pleural space contains fluid or air, (2) a bronchus contains secretions or foreign bodies, or (3) the lungs are hyperinflated. Sounds are more readily transmitted in the presence of consolidation—for example, with pneumonia.

To auscultate breath sounds, use both the bell and diaphragm of a warmed neonatal stethoscope. Begin at the top of the chest and move systematically from side to side (Figure 6-6). Breath sounds in the lower lobes of the lung can be assessed adequately only through the infant's back. Therefore, systematic auscultation of both the anterior and the posterior

chest should be performed and one side of the chest compared with the other.

NORMAL BREATH SOUNDS

Breath sounds should be assessed for pitch, intensity, and duration. Normal breath sounds have been described in adults and older children according to their location in the chest. As previously noted, localization of breath sounds in the neonate is very difficult. The following terms are sometimes used, however, to describe normal sounds within the lungs. These terms are also listed in Table 6-3.

Vesicular

Vesicular (from the Latin for "sac") breath sounds are soft, short, and low pitched during expiration and louder, longer, and higher pitched during inspiration. These sounds are normally found over the entire chest, except over the manubrium and trachea.

Bronchial

The loudest of the breath sounds, bronchial sounds are characterized by a short inspiration and a longer expiration. In adults, these sounds

TABLE 6-3 ▲ Normal Breath Sounds

Sound	Characteristics	Findings
Vesicular	Heard over most of lung fields; low pitch; soft and short expirations	 Low pitch, soft expirations
Bronchovesicular	Heard over main bronchus area and over upper right posterior lung field; medium pitch; expiration equals inspiration	 Medium pitch, medium expirations
Bronchial	Heard only over trachea; high pitch; loud and long expirations	 High pitch, loud expirations

Adapted from: Hagler DA, and Traver GAl. 2002. Respiratory system. In *Mosby's Clinical Nursing*, 5th ed., Thompson JM, et al., eds. Philadelphia: Mosby, 156. Reprinted by permission.

are found over the trachea, but they are seldom heard in the neonate.

Bronchovesicular

Bronchovesicular sounds demonstrate an inspiration and an expiration that are equal in quality, intensity, pitch, and duration. Louder than vesicular but less intense than bronchial sounds, bronchovesicular sounds are normally found over the manubrium and intrascapular regions.

Adventitious Sounds

Adventitious (abnormal) breath sounds are usually a sign of disease and may be superimposed on normal breath sounds. Auscultation shortly after birth frequently demonstrates adventitious sounds resulting from the presence of fetal lung fluid. Adventitious sounds heard at the onset of inspiration are more likely to result from secretions in the larger airways; sounds heard at the end of inspiration represent distal disease.[4] Care should be taken to distinguish sounds arising in the lungs from those arising in the upper airway. This may be achieved by placing the stethoscope over the infant's nose and mouth, which helps to localize upper airway sounds. Suctioning will often clear the upper airway and assist in identifying the presence of referred sounds. Table 6-4 summarizes some adventitious breath sounds.

Crackles

Crackles are defined as a series of brief crackling or bubbling sounds arising from a sudden release of energy—either an airway popping open or a liquid film breaking. In the past, this type of sound has also been referred to as rales.

Fine crackles can be simulated by rubbing together a lock of hair. These sounds commonly originate in the alveoli in the dependent lobes of the lung and are usually heard at the end of inspiration. Frequently heard in the first few hours after birth, fine crackles are also associated with respiratory distress syndrome (RDS) and bronchopulmonary dysplasia (BPD).

Medium crackles can be compared to the fizz of a carbonated drink. Believed to originate in the bronchioles, these sounds are associated with the passage of air through sticky surfaces, such as those found with pneumonia,

TABLE 6-4 ▲ Adventitious Breath Sounds

Sound/Characteristics	Simulation	Pictorial Findings
Crackles: discrete, noncontinuous sounds, sudden energy release		
Fine crackles (rales): high-pitched, discrete, noncontinuous crackling sounds heard during end of inspiration (indicates inflammation or congestion) (RDS)	Lock of hair	
Medium crackles (rales): lower, moister sound heard during midstage of inspiration; not cleared by a cough (edema, pneumonia)	Fizzy drink	
Coarse crackles (rales): loud, bubbly noise heard during inspiration; not cleared by a cough		
Rhonchi: loud, low, coarse sound like a snore heard at any point of inspiration or expiration; coughing may clear sound (usually means mucus or foreign body in trachea or large bronchi)		
Wheeze: musical noise sounding like a squeak; may be heard during inspiration or expiration; usually louder during expiration (BPD)		
Pleural friction rub: dry rubbing or grating sound, usually due to inflammation of pleural surfaces; heard during inspiration or expiration; loudest over lower lateral anterior surface (mechanical ventilation in RDS)	Rubbing cupped hand	

Adapted from: Hagler DA, and Traver GAl. 2002. Respiratory system. In *Mosby's Clinical Nursing*, 5th ed., Thompson JM, et al., eds. Philadelphia: Mosby, 156. Reprinted by permission.

pulmonary congestion, or transient tachypnea of the newborn.

Coarse crackles are loud and bubbly. These sounds are associated with significant accumulations of mucus or fluid in the larger airways.

Rhonchi

When distinguished from wheezes, rhonchi are described as lower in pitch. They are more musical in quality than crackles. Rhonchi are seldom described in the neonate, but may be heard when either secretions or aspirated foreign matter is present in the large airways.

Wheezes

Also referred to as high-pitched rhonchi, wheezes may be heard on inspiration or expiration, but are usually louder on expiration. Seldom heard in the newborn, wheezes may be audible in the infant with BPD because

of narrowing of the airways or presence of bronchospasm.

Rubs

Rubs can be simulated by holding a cupped hand to the ear and rubbing a finger over the cupped hand. Rubs are usually associated with inflammation of the pleura; however, in the neonate, this sound is frequently described during mechanical ventilation.

Stridor

Stridor is a high-pitched, hoarse sound produced during inspiration or expiration at the larynx or upper airways. This sound in a newborn indicates a partial obstruction of the airway and should be investigated promptly. Stridor may also be heard postextubation in infants with edema of the upper airway.

Bowel sounds are occasionally auscultated over the lung fields. These may be referred sounds transmitted from the abdomen. If these

TABLE 6-5 ▲ Common Findings and Their Possible Causes in Infants Receiving Mechanical Ventilation

Finding	Possible Cause
Absence of air entry	Pneumothorax Blocked endotracheal tube (ETT) Accidental extubation Space-occupying lesion
Decreased or unequal air entry	Atelectasis Pneumothorax Intubation of right bronchus
Asymmetric chest movement	Pneumothorax Intubation of right bronchus
Increased chest excursion	Change in compliance resulting in overventilation
Decreased chest excursion	Underventilation Blocked ETT Accidental extubation Air leak

sounds persist over the lung fields, especially on the left side, diaphragmatic hernia should be considered.

PERCUSSION

The small size of the neonatal chest relative to the examiner's hands makes percussion of limited value as a part of the neonatal physical examination. The infant's chest is normally hyperresonant because of the thin chest wall. The experienced examiner may find percussion useful, however, in distinguishing between air and fluid or solid tissue in cases where the infant is in distress and a pneumothorax, pleural effusion, or diaphragmatic hernia is suspected.

The technique for percussion involves placing one finger firmly against the chest wall and tapping that finger with the index finger of the other hand. A change in resonance indicates a change in the consistency of the underlying tissue.

PALPATION

After a thorough inspection of the chest, auscultation of breath sounds, and percussion, if necessary, the examiner next palpates certain areas of the infant's chest.

CLAVICLE

The clavicle is the bone most commonly fractured during the birth process, occurring in 1.9–2.9 percent of term deliveries.[18] Palpate the entire length of the clavicles. Suspect fracture if crepitus, swelling, or tenderness is present. Infants with a fractured clavicle may also demonstrate an incomplete Moro reflex on the affected side (Chapter 11).

BREAST TISSUE

As indicated in the discussion of inspection, the breast buds should be gently palpated to determine the presence of hypertrophy, fissures, secretions, or masses.

STERNUM AND RIBS

Palpate the sternum and the ribs for crepitus or masses. Crepitus may indicate subcutaneous air from an underlying pulmonary air leak. A lump or mass should be investigated for the presence of an underlying fracture. The tip of the xiphoid process often protrudes anteriorly and may be movable with slight pressure.

OVERALL STRUCTURE

The cartilages should be palpated to assess for hypertrophy. The costal cartilages enlarge in rickets and can be palpated as a series of small lumps down the side of the sternum. This phenomenon is known as the "rachitic rosary."

TRANSILLUMINATION

Transillumination is a useful adjunct to physical examination when a pneumothorax is suspected. Place a high-intensity fiberoptic light source perpendicular to the neonate's chest. While moving the light source back and forth from side to side, compare the amount of transillumination between left and right and upper and lower aspects of the chest. In a darkened room, air pockets will present with hyperlucency or a lanternlike glow.[19]

Subcutaneous edema or air may result in a false positive reading. Chest wall edema, dark skin, tape, and equipment may obscure transillumination and result in a false negative finding. In an early study of transillumination, a false positive rate of 4 percent was identified.[20] Diagnoses obtained by transillumination should be confirmed by chest x-ray.

ASSESSMENT DURING MECHANICAL VENTILATION

CONVENTIONAL VENTILATION

The use of mechanical ventilation necessitates increased vigilance in all aspects of physical assessment. Particular attention should be given to assessing the adequacy and symmetry of chest expansion and to the auscultation of breath sounds. Care should be taken to eliminate water in the ventilator tubings before assessing chest sounds because gas bubbling through water produces referred sounds.

Breath sounds may be altered by the presence of an endotracheal tube, which effectively narrows the neonate's airway, and by the flow of gases from the ventilator, which may increase turbulence. Wheezes and rubs are more commonly heard in these cases. Harsh or sandpaper breath sounds are often described in infants receiving mechanical ventilation for RDS. These sounds may result from the forced opening of atelectatic alveoli. Harsh breath sounds may also result from air leaking around the endotracheal tube. Listening with the stethoscope over the infant's mouth may be useful in differentiating sounds produced at the larynx from those produced in the chest. Air leaking around the endotracheal tube may produce a high-pitched sound heard during inspiration. Table 6-5 outlines some common concerns in the neonate receiving mechanical ventilation.

PATIENT-TRIGGERED VENTILATION

Technologic advances in neonatal ventilators have resulted in the development of sensitive indicators of lung compliance and work of breathing. Ventilators that measure tidal volume allow the clinician to assess the neonate's ability to generate a spontaneous breath and to determine the relative size of that breath compared with the size of the breath generated by the ventilator. As the neonate's lung disease improves, he will generate larger tidal volumes, suggesting a readiness for weaning.

Ventilation in which a preset tidal volume is delivered results in breaths that require varying amounts of pressure to deliver the desired volume of gas. As the infant's lung compliance improves, less peak inspiratory pressure is required to deliver the same amount of volume. By monitoring the pressure used, the clinician can assess changes in the infant's lungs.

HIGH-FREQUENCY VENTILATION

High-frequency ventilation techniques require several alterations in the traditional approach to physical assessment of the chest and lungs. The rapid rates used in high-frequency ventilation cause the infant to shake or vibrate, making it impractical to count respiratory rates. Many infants on high-frequency ventilation will be apneic; however, spontaneous respirations that do occur can be recorded in the usual fashion.

The chest should be both observed and palpated to assess the symmetry and quality of vibrations. Excessive movement of the chest or abdomen may indicate overventilation. Decreased or asymmetric movement may indicate complications such as air leak or airway obstruction.

Breath sounds during high-frequency ventilation will be high pitched, with a jackhammer quality. Auscultation should be performed to assess changes in the pitch or quality of sound. Higher pitched or musical sounds may indicate the presence of secretions. Decreases in pitch may indicate the presence of a pneumothorax. Traditional breath sounds can be assessed during periods of manual ventilation or with sighs given during oscillation.

SUMMARY

The respiratory system undergoes rapid and significant changes during the transition to extrauterine life. These changes leave the lungs vulnerable to both transient and more life-threatening maladaptations. Careful scrutiny of the respiratory system is required to identify potential problems for treatment. Findings from the physical examination of the chest and lungs form the basis for further investigations. The findings should be documented using standard terms and reference points to permit comparison of findings with subsequent assessments.

REFERENCES

1. Blackburn ST. 2007 *Maternal, Fetal, and Neonatal Physiology,* 3rd ed. Philadelphia: Saunders, 346–347.

2. Gardner SL, and Johnson JL. 2006. Respiratory diseases. In *Handbook of Neonatal Intensive Care,* 6th ed., Merenstein GB, and Gardner SL, eds. Philadelphia: Mosby, 79–121.

3. Jain L, and Eaton DC. 2006. Physiology of fetal lung fluid clearance and the effect of labor. *Seminars in Perinatology* 30(1): 34–43.

4. Narvey M, and Fletcher MA. 2005. Physical assessment and classification. In *Avery's Neonatology: Pathophysiology and Management of the Newborn,* 6th ed., Macdonald MG, Mullen MD, and Seshia MMK, eds. Philadelphia: Lippincott Williams & Wilkins, 327–350.

5. Bergeson PS, and Shaw JC. 2001. Are infants really obligatory nasal breathers? *Clinical Pediatrics* 40(10): 567–569.

6. Silverman WA, and Andersen DH. 1956. A controlled clinical trial of water mist on obstructive respiratory signs, death rate, and necropsy findings among premature infants. *Pediatrics* 17(1): 1–10.

7. Barrington K, and Finer N.1991. The natural history of the appearance of apnea of prematurity. *Pediatric Research* 29(4 part 1): 372–375.

8. Shaffer TH, and Wolfson MR. 2004. Upper airway structure: Function, regulation, and development. In *Fetal and Neonatal Physiology,* 3rd ed., Polin RA, Fox WW, and Abman SH, eds. Philadelphia: Saunders, 834–841.

9. Greenough A. 2005. Pulmonary disease of the newborn. In *Roberton's Textbook of Neonatology,* 4th ed., Rennie JM, ed. London: Churchill Livingstone, 445–603.

10. Praud JP, and Reix P. 2005. Upper airways and neonatal respiration. *Respiratory Physiology and Neurobiology* 149(1-3): 131–141.

11. Colyar MR. 2003. Assessment of the newborn. In *Well Child Assessment for Primary Care Providers,* Colyar MR, ed. Philadelphia: Davis, 244–262.

12. Hernandez JA, and Glass SM. 2005. Physical assessment of the newborn. In *Assessment and Care of the Well Newborn,* 2nd ed., Thureen PJ, et al., eds. Philadelphia: Saunders, 119–122.

13. Greenspan JS, Miller TL, and Shaffer TH. 2005. The neonatal respiratory pump: A developmental challenge with physiologic limitations. *Neonatal Network* 24(5): 15–22.

14. Fuloria M, and Kreiter S. 2002. The newborn examination: part I. Emergencies and common abnormalities involving the skin, head, neck, chest, and respiratory and cardiovascular systems. *American Family Physician* 65(1): 61–68.

15. Grotto I, et al. 2001. Occurrence of supernumerary nipples in children with kidney and urinary tract malformations. *Pediatric Dermatology* 18(4): 291–294.

16. Elliott MR, et al. 2004. Frequency of newborn behaviours associated with neonatal abstinence syndrome: A hospital-based study. *Journal of Obstetrics and Gynaecology Canada* 26(1): 25–34.

17. Venkatesh M, et al. 2006. Infection in the neonate. In *Handbook of Neonatal Intensive Care,* 6th ed., Merenstein GB, and Gardner SL, eds. Philadelphia: Mosby, 569–593.

18. Joseph PR, and Rosenfeld W. 1990. Clavicular fractures in neonates. *American Journal of Diseases of Children* 144(2): 165–167.

19. Hagedorn MIE, et al. 2006. Respiratory diseases. In *Handbook of Neonatal Intensive Care,* 6th ed., Merenstein GB, and Gardner SL, eds. Philadelphia: Mosby, 595–698.

20. Kuhns LR, et al. 1975. Diagnosis of pneumothorax or pneumomediastinum in the neonate by transillumination. *Pediatrics* 56(3): 355–360.

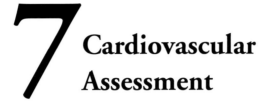

7 Cardiovascular Assessment

Lyn Vargo, PhD, RN, NNP-BC

Cardiovascular assessment of the newborn requires great skill in the techniques of inspection, palpation, and auscultation. Inspection of the general activity of the neonate, breathing patterns, presence or absence of cyanosis, and activity of the precordium are all important. Palpation of pulses, apical impulse, and thrills is also imperative. Auscultation, however, is the main focus of the cardiovascular exam. Through auscultation, the examiner assesses heart rate, rhythm, regularity, and heart sounds (especially murmurs). A pediatric or neonatal stethoscope with a diaphragm and a bell is very helpful for auscultation. The bell conducts sound without distortion (although it can be difficult to maintain an airtight seal). The bell is useful for low-pitched sounds. If properly sized, the diaphragm maintains its own seal and is useful for high-pitched sounds.

The dynamic properties of the newborn heart make cardiovascular assessment of the neonate challenging. The change from "fetal-placental" to "newborn-lung" circuitry means that the findings of the cardiovascular exam constantly change over the first few hours, days, and weeks of life. Practitioners performing cardiovascular assessments must be aware of these alterations and

their timing and incorporate this knowledge into their examinations.

Because changes in ductal flow, decreasing pulmonary vascular resistance, and increasing systemic vascular resistance occur over the first few hours and days of life, cardiovascular assessments ideally should be done shortly after birth, at 6 to 12 hours of age, at 1 and 3 days of age, and at regular intervals thereafter. Because this is rarely possible in the normal newborn, it is recommended that, at a minimum, examinations be done shortly after birth, at one day of age, and at regular pediatric office visits thereafter.

REVIEWING MATERNAL, FAMILY, AND BIRTH HISTORIES

The first consideration in a complete cardiovascular assessment is a thorough maternal history. Several maternal conditions can affect the neonate's cardiovascular system. These include maternal diabetes, systemic lupus erythematosus, and a maternal history of congenital heart disease (CHD). Maternal diabetes can increase the risk of CHD in the neonate to three to four times that for the general population.[1] The prevalence of CHD (for truncus arteriosus, transposition of the great arteries, tetralogy of Fallot, atrioventricular [AV] canal, and

TABLE 7-1 ▲ Environmental Factors Associated with Congenital Heart Defects

Teratogenic Influence	Risk of Cardiac Defect (%)	Common Types of Defects
Maternal rubella	35	PDA, PPS, septal defects
Maternal diabetes	3–5	VSD, coarc, complete transposition
Maternal phenylketonuria	25–50	TET
Systemic lupus erythematosus	20–40	Complete heart block
Maternal alcohol abuse	25–30	Septal defects
Hydantoin	2–3	Pulmonary and aortic stenosis, coarc, PDA
Lithium	10–20	Ebstein's malformation, TA, ASD
Retinoic acid	?	Defects of ventricular outflow tracts
Trimethadione (historical)	15–30	TET, complete transposition, HLHS
Thalidomide (historical)	<5	TET, septal defects, truncus arteriosus

Key: ASD, atrial septal defect; coarc, coarctation of the aorta; HLHS, hypoplastic left heart syndrome; PDA, patent ductus arteriosus; PPS, peripheral pulmonary artery stenosis; TA, tricuspid atresia; TET, tetralogy of Fallot; VSD, ventricular septal defect.

Adapted from: Burn J. 2002. The aetiology of congenital heart disease. In *Paediatric Cardiology,* 2nd ed., Anderson RH, et al. eds. New York: Churchill Livingstone, 151. Reprinted by permission.

hypoplastic left heart syndrome) in national estimates for the U.S. between 1999 and 2001 was between 0.82 and 4.73 per 10,000 live births.[2]

Ventricular septal defects and transposition of the great arteries are common defects seen in infants of diabetic mothers. There is also a specific cardiomyopathy commonly found in infants of diabetic mothers.[3]

Systemic lupus erythematosus in the mother has been shown to increase the incidence of congenital complete AV block in the neonate.[4] These infants present with low resting heart rates, sometimes while *in utero.*

As women with CHD are living longer and reaching childbearing age, new information has become available. It has been documented that there is a 10 to 15 percent risk of CHD in the offspring of mothers with CHD.[3,5]

Even though only a small percentage of CHD can be related to environmental factors, a history of the pregnancy (especially of the first two months, when the heart is forming) is important. Environmental factors known to increase the risk of congenital heart defects are listed in Table 7-1. Drugs known to cause heart defects include amphetamines, lithium, phenytoin sodium, thalidomide, retinoic acid, valproic acid, and alcohol.[5,6] In addition, viral infections during the last two weeks of pregnancy may cause acute myocarditis in the neonate.

Because of the influence of genetic factors, family history is an important feature of a cardiovascular assessment. Details about other siblings with CHD should be identified. If one parent is affected or if an older sibling had a specific defect, there is a 1 to 5 percent risk of recurrence.[3] Also, several specific disorders that might demonstrate dominant or recessive inheritance patterns are associated with specific congenital heart defects (Table 7-2). If any of these disorders is identified in the family history, the neonatal assessment should be even more rigorous than usual.

Details of the labor and delivery history must be considered during the cardiovascular examination. Knowledge of any causal factors, such as perinatal hypoxia, maternal infection, or drugs given to the mother during labor, will help the examiner determine whether CHD is a likely explanation for abnormal physical findings.

Finally, birth weight, gestational age, and sex must be taken into consideration. There is

TABLE 7-2 ▲ Disorders Associated with Congenital Heart Defects

Disorder	% Patients with Cardiac Disease	Types of Cardiac Abnormalities
de Lange syndrome	30	VSD, ASD, PDA, AS, EFE
Holt-Oram heart-hand syndrome	100	ASD-2, VSD or PDA in 2/3, conduction block, HLHS, TAPVC, truncus arteriosus
Marfan syndrome	Up to 100	Aortic aneurysm, AR, MR, TR, prolapse
Noonan syndrome		PS/dysplasia, hypertrophic cardiomyopathy, PDA, coarc
Carpenter syndrome	33	PDA, PS, VSD, TF, TGA, ASD
Ellis van Creveld	50–60	Single atrium, primum ASD, coarc, HLHS
Mucopolysaccharidosis type 1	>50	Valvular disease in all types
Trisomy 21 (Down syndrome)	40–50	AV canal, VSD, PDA, ASD-1 and -2, TF
Trisomy 18 (Edwards syndrome)	90–100	VSD, polyvalvular disease, ASD, PDA
Trisomy 13 (Patau syndrome)	80	PDA, VSD, ASD, coarctation of the aorta, AS, PS
XO (Turner syndrome)	>50	Coarc, bicuspid aortic valve, aortic aneurysm, AS, VSD
Beckwith-Wiedemann syndrome	15 ?	Hypertrophic cardiomegaly, ASD, VSD, PDA, TF
CHARGE association	65–75	TF, DORV, ASD, VSD, PDA, coarc, AV canal
DiGeorge syndrome	>50	Interrupted aortic arch, truncus arteriosus, TF, right aortic arch
VACTERL association	10	VSD, ASD, TF
Williams-Beuren syndrome	50–80	Supravalvar AS, stenosis of left coronary artery, small aorta, multiple pulmonary arteries, cerebral and renal arteries
Cleft lip and palate	25	VSD, PDA, TGA, TF, SV
Diaphragmatic hernia	25	TF
Omphalocele	20	TF, ASD
Intestinal atresia	10	VSD
Renal agenesis unilateral/ bilateral	17/75	VSD

Key: AR, aortic regurgitation; AS, aortic stenosis; ASD, atrial septal defect; ASD-1, primum atrial septal defect; ASD-2, secundum atrial septal defect; AV, atrioventricular; coarc, coarctation of the aorta; DORV, double outlet right ventricle; EFE, endocardial fibroelastosis; HLHS, hypoplastic left heart syndrome; MR, mitral regurgitation; PDA, patent ductus arteriosus; PS, pulmonic stenosis; SV, single ventricle; TAPVC, total anomalous pulmonary venus connection; TF, tetralogy of Fallot; TGA, transposition of the great arteries; TR, tricuspid regurgitation; VSD, ventricular septal defect.

Adapted from: Flanagan MF, Yeager SB, and Weindling SN. 2005. Cardiac disease. In *Avery's Neonatology: Pathophysiology and Management of the Newborn,* 6th ed., MacDonald MG, Mullett MD, and Seshia MMK, eds. Philadelphia: Lippincott Williams & Wilkins, 636–637. Reprinted by permission.

an increased incidence of CHD in low birth weight infants, and premature infants have an increased risk of patent ductus arteriosus. Several congenital heart defects are more common in one sex than in the other.

OBSERVING APPEARANCE AND BEHAVIOR

Because of the central role the heart plays, a complete cardiovascular assessment encompasses most of the other systems. The cardiovascular exam cannot be considered in isolation from the neurologic, respiratory, abdominal, and skin examinations.

The initial cardiovascular assessment of the neonate should include general observation of the infant's overall appearance and behavior. A newborn with CHD may exhibit decreased activity and/or appear flaccid. Notation of extracardiac anomalies is important because CHD is associated with such abnormalities in approximately 25 percent of infants.[7] Increased incidence of CHD is seen with neurologic and gastrointestinal anomalies, tracheoesophageal fistulas, renal and urogenital irregularities, and diaphragmatic hernia.[5]

INSPECTING SKIN AND MUCOUS MEMBRANES

The next step in the neonatal cardiovascular exam is inspection of the infant's color. Accurate assessment of skin color depends on the observer's astuteness and on ambient temperature and lighting conditions.[8] A cyanotic Caucasian infant may look pink under bright lighting, and a centrally pink infant may look cyanotic under dim lighting. In a well-lit room, the infant should be centrally pink—that is, not only should his general color appear pink, but his lips, tongue, earlobes, and (in males) scrotum should also appear pink. The best indicator of determining central cyanosis is generally the tongue, due to its rich vascular supply and lack of pigmentation.[5,9]

POLYCYTHEMIA

Many infants appear pink at rest but become deep red to purplish with crying. This is usually related to polycythemia, a condition found when the infant's central hematocrit is greater than 65 percent. Although polycythemic/plethoric infants may appear cyanotic, as neonates, they rarely are. The ruddy or reddish color may be mistaken for cyanosis simply because newborns who have increased amounts of hemoglobin usually have a larger percentage of that hemoglobin unsaturated. This unsaturated hemoglobin masks the saturated hemoglobin, and the infants appear purplish in color.

CYANOSIS

Central cyanosis refers to the bluish color of the skin, lips, tongue, earlobes, scrotum (in males), and nail beds seen in the neonate with significant arterial oxygen desaturation. Central cyanosis becomes visible when there are at least 5 g of hemoglobin per 100 mL of blood not bound to oxygen.[5,9] Central cyanosis must be differentiated from peripheral cyanosis (acrocyanosis), which is blue color in the hands and feet, and circumoral cyanosis, which is blue color around the mouth. Peripheral cyanosis is normal in newborns until about two days of age and is thought to be caused by vasomotor instability. No treatment is necessary for peripheral cyanosis. When in doubt whether cyanosis is central or peripheral, check the infant's arterial saturation via a pulse oximeter.[5,10] Central cyanosis is difficult to detect unless the arterial desaturation is 80–85 percent or lower in an infant with a normal hemoglobin level.[5,9,10]

Central cyanosis can be the result of many things: lung disease, sepsis, persistent pulmonary hypertension, or neurologic disease. Cyanosis is also one of the two best indicators of CHD (symptoms of congestive heart failure is the other). It is therefore important to carefully assess cyanosis and the infant's response to oxygen. Cyanosis that does not improve upon administration of 100 percent oxygen is most likely the result of cardiac causes, as is cyanosis that increases with crying.[11]

PALLOR/MOTTLING/PERFUSION

Pallor and mottling of the skin should also be considered in assessing cardiac status, as should the infant's general overall perfusion. Infants with compromised cardiac status may appear pale as a result of vasoconstriction and the shunting of blood away from the skin to more vital organs. Mottling, if present, must be evaluated with any other signs and symptoms associated with it. It may be a sign of cardiogenic shock when associated with hypovolemia or decreased cardiac output. Mottling can also be seen in normal infants under certain

FIGURE 7-1 ▲ Radial and brachial pulses.

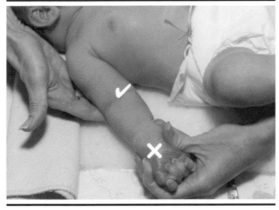

Demonstrates the location of radial pulse (✗), palpable on the flexor surface of the wrist just medial to the distal end of the radius. Demonstrates the location of the brachial pulse (✔) in and above the groove of the elbow, medial to the biceps muscle and tendon.

FIGURE 7-2 ▲ Femoral pulses.

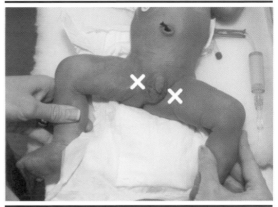

Demonstrates the location of the femoral pulses (✗), palpable just below the inguinal ligament, an equal distance between the pubic tubercle and the anterior superior iliac spine.

circumstances, such as in the stressed or cold neonate, when it is then referred to as cutis marmorata. A hypoxic, anemic infant may not appear cyanotic because hemoglobin levels may be too low to produce a bluish color.[3,5]

Capillary filling time can give valuable information about the infant's cardiac perfusion to the skin and should be determined by pressing a finger against the infant's skin in both a central and a peripheral area. When blanching is noted, the examiner counts the seconds required for the color to return to the skin. Capillary filling time of greater than three to four seconds is usually considered abnormal.

EDEMA

In the infant, edema is rarely associated with cardiac problems, as it is in older patients. Isolated peripheral edema is a hallmark sign of Turner syndrome, however. Infants with this syndrome show a high incidence of coarctation of the aorta.

OBSERVING BREATHING PATTERNS

Respiratory activity must be observed in relation to the cardiac examination. Respiratory

rate and effort should be documented (as addressed in Chapter 6). Signs of respiratory distress—such as grunting, flaring, retractions, tachypnea, and crackles—may be signs of congestive heart failure. It is also important to keep in mind that an infant with nonlabored respiratory effort who is cyanotic is most likely cyanotic as a result of a congenital heart defect that restricts pulmonary blood flow.[12]

PALPATING PERIPHERAL PULSES

The character of the peripheral pulses should be assessed next. This is best done with the infant quiet. Pulse rate, rhythm, volume, and character should all be examined. Pulses represent an approximate determination of cardiac output. The axillary, palmar, brachial, radial, femoral, popliteal, posterior tibial, and dorsalis pedis may be palpated using the index finger (Figures 7-1 through 7-4). (Note that the dorsalis pedis may not be felt in newborns; this is considered normal.)

PULSE RATE

On initial palpation, the pulse rate should be noted. The significance of rate is discussed later in this chapter. After determining the

FIGURE 7-3 ▲ Posterior tibial pulse.

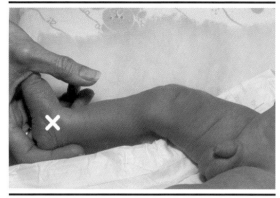

Demonstrates the location of the posterior tibial pulse (**✗**), palpable just behind and slightly below the medial malleolus.

FIGURE 7-4 ▲ Dorsalis pedis pulse.

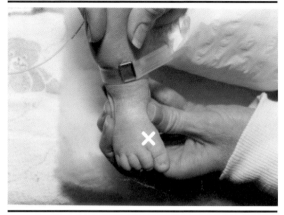

Demonstrates the location of the dorsalis pedis pulse (**✗**), palpable on the dorsum of the foot by following an imaginary line that traces the groove between the first and second toes.

rate, document any irregularities in rhythm or skipped beats. A pulse deficit (a difference between the heart rate counted with a pulse and that counted by auscultation) is frequently seen with ectopic rhythms.

PULSE VOLUME/CHARACTER

Probably the most important determinations in neonatal pulse evaluation are those assessing volume and character. Volume of peripheral pulses is assessed on a scale of 0 to +4, with +4 being the strongest and 0 representing an absent or nonpalpable pulse (Table 7-3).[13]

At a minimum, the femoral and brachial pulses should be palpated bilaterally, and then one femoral and the right brachial should be palpated simultaneously.[5,9] (The right brachial should be palpated instead of the left because the right subclavian artery is always preductal, but the left subclavian artery may or may not be preductal.) Absent or weak femoral pulses—especially in comparison to the right brachial pulse—are abnormal and may indicate decreased aortic blood flow as seen with coarctation of the aorta, aortic stenosis, and hypoplastic left heart syndrome.

Bounding pulses in any extremity should be noted. Bounding pulses are usually present with patent ductus arteriosus and other aortic-runoff lesions (truncus arteriosus, aortic regurgitation, systemic arteriovenous fistula).[5,9] Normal premature infants have prominent peripheral pulses, but strong palmar or digital pulses indicate a wide pulse pressure such as that seen with patent ductus arteriosus.[14] Weak or absent peripheral pulses occur in the presence of low cardiac output from any cause, especially left heart obstructive lesions.[15]

TABLE 7-3 ▲ Grading of Pulses

Grade	Description
0	Not palpable
+1	Difficult to palpate, thready, weak, easily obliterated with pressure
+2	Difficult to palpate, may be obliterated with pressure
+3	Easy to palpate, not easily obliterated with pressure (normal)
+4	Strong, bounding, not obliterated with pressure

From: Hockenberry MJ, and Barrera P. 2007. Communication and physical developmental assessment of the child. In *Wong's Nursing Care of Infants and Children,* 8th ed., Hockenberry MJ, and Wilson D, eds. Philadelphia: Mosby, 173. Reprinted by permission.

Inspecting and Palpating the Chest

Precordium

In the cardiac exam, assessment of the chest should begin with inspection of the precordium, the area on the anterior chest under which the heart lies (Figure 7-5). Generally, except during the first few hours of life, the precordium of a term neonate should be quiet. During the first few hours of life, there may be a visible impulse noted along the lower left sternal border in normal newborns because of the right ventricular predominance common to transitional circulation. As the transitional circulatory pattern changes, this sign will generally disappear in the normal newborn. When seen in the term neonate after the first hours of life, a bounding precordium is characteristic of heart disease, typically defects with increased ventricular volume work such as left-to-right shunt lesions (patent ductus arteriosus or ventricular septal defect), or severe valvular regurgitation.[5,9] Premature infants may have an active precordium because of their decreased subcutaneous tissue.

Apical Impulse

After general assessment of the precordium, the examiner should inspect for position and character of the apical impulse, the forward thrust of the left ventricle during systole. The apical impulse is usually seen in the neonate in the fourth intercostal space, either at or to the left of the midclavicular line (Figure 7-6). It can be further localized and examined with light palpation using the fingertips. An apical impulse placed downward and to the left suggests left ventricular dilation. A very sharp apical impulse is found with high cardiac output or left ventricular hypertrophy.

The point of maximum impulse (PMI) and the apical impulse are usually the same, but this is not always true in neonates during the

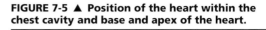

FIGURE 7-5 ▲ Position of the heart within the chest cavity and base and apex of the heart.

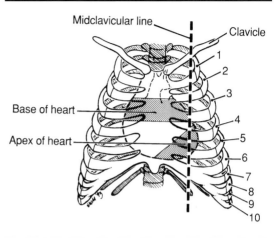

first few hours or days of life. During that time, an impulse stronger than the apical impulse can be found in the fifth intercostal space at the lower sternal border or even substernally. This then represents the PMI and is normal because of the right ventricular predominance found in the newborn (see Figure 7-6). The PMI or the apical impulse may be displaced in several situations, such as dextrocardia, tension pneumothorax, and diaphragmatic hernia.

Heaves, Taps, and Thrills

Further palpation of the precordium will yield other valuable information. Heaves, taps,

FIGURE 7-6 ▲ Areas of cardiac inspection and palpation.

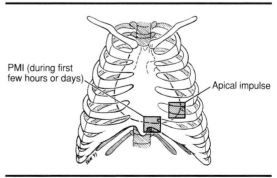

FIGURE 7-7 ▲ Four auscultatory areas of the heart.

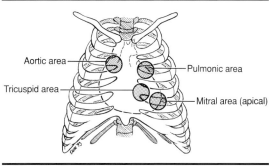

and thrills can all be palpated. These findings are usually best felt by palpating with the portion of the palm at the base of the fingers rather than with the fingertips. This is because certain parts of the hand are more discriminatory than others for specific sensations. Vibratory sensations are best felt with the ulnar surface of the hand.

A heave (or lift) is a point of maximum impulse that is slow rising and diffuse. Heaves are associated with volume overload.[5]

A sharp, well-localized PMI is called a tap. Taps are usually associated with pressure overload.[5] A hypertrophied but not dilated right ventricle produces a distinct parasternal tap.[3]

Thrills are low-frequency, palpable murmurs that feel similar to touching a purring cat. A thrill denotes a loud murmur (at least a Grade IV murmur). In the neonate, thrills are not common. When present, they can provide useful information about cardiac problems. A thrill in the upper left sternal border originates from the pulmonary valve or pulmonary artery and may be associated with pulmonary stenosis, tetralogy of Fallot, or rarely a patent ductus arteriosus.[5]

AUSCULTATING TO ASSESS CARDIOVASCULAR STATUS

Expert auscultation of the neonatal heart requires much practice over time. An experienced mentor can help the fledgling examiner learn to identify and distinguish heart sounds. The neonatal heart should be auscultated with the infant inactive and quiet.

At a minimum, the four traditional auscultatory areas should be examined. These are the aortic area (second intercostal space, right sternal angle), pulmonic area (second intercostal space, left sternal angle), tricuspid area (fourth intercostal space, left sternal angle), and mitral area (fourth intercostal space, left midclavicular line) (Figure 7-7). A more thorough examination is recommended, however. It should include right and left infraclavicular areas, both sides of the back, the right anterior chest, both axillae, the anterior fontanel (examining for cerebral arteriovenous fistulas), and the liver (examining for hepatic arteriovenous fistulas).

HEART RATE

Heart rate should be auscultated first and counted. A term neonate's heart rate at rest should be 100 to 160 beats per minute (bpm), although brief fluctuations above and below these values can be anticipated in a normal newborn.[12] (Some healthy neonates in deep sleep will have heart rates as low as 70 bpm.) Premature infants have a slightly higher mean heart rate than that seen in term infants.

Sinus bradycardia, or a heart rate less than normal for age (usually less than 80 bpm), is a common transient finding in both term and premature infants. The reason for this is the predominance of the parasympathetic system. Any stimulus—such as yawning, stooling, or suctioning—may result in vagal stimulation and subsequent bradycardia. These episodes are usually transient, require no treatment, and are self-correcting. Some episodes, especially in premature infants, may require stimulation or treatment of the underlying cause, such as treatment for apnea of prematurity with methylxanthines.

FIGURE 7-8 ▲ ECG rhythm strip of infant with supraventricular tachycardia with a ventricular rate of approximately 300 bpm.

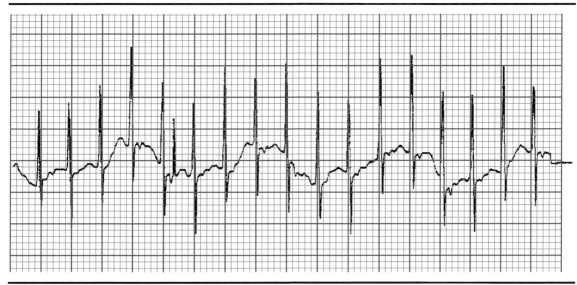

Sinus tachycardia is defined as a heart rate greater than normal for age (usually greater than 180 to 200 bpm). It is generally considered the most common form of rapid heart rate in the neonate.[16] It normally occurs with any stimulus—such as crying, feeding, fever, or activity—that causes increased demands on the heart. Normally, with removal of the stimulus, the heart rate slowly returns to baseline. Sinus tachycardia rarely requires treatment.

Variation in the heart rate is the norm among neonates and is seen as a positive sign of the infant's ability to react to the environment.[16] Infants who do not respond to stimuli with an increase in heart rate are clearly abnormal and should be observed very closely.

Although sinus tachycardia with rates up to 200 bpm can be tolerated by the neonate, heart rates greater than 200 bpm or supraventricular tachycardia (SVT) cannot. SVT encompasses paroxysmal atrial tachycardia and atrial flutter and fibrillation. Figure 7-8 is a rhythm strip of SVT. In the neonate, SVT represents a medical emergency and requires immediate intervention. At such rapid heart rates, cardiac output is extremely compromised because of short diastolic filling time. Without treatment, decreased cardiac output will cause congestive heart failure within 48 hours and possibly death. Treatment for SVT depends on the cause, but the condition may respond to vagal stimulation (such as applying a cold washcloth or ice to the face), drugs, or cardioversion.

CARDIAC RHYTHM AND REGULARITY

After assessing heart rate, evaluate cardiac rhythm and regularity. Listen carefully to the rhythm of the heart sounds, and determine if there is any irregularity. Noting patterns and frequencies of the irregularity helps identify the type of arrhythmia. Whenever an arrhythmia is suspected, an electrocardiogram (ECG) and/or continuous heart monitoring is indicated to establish a diagnosis. Arrhythmias are not uncommon in the neonate. Fortunately, they are usually benign and require no treatment. Those most commonly found in the neonate include the following:

▶ *Sinus arrhythmia.* This is a very common, normal variant in most newborns that is associated with respirations.[5] Sinus arrhythmia is characterized by irregularity of the R-R interval, with an otherwise normal cardiac cycle. No treatment is required for this rhythm.

▶ *Premature atrial beats.* This arrhythmia is marked by an early beat arising from supraventricular focus. Ventricular conduction is usually normal. The arrhythmia is almost always benign in the newborn, but can be abnormal when seen with CHD, sepsis, hypoxia, hyperthyroidism, cardiac tumors, myopathies, electrolyte abnormalities, digoxin toxicity, administration of caffeine, atropine, theophylline, or inotropic agents, and severe respiratory distress.[17] If significant, the underlying cause may require treatment (especially if related to digitalis toxicity), but these beats are usually well tolerated, and no treatment is indicated.[5]

▶ *Premature ventricular beats.* With this early beat arising from an irritable ventricular focus, ventricular conduction will be abnormal, giving rise to a wide and bizarre QRS complex. The arrhythmia may result from hypoxia, irritation by an invasive catheter or surgical procedure, or CHD. Treatment is unnecessary if the phenomenon is infrequent.

HEART SOUNDS

Traditional cardiac physiology teaches that the first heart sound (S1) is produced by closure of the mitral and tricuspid valves, and the second heart sound (S2) is produced by closure of the aortic and pulmonic valves. More recent literature debates this, however, and the true origin of heart sounds remains unclear. Despite this uncertainty, the traditional concept can be helpful in conceptualizing and learning to recognize heart sounds and therefore continues to be used.[3]

S1

The first heart sound, if thought of as representing closure of the mitral and tricuspid valves at the onset of ventricular systole, should be heard most loudly at the apex of the heart. (See Figure 7-5 for location of the apex and base of the heart.) Indeed, S1 is best heard at the mitral or tricuspid area. The first heart sound is usually loud at birth, decreasing in intensity during the first 48 hours of life. Any factor that increases cardiac output also increases the intensity of S1.

Splitting is defined as hearing two distinct components of a heart sound. It is caused by the asynchronous closure of the two valves that create the heart sound. The neonate's rapid heart rate usually makes splitting difficult to distinguish. Although some studies have documented splitting of S1 in the newborn, splitting is not commonly heard; S1 is usually described as being single.

S2

The second heart sound, if thought of as representing closure of the aortic and pulmonic valves, should be heard most loudly at the base of the heart. Indeed, S2 is best heard at the aortic or pulmonic area. S2 is usually single at birth, but it is split in two-thirds of infants by 16 hours of age and in 80 percent of infants by 48 hours of age.[3] With practice, the trained examiner should be able to recognize the splitting of S2 despite the infant's rapid heart rate.

Wide splitting of S2 should be considered abnormal in newborns. It can occur with atrial septal defect, pulmonary stenosis, Ebstein's anomaly, partial anomalous pulmonary venous return, mitral regurgitation, or right bundle branch block.[5]

S3

In addition to S1 and S2, extra heart sounds can potentially be heard in the neonate. Again, because of the infant's rapid heart rate, they may be difficult to distinguish. A third heart sound (S3) can occasionally be heard in infancy; if present, it is best heard at the apex of the heart during early diastole. S3 most often signifies rapid or increased flow across the AV valves (rapid ventricular filling) and is commonly heard in premature infants with patent ductus arteriosus. Rarely is it heard in the newborn with overt congestive heart failure.[18]

S4

A fourth heart sound (S4) should rarely be heard in neonates. If present, it is heard at the apex of the heart and is a low-pitched sound of late diastole. S4 is always pathologic and is heard in conditions characterized by decreased compliance (especially cardiomyopathy) or congestive heart failure.[5] The term *decreased compliance* refers to myocardium that is relatively stiff and therefore does not expand well as the blood enters the chambers. This affects the volume of blood that is ejected by the heart with contraction.

Ejection Clicks

Ejection clicks (snappy, high-frequency sounds) can, if they are present, best be heard just after the first heart sound. Ejection clicks occur at the time of ventricular ejection and resemble in timing, but not in quality, a widely split first heart sound. Ejection clicks are commonly heard during the first 24 hours of life and are usually normal during that time (related to the pulmonary hypertension seen in the newborn at that time).[5] Any time after the first 24 hours of life, ejection clicks are always considered abnormal. The most frequent findings associated with these clicks are aortic or pulmonic stenosis, idiopathic dilation of the pulmonary artery, systemic or pulmonary hypertension, truncus arteriosus, or tetralogy of Fallot.[5]

Murmurs

Murmurs are caused by turbulent blood flow. They are often described as prolonged heart sounds. There are two kinds of murmurs: innocent and pathologic. Pathologic murmurs result from underlying cardiovascular disease; innocent murmurs do not.

Whenever an examiner detects a murmur, the question of its origin arises. The murmur must therefore be fully evaluated as to its timing, location, intensity, radiation, quality, and pitch. The neonate's age in hours and days is also especially significant because of the dynamic properties of the newborn heart. Putting all this information together with the other findings of the physical examination should help the examiner determine the significance of the murmur.

The *timing* of the murmur is the first quality the examiner must listen for. To evaluate timing, the examiner needs to understand what is happening to the heart during systole and diastole. Systole is the period when the heart contracts and the heart chambers eject blood. Systole occurs following closure of the mitral and tricuspid valves, and its onset occurs just after S1. Diastole is the period when the heart is relaxed and the chambers are filling with blood. Diastole occurs following closure of the aortic and pulmonic valves, and its onset occurs just after S2. When establishing the timing of a murmur, the examiner must ask: Does it occur in systole or diastole? That is, does the murmur occur after S1 or after S2? Is the murmur early, mid, or late in systole or diastole? Does it occur throughout systole (holosystolic or pansystolic) or during midsystolic ejection? Continuous murmurs are heard through both systole and diastole.

Loudness, or intensity, of the murmur should be determined next. Murmurs are graded from I to VI, as follows:

Grade I: Barely audible, audible only after a period of careful auscultation

Grade II: Soft, but audible immediately

Grade III: Of moderate intensity (but not associated with a thrill)

Grade IV: Louder (may be associated with a thrill)

Grade V: Very loud, can be heard with the stethoscope rim barely on the chest (may be associated with a thrill)

Grade VI: Extremely loud, can be heard with the stethoscope just slightly removed from the chest (may be associated with a thrill)

Sometimes the intensity of a murmur will vary from exam to exam. The reason may be changing pulmonary vascular resistance or anything else that alters the status of cardiac output, such as anemia, activity, or changing ventilatory requirements.

Location of the place on the chest wall where the murmur is heard at maximum intensity is another important feature to evaluate. Location is usually described in terms of the interspace and the midsternal, midclavicular, or anterior axillary lines (see Figure 6-3) because the anatomic site of most murmurs is usually found at the location below where they are best heard. Describing murmurs in terms of aortic, pulmonary, tricuspid, or mitral areas is not recommended in neonates because malposition of valves and vessels may be found in CHD.

Other locations where a murmur is heard should also be documented. This is described as *radiation* or transmission of the murmur. Radiation from the normally positioned pulmonary outflow tract is to the left upper back; radiation from the normally positioned aortic outflow tract is to the carotid arteries.

Quality and *pitch* of the murmur are the final two features that should be assessed. Pitch is described as high, medium, or low. High-pitched murmurs occur when there is turbulence from a high-pressure to a low-pressure area.[14] This can happen with aortic or mitral insufficiency. Low-pitched murmurs occur when there is a low-pressure difference in the turbulent flow. An example of this is mitral stenosis. Identifying the quality of a murmur

(terms include *harsh, rumbling,* or *musical*) also helps to describe it.

Innocent murmurs. During the first 48 hours of life, many newborns have murmurs, the majority of which are innocent. They are usually associated with the decreasing pulmonary vascular resistance occurring at this time and with the gradual closure of the patent ductus arteriosus. Innocent murmurs, sometimes called flow murmurs, are most often Grade I or II, are associated with normal ECG and chest x-ray findings, are usually systolic murmurs, and are not associated with any other symptoms. Some of the more common innocent murmurs heard during the first 48 hours of life include the following:

▶ *Systolic ejection murmur.* This is the most common innocent murmur (heard in up to 56 percent of newborns).[14] Usually Grade I–II/VI, it is best heard along the mid- and upper left sternal border and described as vibratory. Systolic ejection murmurs present within the first day of life, may last as long as one week, and are most likely the result of the significant increase in flow across the pulmonary valve associated with rapidly decreasing pulmonary vascular resistance.[18]

▶ *Continuous systolic or crescendo systolic murmur.* This murmur occurs in up to 15 percent of normal infants with a usual intensity of Grade I–II/VI; it is best heard in the upper left sternal border. Presenting within the first eight hours of life, this murmur is caused by the transient left-to-right flow through the ductus arteriosus during the period when pulmonary vascular resistance is falling but ductal closure has not yet been accomplished.[18]

▶ *Early soft midsystolic ejection murmur* (also called peripheral pulmonic stenosis, pulmonary flow murmur, or pulmonary branch murmur). Heard often in newborns, especially premature infants, its intensity is usually Grade I–II/VI, and it is medium to high pitched. This murmur is best heard in the upper left sternal border, with wide radiation to both lung fields, axillae, and back. It presents within the first week or two of life.[19] Early soft midsystolic ejection murmurs last for weeks to months, but generally disappear by three to six months of age.[5] They result from turbulence produced at the relatively acute angle of the bifurcation of the pulmonary artery.[5,20]

Pathologic murmurs. Pathologic murmurs in the neonate occur at varying times, depending on the anatomic abnormality causing them and on normal changes associated with transitional circulation. For example, pathologic murmurs heard in the delivery room are almost always caused either by stenosis or by regurgitation; they are almost never the result of shunting because vascular resistances in the lungs and the body are equal at birth.[5] Many specific defects do not present with a murmur until three days, one week, or four to six weeks of age, when the pulmonary vascular resistance has fallen sufficiently. Atrial septal defects sometimes do not present until one to two years of age.[5] The absence of a murmur does not rule out the potential for serious CHD. As many as 20 percent of infants who die from congenital heart defects during the first month of life do not have heart murmurs.[18] In fact, the absence of a murmur may be an ominous sign in both acyanotic and ductal-dependent lesions.

The examiner should approach all murmurs cautiously. Soft murmurs heard in otherwise asymptomatic infants can be observed carefully by the experienced practitioner for the first 48 hours of life. But any murmur that persists beyond this time, is louder than a Grade I or II, or occurs in a symptomatic neonate requires further investigation. The cardiovascular workup should include a chest x-ray, an echocardiogram, and a consultation with a cardiologist. Many cardiologists also believe that an ECG is an important component of a complete cardiac evaluation.

Pathologic murmurs are more difficult to categorize than innocent murmurs. The following commonly occur in the immediate neonatal period:

▶ *Loud systolic ejection murmur.* Usually Grade II–V, this murmur appears within hours of birth and is almost always the result of aortic or pulmonary stenosis or coarctation of the aorta.[5]

▶ *Continuous murmur.* Occurring in one-third of premature infants with a patent ductus arteriosus (may only be systolic and difficult to hear in infants who are on ventilators), this type of murmur is also heard in infants with AV fistulas, regardless of gestational age.[5]

In addition, pathologic systolic murmurs may occasionally be heard with mitral and tricuspid insufficiency of various causes (especially with left ventricular failure in infants with critical left ventricular outlet obstruction and tetralogy of Fallot). Pathologic murmurs associated with ventricular septal defect and patent ductus arteriosus in term neonates do not present until pulmonary vascular resistance has fallen—often not until after discharge from the nursery or at several weeks of age.

PALPATING THE LIVER

Palpation of the liver (described in Chapter 8) is a significant part of the cardiovascular assessment. The liver becomes engorged when central venous pressure increases. A liver located more than 3 cm below the right costal margin is a good indicator of right-sided heart failure in a term infant.

FIGURE 7-9 ▲ Diagram showing how to select accurate BP cuff size.

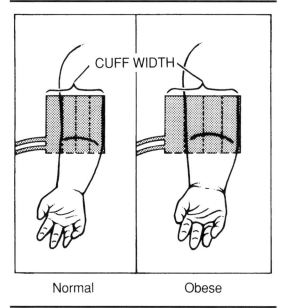

CUFF WIDTH

Normal   Obese

The end of the cuff is at the top. Note that the cuff width should be 25 to 55 percent wider than the diameter of the limb being measured.

EVALUATING BLOOD PRESSURE

Evaluation of the neonate's blood pressure (BP) should be done with the infant quiet. This assessment should be left until the end of the examination because the pressure of the cuff inflating may make the infant cry. Although the American Academy of Pediatrics does not recommend universal screening of blood pressure, systemic BP should be measured in every neonate with suspected CHD, renal disease, or clinical signs of hypotension.[5,21]

A cuff of the proper size must be used when obtaining a BP measurement. Indeed, the most frequent reason for a hypertensive BP is the use of a BP cuff that is too small for the infant. Using limb length as the sole criterion for establishing cuff size for BP monitoring can be misleading. This method does not take into consideration large-for-gestational-age infants with excessive subcutaneous fat. These infants will show falsely elevated BPs if cuff size is inappropriate. It is therefore recommended that the cuff width (not the cuff length) be 40 to 50 percent of the circumference of the extremity or 25 to 55 percent wider than the diameter of the limb being measured (Figure 7-9).[5] In addition, the inflatable bladder should entirely encircle the extremity without overlapping.[13]

MONITORING METHODS

There are several methods for monitoring systemic BP in neonates: flush, palpation, ultrasound Doppler, and oscillometric measurements. BP obtained by auscultation is not appropriate for neonates.

Flush

The flush method, now rarely used, is simple to do and can be useful in certain situations. With this method, the hand or foot is squeezed to blanch it, and the BP cuff is rapidly inflated. The pressure in the cuff is released, and the pressure point at which the extremity suddenly flushes is documented. The pressure obtained by this method represents the mean arterial pressure.

Palpation

BP can also be obtained by palpatory methods in infants. While releasing the pressure in the cuff, the examiner palpates the pulse distal to the cuff. The pressure point at which the pulse reappears upon deflation approximates the systolic blood pressure.

Ultrasound Doppler

A more accurate method, similar to the palpatory method of BP measurement, is done with an ultrasonic Doppler. A transducer is placed over the artery distal to the BP cuff after a conductive gel is applied, and an audible pulse is listened for as the BP cuff is deflated. The pressure point at which the pulse is heard is documented. This method also approximates the systolic BP.

Oscillometric Measurement

Most centers now use oscillometric methods to document BP in neonates. Systolic,

FIGURE 7-10 ▲ Systolic, diastolic, mean, and pulse pressures for newborns (based on birth weight) during the first 12 hours of life.

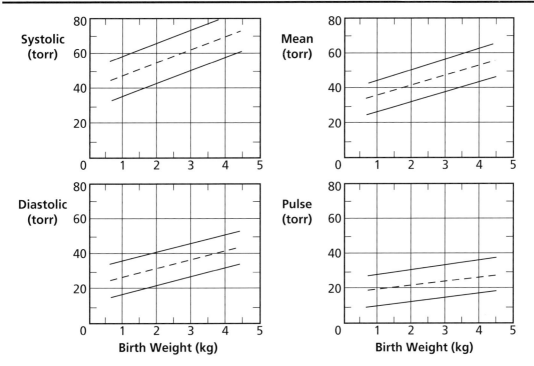

Linear regressions (broken lines) and 95 percent confidence limits (solid lines) of systolic (top left) and diastolic (bottom left) aortic blood pressures and mean pressure (top right) and pulse pressure (bottom right) on birth weight in healthy newborn infants during the first 12 hours after birth.

Adapted from: Versmold HT, et al. 1981. Aortic blood pressure during the first 12 hours of life in infants 610 to 4,220 grams. *Pediatrics* 67(5): 611. Reprinted by permission.

diastolic, and mean arterial BP and heart rate are all digitally recorded using special cuffs and oscillometric systems. These systems have been found to be fairly reliable.

Catheter

Finally, indwelling arterial catheters also provide systolic, diastolic, and mean blood pressures. These catheters provide minute-by-minute readings of BP values. Accuracy of this type of monitoring requires a knowledge of the system and the variables that will affect it. Some of these variables include transducer position, air bubbles in the system, and equipment calibration.

NORMAL VALUES

Normal blood pressure values in newborns vary, depending on body weight and postnatal age. In the first few hours of life, BP can be significantly affected by type of delivery, birth asphyxia, and placental transfusion. The newborn's initial BP decreases during the first 3 to 4 hours of life, presumably because of fluid shifts into and out of the vascular space.[18] The systolic pressure reaches a minimum at 3 to 4 hours of age and then gradually increases to reach a plateau at about four to six days of age to a level closer to the initial postpartum level.[22] Blood pressures in neonates are also affected by activity, temperature, and behavioral state.

Figure 7-10 documents confidence limits for newborns (based on birth weight) during the first 12 hours of life.

Whenever there is any question of CHD, there is difficulty obtaining blood pressures, a murmur is heard, or there is an absence of femoral pulses on the physical exam, four extremity blood pressures must be obtained. Pressures obtained in the legs are often slightly higher than those in the arms, but they can be equal or slightly lower. A systolic blood pressure in the upper extremities more than 20 mmHg higher than that in the lower extremities strongly suggests coarctation of the aorta.[5,18] This pressure difference can sometimes be masked in the left arm by a patent ductus arteriosus that allows blood to pass around the restricted area; therefore, the right arm will yield the most valuable information because it is always preductal.

In addition to systolic, diastolic, and mean BP readings, the *pulse pressure* can provide other valuable information. The pulse pressure is defined as the difference between the systolic and the diastolic blood pressures. Averages for term neonates are between 25 and 30 mmHg; for premature infants, they are between 15 and 25 mmHg.[18] Wide pulse pressures may be a sign of a large aortic runoff, as seen with patent ductus arteriosus. Narrow pulse pressures are documented in neonates with peripheral vasoconstriction, heart failure, or low cardiac output.

SUMMARY

Properly executed, the cardiovascular assessment provides a great deal of information about the overall health of the newborn, as well as valuable information about congenital heart defects that might be present. Time, patience, and experience with inspection, palpation, and auscultation are all necessary to develop the skills essential to a thorough cardiac examination.

REFERENCES

1. Nora JJ, and Nora AH. 1978. The evolution of specific genetic and environmental counseling in congenital heart diseases. *Circulation* 57(2): 205–213.

2. Centers for Disease Control and Prevention. 2006. Improved national prevalence estimates for 18 selected major birth defects—United States, 1999–2001. *MMWR* 54(51): 1301–1305.

3. Duff DF, and McNamara DG. 1998. History and physical examination of the cardiovascular system. In *The Science and Practice of Pediatric Cardiology*, 2nd ed., Garson A Jr, et al., eds. Baltimore: Lippincott Williams & Wilkins, 693–713.

4. Hull D, Binns BA, and Joyce D. 1966. Congenital heart block and widespread fibrosis due to maternal lupus erythematosus. *Archives of Disease in Childhood* 41(220): 688–690.

5. Park MK. 2008. *Pediatric Cardiology for Practitioners*, 5th ed., Philadelphia: Mosby, 3–8, 140–157, 9–39, 417–444, 161–191.

6. Hoffman JI. 2002. Incidence, mortality, and natural history. In *Paediatric Cardiology*, 2nd ed. Anderson RH, et al., eds. New York: Churchill Livingstone, 111–139.

7. Greenwood RD, et al. 1975. Extracardiac abnormalities in infants with congenital heart disease. *Pediatrics* 55(4): 485–492.

8. Hazinski MF. 1984. Congenital heart disease in the neonate. Part 7: Common congenital heart defects producing hypoxemia and cyanosis. *Neonatal Network* 2(6): 36–51.

9. Allen HD, Phillip JR, and Chan DP. 2007. History and physical examination. In *Moss and Adams' Heart Disease in Infants, Children, and Adolescents: Including the Fetus and Young Adult,* 7th ed., Allen HD, et al., eds. Baltimore: Lippincott, Williams & Wilkins, 58–65.

10. Rennie JM. 2005. *Roberton's Textbook of Neonatology,* 4th ed. Philadelphia: Churchill Livingstone, 249–266.

11. Spilman LJ, and Furdon SA. 1998. Recognition, understanding, and current management of cardiac lesions with decreased pulmonary blood flow. *Neonatal Network* 17(4): 7–18.

12. Southgate WM, and Pittard WB III. 2001. Classification and physical examination of the newborn infant. In *Care of the High-Risk Neonate,* 5th ed., Klaus MH, and Fanaroff AA, eds. Philadelphia: Saunders, 100–129.

13. Monett ZJ, and Moynihan PJ. 1991. Cardiovascular assessment of the neonatal heart. *Journal of Perinatal & Neonatal Nursing* 5(2): 50–59.

14. Moller JH. 1992. Physical examination. In *Fetal, Neonatal, and Infant Cardiac Disease,* Moller JH, and Neal WA, eds. Norwalk, Connecticut: Appleton & Lange, 167–177.

15. Tynan M. 2002. Clinical presentation of heart disease in infants and children. In *Paediatric Cardiology*, 2nd ed. Anderson RH, et al., eds. New York: Churchill Livingstone, 275–283.

16. Theorell C. 2002. Cardiovascular assessment of the newborn. *Newborn and Infant Nursing Reviews* 2(2): 111–127.

17. Pilcher J. 2004. *Pocket Guide to Neonatal EKG Interpretation,* 2nd ed. Santa Rosa, California: NICU INK, 15–37.

18. Johnson GL. 1990. Clinical examination. In *Fetal and Neonatal Cardiology,* Long WA, ed. Philadelphia: Saunders, 223–235.

19. Danford DA, and McNamara DG. 1998. Innocent heart murmurs and heart sounds. In *Science and Practice of Pediatric Cardiology,* Garson A, et al., eds. Philadelphia: Lea & Febiger, 2203–2212.

20. Danilowicz DA, et al. 1972. Physiologic pressure differences between main and branch pulmonary arteries in children. *Circulation* 45(2): 410–419.

21. American Academy of Pediatrics, Committee on Fetus and Newborn. 1993. Routine evaluation of blood pressure, hematocrit, and glucose in newborns. *Pediatrics* 92(3): 474–476.

22. Scanlon JW, et al. 1979. *A System of Newborn Physical Examination.* Baltimore: University Park Press, 67–73.

NOTES

NOTES

8 Abdomen Assessment

Martha Goodwin, MSN, RN, NNP-BC

Assessment of the newborn abdomen is best performed during the first few hours of life, when the bowel is not yet filled with gas. The ideal time to perform the examination is when the infant is in a quiet state and the abdominal muscles are relaxed. Techniques used include observation, auscultation, and palpation. Although percussion is used to examine the adult abdomen, it is of limited usefulness when examining the newborn. Common variations and abnormal findings in the newborn abdominal assessment are addressed as the examination techniques are discussed.

REVIEW OF PREGNANCY AND DELIVERY HISTORY

Evaluation of the maternal history is discussed in detail in Chapter 2; however, specific findings are of interest when examining the abdomen and gastrointestinal (GI) tract. Any antenatal ultrasound finding of abnormalities, such as enlarged kidneys, dilated bowel, or unusual masses, will alert the examiner to evaluate thoroughly these areas on the initial examination.[1] Polyhydramnios by history or noted at delivery must be evaluated because approximately 20–30 percent of these fetuses have major structural malformations. The risk of anomaly increases with greater amounts of amniotic fluid. A maximum vertical pocket of amniotic fluid >16 cm increases the chance of anomaly to 90 percent.[2,3] The most common GI abnormalities associated with polyhydramnios are esophageal atresia and duodenal atresia.

The history of the events surrounding delivery should be reviewed as well. The finding of an extremely large amount of amniotic fluid in the stomach at delivery may indicate the presence of duodenal atresia. The presence of copious oral secretions coupled with the inability to pass a soft catheter to the stomach may indicate an esophageal atresia, usually associated with a tracheoesophageal fistula. The presence of bilious gastric secretions at delivery is also abnormal and should alert the examiner to the possibility of intestinal obstruction.

INSPECTION

SKIN

The skin of the abdomen should be pink. Newborn rash may be present, and there may be bruising from the process of delivery, although this is rare. A few large veins may be visible, especially on a light-skinned infant, but marked venous distention should not be present. The normal preterm infant will have

FIGURE 8-1 ▲ Congenital deficiency of the abdominal musculature, showing typical "prune" (wrinkled) belly appearance.

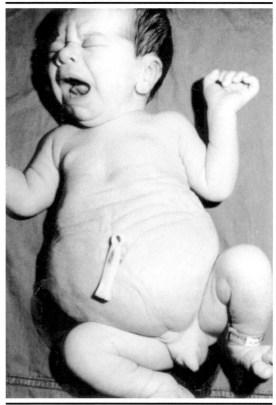

Courtesy of Dr. David A. Clark, Albany Medical Center.

more visible vasculature because of decreased subcutaneous tissue. The postterm baby may have superficial cracking and peeling of the skin over the abdomen.

Shape and Movement

The abdomen of the term newborn is soft and rounded, with easy movements associated with respirations. The abdominal and diaphragmatic muscles work together during respiration, causing the chest and abdomen to move parallel with each other. Asynchronous movements—that is, the chest and abdomen moving in opposition to each other—can indicate respiratory distress.

The abdomen can vary from nearly flat to slightly distended, depending on how recently the infant has been fed and if he has swallowed air with crying. The abdominal circumference measured at the greatest diameter (just above the umbilicus) is normally less than the head circumference up until 30–32 weeks of gestational age. From 32 to 36 weeks gestational age, the abdominal and head circumferences will be equal. After 36 weeks gestational age, the abdominal circumference will be greater than the head circumference.[4]

A sunken, or scaphoid, abdomen may indicate a diaphragmatic hernia. The abdomen of a normal preterm infant may appear distended because of lack of muscle tone; a term infant may have decreased muscle tone related to maternal medications received in labor. This is easily distinguished from the flaccid, lumpy abdomen of the infant with congenital absence of the abdominal musculature, also called "prune belly" syndrome (Figure 8-1). This very rare syndrome, discussed further in Chapter 9, occurs mostly in males and is associated with severe renal and urinary tract abnormalities.[5] A markedly distended abdomen in any infant warrants further investigation. Bowel obstruction presents with distention and vomiting, the timing and character of which vary, depending on the location of the obstruction. Isolated distention of the lower abdomen may be associated with bladder distention, genitourinary (GU) abnormalities, anomalies of the female reproductive tract, or teratomas.

Obstructions of the upper GI tract, such as esophageal and duodenal atresia, tend to present with excessive salivation and nonbilious vomiting. As the level of obstruction progresses down the intestinal tract, symptoms shift to abdominal distention and bilious vomiting. Bilious vomiting is the result of obstruction beyond the level of the ampulla of Vater, where bile from the gallbladder enters the small intestine.[6] Meconium ileus is the only bowel obstruction that can present with abdominal distention at birth. It is the result of abnormal pancreatic enzyme function seen with cystic fibrosis.[6] Abdominal distention otherwise presents only after the infant has swallowed air to fill the bowel.

The presence of bilious emesis in any infant, with or without abdominal distention, requires immediate investigation to rule out a malrotation with midgut volvulus. A malrotation results from abnormal fixation of the intestine in the abdomen; midgut volvulus is the abnormal rotation of the bowel around the mesentery and subsequent obstruction of blood flow to the bowel. This is one of the most urgent emergencies in neonatal surgery. *Immediate intervention is required to avoid irreversible infarction of the intestine.*[3]

The shape of the abdomen should be symmetric, without obvious swellings or depressions. Occasionally, a loop of bowel may be visible beneath the abdominal skin. This is more common in the preterm infant and is of concern only if it remains fixed in one spot or is associated with generalized distention and symptoms of bowel obstruction. Diastasis recti is a midline separation of the rectus abdominus muscles and can be seen as a midline, elevated ridge extending from below the sternum to the umbilicus when the infant is crying. This is a normal finding and will resolve without intervention.

An umbilical hernia may also be seen on examination. It is a common finding in 30 percent of term African American infants and is also seen in low birth weight males. An umbilical hernia is often seen in hypothyroidism, a relatively rare condition. There is protrusion of abdominal contents into the hernia, which is soft and easily reducible (Figure 8-2). Umbilical hernias usually close spontaneously by two years of age.[7]

An epigastric hernia is a small, firm, palpable nodule seen between the umbilicus and the xiphoid process. It results from fat

FIGURE 8-2 ▲ Umbilical hernia.

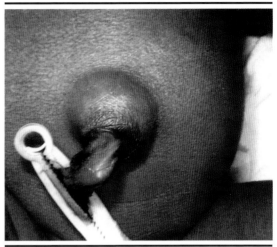

From: Clark DA. 2000. *Atlas of Neonatology.* Philadelphia: Saunders, 17. Reprinted by permission.

protruding through a small opening in the muscle. Surgical intervention is necessary for this uncommon hernia.

UMBILICAL CORD

The umbilical cord of the healthy newborn is shiny, pearly white, and gelatinous. It contains two arteries and one vein. The average size is 1.5 to 2 cm at the base. The umbilical cord contains Wharton's jelly, which protects the vessels and also is an indicator of the infant's nutritional status. A thick cord is often seen in large-for-gestational-age infants, whereas a small, thin cord is often seen in babies who are small for gestational age, postmature, or who had placental insufficiency. Any unusual bulging or herniation in the cord requires further investigation and could indicate the presence of a small omphalocele.

The cord is clamped and cut proximal to the placental insertion when unusual areas are present to avoid damage to structures such as the bowel or bladder. When the cord is cut, the vessels should be visible. The paired arteries are small, thick walled, and constricted. The vein is large, thin walled, and open. The absence of one of the arteries is seen in 1 percent of

FIGURE 8-3 ▲ Malformations of the urachus.

A. Urachal cysts. The most common site is in the superior end of the urachus just inferior to the umbilicus. **B.** Two types of urachal sinus are shown: One opens into the bladder and the other opens at the umbilicus. **C.** Patent urachus or urachal fistula connecting the bladder and the umbilicus.

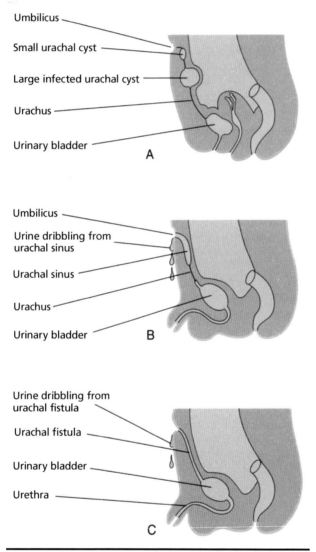

From: Moore KL, and Persaud TVN. 2008. *The Developing Human: Clinically Oriented Embryology,* 8th ed. Philadelphia: Saunders, 259. Reprinted by permission.

infants. It is associated with fetal abnormalities of the cardiovascular, GI, or GU systems or may be an isolated finding in an otherwise normal baby.[8]

The cord is normally white. A yellow or green cord may be seen when meconium staining has occurred 6 to 12 hours prior to delivery. Green color may rarely be an indicator of infection. Redness encircling the cord and extending onto the abdomen can be a sign of omphalitis (infection of the umbilical cord). Omphalitis must be treated promptly and properly because it can spread rapidly to underlying structures, causing severe systemic disease and even death.

The cut surface of the cord may initially ooze a small amount of clear, sticky fluid, but it will dry quickly. In normal situations, the cord will begin to dry soon after birth and will shrivel and fall off within 10 to 14 days.

Purulent drainage may indicate the presence of an abscess. Excessive amounts of clear drainage may indicate the presence of a patent urachus (persistence of an embryologic connection from the bladder to the umbilicus) (Figure 8-3). Persistence of the embryologic tract connecting the ileum to the umbilicus is called an omphalomesenteric duct. An infant with this defect will have leakage of ileal contents through the umbilical cord. A small, red, raw-appearing granuloma will occasionally form at the site of the separation of the umbilical cord. It is also called an umbilical polyp.

ABDOMINAL WALL DEFECTS

Defects in formation of the abdominal wall may occur during embryonic life, resulting in abnormal externalization of the abdominal contents. Three such defects are omphalocele, gastroschisis, and exstrophy of the bladder.

Omphalocele

An omphalocele is the herniation of abdominal contents into the umbilical cord

FIGURE 8-4 ▲ Omphalocele.

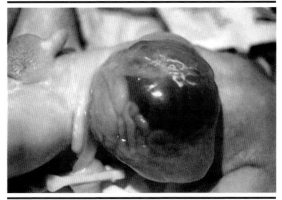

From: Clark DA. 2000. *Atlas of Neonatology.*
Philadelphia: Saunders, 190. Reprinted by permission.

FIGURE 8-5 ▲ Gastroschisis.

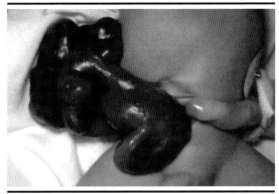

From: Clark DA. 2000. *Atlas of Neonatology.*
Philadelphia: Saunders, 190. Reprinted by permission.

(Figure 8-4). The hernia is contained in a translucent sac that is contiguous with the umbilical cord. The sac may rupture at or before delivery, so careful examination is necessary. Omphalocele is thought to result from failure of the bowel to reenter the abdominal cavity after its normal extrusion into the cord before the tenth week of gestation. This failure results from faulty migration and fusion of embryonic tissues and is associated with cardiac, neurologic, genitourinary, skeletal, or chromosomal abnormalities in 67 percent of infants.[3] Omphalocele is frequently associated with Beckwith-Wiedemann syndrome and with trisomies 13, 18, and 21.[3,9]

Gastroschisis

Gastroschisis is a defect in the abdominal wall through which the viscera protrude. There is no sac covering this defect, and the umbilical cord is discrete from it. The gastroschisis is usually to the right of midline (Figure 8-5). The etiology of gastroschisis remains controversial. There is increasing acceptance of the theory that it is the *in utero* rupture of an umbilical cord hernia.[3] Another theory is of a vascular accident interfering with normal formation of abdominal musculature. There is a lower incidence of associated anomalies with gastroschisis than with omphalocele, although

atresias of the bowel and ischemic enteritis may result from constriction of mesenteric blood flow. Both gastroschisis and omphalocele vary greatly in size, from smaller than a golf ball to so large that all of the abdominal contents (including the liver) are externalized.

Exstrophy of the Bladder

Exstrophy of the bladder (Figure 8-6) is a very rare defect. It is a malformation sequence resulting from lack of normal formation of the lower abdominal wall early in gestation. The posterior wall of the bladder is exposed, and urine drains onto the abdomen. Exstrophy of the bladder is more common in males, and there may be associated urogenital abnormalities in both males and females.[9] This condition is discussed further in Chapter 9.

Perianal area

The perianal area should be inspected for presence and placement of an anus, for anal sphincter tone, and for abnormalities such as fistulas. Sphincter tone can be assessed by gently stroking the anal area. An anal wink will occur. Absence of an anal wink suggests an abnormality of the central nervous system.

If the anus is completely absent, or imperforate, this may be evident immediately (Figure 8-7). However, atresia and stenosis can occur at any level of the anorectal canal, so patency

FIGURE 8-6 ▲ **Exstrophy of the urinary bladder.**

FIGURE 8-6 ▲ Exstrophy of the urinary bladder.

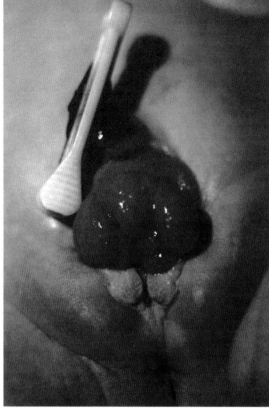

From: Clark DA. 2000. *Atlas of Neonatology.*
  Philadelphia: Saunders, 201. Reprinted by permission.

FIGURE 8-7 ▲ Imperforate anus.

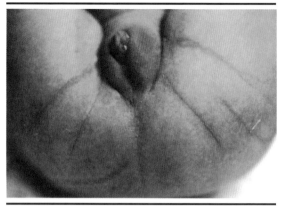

From: Clark DA. 2000. *Atlas of Neonatology.*
  Philadelphia: Saunders, 173. Reprinted by permission.

of the anus cannot be established until the passage of meconium. Digital examination of the rectum or the insertion of instruments is not recommended because of the risk of damage to the anal canal. Passage of stool usually occurs within 24 hours of birth, often within 12 hours, but a normal infant may not stool until 48 hours of life. In infants showing no other signs of problems, investigation is not warranted until this point. Continued absence of stool suggests anal atresia. Passage of very small caliber stools suggests stenosis.

A fistula is an anomalous connection between the intestinal tract and the GU tract. Presence of meconium in the vagina suggests a rectovaginal fistula (Figure 8-8). Meconium

in the urethral orifice indicates a rectourethral fistula.

AUSCULTATION

Auscultation should be performed before palpation because palpation can interfere with normal bowel sounds as well as cause agitation in the infant. Auscultation should be performed with a warmed stethoscope while the infant is quiet. The examiner should patiently listen to all four quadrants of the abdomen.

Bowel sounds will be audible beginning about 15 minutes after birth, although they are relatively quiet until feedings have begun. Their presence, quality, and intensity should be noted. Normal bowel sounds have a metallic, tinkling quality and are heard every 15 to 20 seconds. If bowel sounds are infrequent, the examiner should listen for a full 5 minutes before diagnosing them as absent. This part of the exam must be correlated with other clinical findings. Hyperactive bowel sounds in a healthy-appearing baby who has just fed may be normal. The same finding in an ill-appearing infant with a distended abdomen is not normal and could indicate obstruction. Maternal sedation can result in hypoactive bowel sounds.[4]

FIGURE 8-8 ▲ Rectovaginal fistula.

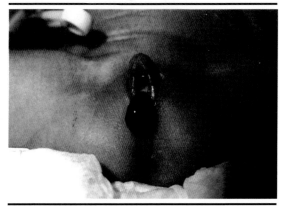

From: Clark DA. 2000. *Atlas of Neonatology.*
Philadelphia: Saunders, 173. Reprinted by permission.

FIGURE 8-9 ▲ Abdominal organs of the infant.

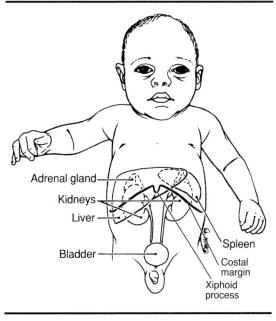

Breath sounds may be audible when the upper abdomen is auscultated. This is a normal finding because sounds transmit easily throughout an infant's body. Vascular sounds are not normally auscultated over the abdomen of the term infant. Rarely, a bruit will be found on abdominal exam. A bruit is the sound of blood flow through a restricted or tortuous vessel. It is heard as a swooshing sound similar to a cardiac murmur. Bruits may be heard anywhere over the abdomen and can indicate malformations of hepatic and renal vessels or hemangiomas.

PALPATION

Palpation is the last step in the abdominal examination because it often results in the infant becoming upset. Palpation can be performed with the baby in any state, but it is easiest when the infant is quiet. If the baby is fussy, flexing the infant's hip to relax the abdominal muscles during the exam may help.

The skin of the abdomen should be warm and pink, with brisk capillary refill. Muscle tone should be assessed at this point in the examination. Hypertonicity of the abdominal musculature may indicate pain or peritoneal irritation. Hypotonicity may be present in neuromuscular disease, perinatal depression,

or if the mother has taken medications that cause neonatal depression.

ORGANS

Palpation should begin with the superficial structures and then progress to the deeper organs (Figure 8-9). The shape of the thorax in the newborn is such that the upper abdominal organs are not as thoroughly covered by the anterior rib cage and can be easily felt on exam. The liver is a superficial organ and should be identified first. The normal newborn liver occupies a wide area of the upper abdomen, extending well into the left upper quadrant. It extends 1 to 2 cm below the right costal margin. To palpate the liver, the examiner should begin just above the iliac crest on the right. Using the palmar surface of the fingers parallel to the costal margin, the examiner gently palpates in a progressively caudal fashion. The abdomen should be depressed 1 to 2 cm. Care should be taken not to lift the hands completely off the abdomen because this may result in missing the edge of an enlarged liver.

FIGURE 8-10 ▲ The femoral triangle.

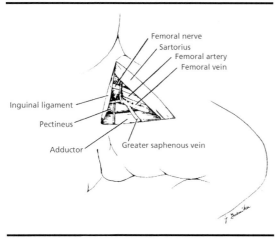

Adapted from: Plaxico DT, and Bucciarelli RL. 1978.
Greater saphenous vein venipuncture in the
neonate. *Journal of Pediatrics* 93(6): 1025. Reprinted
by permission.

The liver edge is normally smooth, firm, and sharp. A boggy liver is a sign of congestion and may indicate congestive heart failure. A hard or nodular liver edge is also abnormal.[4]

Using the technique just described, the practioner then examines the left side of the abdomen for the presence of the spleen. The tip of the spleen may be felt, but in many cases, it is not palpable at all. A spleen that is palpable more than 1 cm below the costal margin may be enlarged and warrants further investigation. No spleen will be found in those infants with certain cardiac conditions involving asplenia.

Rarely, the liver will be found on the left and the spleen on the right. This condition is known as *situs inversus*. Complete *situs inversus* is reversal of position of all the thoracic and abdominal organs, a "mirror image" of normal positioning. Partial *situs inversus* is the reversal of the positions of some but not all of the abdominal organs. Both types of *situs inversus* may be associated with cardiac defects, but such defects are more common in partial *situs inversus*.[10]

Palpation of the kidneys can be difficult, but it is easiest when done early, before the infant has eaten or begun prolonged crying. The kidneys are found using deep palpation, at a 45-degree angle caudal and lateral to the umbilicus. This can be most easily accomplished with one hand under the infant's back and the other pressing downward on the abdomen (see Figure 9-2). The normal newborn kidney is 4.5 to 5 cm from the upper to lower pole. On examination, the kidneys have the size and consistency of a large ripe olive. The right kidney is normally situated slightly lower than the left. A very easily palpated kidney is usually enlarged and may indicate hydronephrosis or a cystic kidney. Any texture other than smooth and firm is abnormal and should be investigated further as well.

The bladder is situated from 1 to 4 cm above the symphysis pubis. Palpation of the bladder should begin at the level of the umbilicus and progress downward until the smooth upper aspect of the bladder is felt. The bladder may also be percussed. A dull sound indicates the presence of urine in the bladder. Continuous bladder distention is abnormal and may indicate a urinary tract obstruction or central nervous system abnormality.

MASSES

Once the abdominal organs have been examined, the entire abdomen should be palpated for the presence of masses. In a systematic fashion, the examiner should explore each quadrant using first light and then deeper palpation. Normal findings include stool in the colon, felt as a sausage shape in the right and left lower quadrants. Gaseous distention may also be palpated in an infant who has swallowed air. Serial examinations will differentiate between normal stool in the colon that progresses and an abnormal mass that is fixed. A firm, oval-shaped mass may be felt in the upper midabdomen with pyloric stenosis, although this does not usually present in the newborn period. Most abdominal masses in the newborn involve the urinary tract and are cystic or solid on examination. Neoplasia is very rare in the newborn.

Groin and Femoral Area

As the final step in the examination, the groin and femoral region should be inspected and palpated (Figure 8-10). Ideally, this should be done both while the infant is quiet and while he is crying. The groins are normally flat. A visible femoral pulse may be present in a preterm infant or a thin term infant. The femoral artery pulses must be palpated and their character evaluated. The pulses are usually evaluated during the earlier part of the exam, when the infant is quiet and prior to deep palpation of the abdomen. The pulses should be compared bilaterally and also compared with the brachial pulse. Any difference in quality should be noted. An absent or weak femoral pulse may be noted with coarctation of the aorta or an interrupted aortic arch. Full and bounding femoral pulses may indicate a patent ductus arteriosus. When a pulse discrepancy is discovered, blood pressure readings should be obtained in the upper and lower extremities. A difference of 20 mmHg or greater should be investigated further. Complete evaluation of pulses is discussed in detail in Chapter 7.

The groin should also be observed for bulges in the inguinal and femoral areas. An inguinal hernia is a defect in the muscle wall that allows the intestine to slip into the scrotum in males and into the soft tissue in females (Figure 8-11). A bulge in the labia majora may be a hernia or an abnormal gonad. The presence of a hernia is most easily evaluated when the infant is crying because intra-abdominal pressure increases. Inguinal hernias are more common in males than in females, and they are very common in the extremely preterm male. The hernia should be soft and capable of being pushed back into the body cavity without difficulty. Surgical repair is required for inguinal

FIGURE 8-11 ▲ Inguinal hernia.

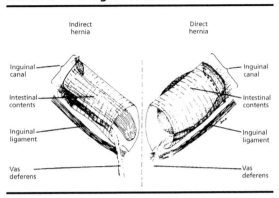

From: Alexander MM, and Brown MS. 1979. *Pediatric History Taking and Physical Diagnosis for Nurses*, 2nd ed. New York: McGraw-Hill, 223. Reprinted by permission of the authors.

hernias. It is done emergently if any evidence of strangulation is noted.

A small bulge adjacent and medial to the femoral artery may be a femoral hernia. Although it is an uncommon finding in an infant, it is seen more often in females than in males.

Summary

The examination of the abdomen involves observation, auscultation, and palpation. Following a systematic routine and doing everything possible to keep the infant quiet and cooperative will facilitate the exam. With practice, the examiner will learn to differentiate normal variations from abnormal findings, permitting timely intervention when abnormalities are found.

References

1. Garry DJ, and Figueroa R. 2005. Ultrasound evaluation of the uncomplicated pregnancy. In *Intensive Care of the Fetus and Neonate*, 2nd ed, Spitzer AR, ed. Philadelphia: Mosby, 37–56.
2. Wolf RB, and Moore TR. 2006. Amniotic fluid and nonimmune hydrops fetalis. In *Neonatal-Perinatal Medicine: Diseases of the Fetus and Infant*, 8th ed., Martin RJ, Fanaroff AA, and Walsh MC, eds. Philadelphia: Mosby, 409-428.

3. Magnuson DK, Parry RL, and Chwals WJ. 2006. Selected abdominal gastrointestinal anomalies. In *Neonatal-Perinatal Medicine: Diseases of the Fetus and Infant,* 8th ed., Martin RJ, Fanaroff AA, and Walsh MC, eds. Philadelphia: Mosby, 1381–1403.

4. Fletcher MA, 1998. *Physical Diagnosis in Neonatology.* Lippincott Williams & Wilkins, 349–369.

5. Kaplan GW, and McAleer IM. 2005. Structural abnormalities of the genitourinary tract. In *Avery's Neonatology: Pathophysiology and Management of the Newborn,* 6th ed., McDonald MG, Mullett MD, and Seshia MMK, eds. Philadelphia: Lippincott Williams & Wilkins, 1066–1096.

6. Arthur LG, and Schwartz MZ. 2005. Congenital anomalies of the gastrointestinal tract. In *Intensive Care of the Fetus and Neonate,* 2nd ed., Spitzer AR, ed. Philadelphia: Mosby, 1017–1025.

7. Thureen P, et al. 2005. *Assessment and Care of the Well Newborn,* 2nd ed. Philadelphia: Saunders, 119–172.

8. Blackburn ST. 2007. *Maternal, Fetal, and Neonatal Physiology: A Clinical Perspective,* 3rd ed. Philadelphia: Saunders, 70–124.

9. Jones KL. 2006. *Smith's Recognizable Patterns of Human Malformation,* 6th ed. Philadelphia: Saunders, 174–177, 18–21, 794.

10. Zahka KG, and Bengur AR. 2006. Cardiovascular problems of the neonate. In *Neonatal-Perinatal Medicine: Diseases of the Fetus and Infant,* 8th ed., Martin RJ, Fanaroff AA, and Walsh MC, eds. Philadelphia: Mosby, 1242–1252.

BIBLIOGRAPHY

Bolender DJ, and Kaplan S. 2004. Basic embryology. In *Fetal and Neonatal Physiology,* 3rd ed., Polin RA, Fox WW, and Abman SH, eds. Philadelphia: Saunders, 37–40.

Burrin DG. 2004. Physiology of the gastrointestinal tract in the fetus and neonate. In *Fetal and Neonatal Physiology,* 3rd ed., Polin RA, Fox WW, and Abman SH, eds. Philadelphia: Saunders, 1095–1110.

NOTES

9 Genitourinary Assessment

Terri A. Cavaliere, DNP, RN, NNP-BC

A comprehensive physical assessment of the newborn includes evaluation of the genitourinary (GU) system, which consists of the kidneys, the urinary tract, and the reproductive tract. Because these organs are closely related both anatomically and embryologically, they are discussed together. This chapter focuses on examination of the GU system in the neonate using the techniques of inspection, palpation, and occasionally, percussion. Normal newborn characteristics and simple variations from normal are presented first, followed by a discussion of abnormalities and malformations.

HISTORY REVIEW

A review of the prenatal history is part of any neonatal physical examination. A history of polyhydramnios or oligohydramnios during pregnancy should alert the examiner to the possibility of abnormalities of the GU tract or renal impairment.[1,2] Antenatal sonography often assists in the diagnosis of disorders before the onset of signs and symptoms in the neonate. Variations in the amount of amniotic fluid and structural abnormalities may have been detected by ultrasound. Family history is an important consideration because certain GU anomalies are associated with a genetic predisposition.[2,3] Parents of newborns with GU disorders should be questioned as to the occurrence of anomalies in other family members. Genetic counseling may be appropriate in some instances.

RELATED FINDINGS

Even without a documented history of oligohydramnios, physical signs of intrauterine compression in the newborn, such as flattened facies, malformed ears, and contraction deformities of the limbs (Figure 9-1), suggest urogenital defects. Pulmonary hypoplasia, presenting as respiratory distress, may occur secondary to oligohydramnios or to limited excursion of the diaphragm caused by an intraabdominal mass.[1,2,4]

There is a well-established association between GU anomalies and abnormalities of other systems: cardiovascular, neurologic, gastrointestinal, and musculoskeletal, as well as those that are genetic in origin. Careful evaluation of the GU system is warranted in neonates with other congenital anomalies such as myelomeningocele, complex congenital heart disease, and VACTERL (**v**ertebral anomalies, **a**nal atresia, **c**ardiac abnormalities, **t**racheoesophageal abnormalities, **r**enal abnormalities, and **l**imb anomalies) association.

FIGURE 9-1 ▲ Compression effects of oligohydramnios, which may signal possible GU or renal abnormalities.

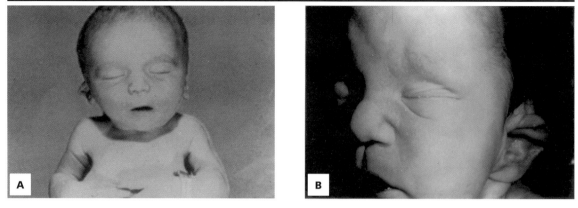

A. Joint contractures, narrow thorax, malformed ear. **B.** Typical facies: flattened nose, epicanthal fold, furrowed brow.

Courtesy of J. Hernandez, MD, The Children's Hospital, Denver, Colorado.

The presence of oliguria and anuria may indicate underlying urologic disease. Thirteen percent of full-term and 21 percent of premature neonates void at delivery.[5] This event frequently goes unnoticed. By 24 hours of age, 92 percent of all healthy newborns will have voided for the first time; 98 percent of newborns void by 48 hours.[6] Lack of urine output in the first 48 hours of life in an otherwise healthy neonate should not be a cause for alarm. However, diagnostic evaluation and/or intervention are necessary if there are any signs of illness or abnormalities (palpable bladder, abdominal mass, renal disease) or if more than 48 hours pass without urination.[7] Anuria or oliguria that develops after the first 48 hours of life can also be a sign of malformation or obstruction of the urinary tract.

Urine output is normally low during the first two days of life: Full-term neonates may void between one to four times, whereas premature neonates void more frequently. The volume of urine production rises as intake increases.[8] Documentation of adequate urinary output is important, especially with early hospital discharge of newborns. Parent counseling and adequate follow-up care are essential.

NORMAL PHYSICAL EXAMINATION

ABDOMEN

A comprehensive abdominal examination is described in Chapter 8. Those details pertinent to the GU system are presented here.

On inspection, the abdomen of a term neonate is rounded and symmetric, with smooth, opaque skin. A preterm newborn has a more protuberant abdomen because of immature muscle development, and the skin covering the abdomen may be thinner, with more prominent blood vessels.

The umbilical cord should be evaluated for appearance, length, diameter, number of vessels, and insertion site. At birth, it is gelatinous and bluish white in color and contains three vessels: two arteries and one vein. There should be no exudate or discharge from the umbilicus. Normal cord length is 30–100 cm, with an average diameter of 1.5–2 cm.[6]

Palpation of the abdomen is easiest in the first 24–48 hours of life, before air fills the entire gastrointestinal tract and before abdominal tone increases.[3,7] It is best performed on a quiet neonate lying in a supine position with knees and hips maintained in flexion by the examiner's hand. Providing a pacifier to

FIGURE 9-2 ▲ One technique for palpating the kidneys.

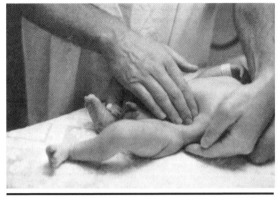

From: Coen RW, and Koffler H. 1987. *Primary Care of the Newborn.* Boston: Little, Brown, 30. Reprinted by permission.

FIGURE 9-3 ▲ Alternate method for palpating the kidneys.

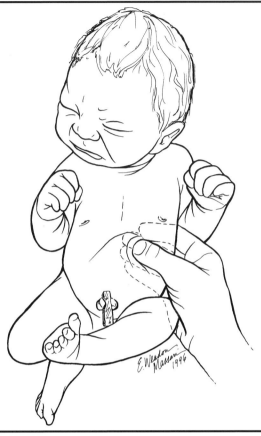

evoke the sucking reflex may help to relax the abdominal musculature.

All four quadrants should be examined to detect any masses. The neonate's kidneys are in a lower position in the abdomen than they will be later in life. Normally, the inferior poles of both kidneys can be felt; the right kidney is usually lower than the left.[2] Kidneys should be approximately equal in size and smooth to the touch. Ureters are not palpable.

The presence of stool-filled intestines or a fussy, crying infant may make this portion of the exam somewhat difficult. If the examiner is unable to palpate the kidneys, the fact that the neonate has voided ensures the presence of some renal tissue. Enlarged kidneys are easy to detect; this finding should prompt further investigation.

Figure 9-2 illustrates one technique for palpating the kidneys. The upper hand palpates the upper and lower quadrants while the other hand supports the flank. The process is repeated on the opposite side. An alternate method is depicted in Figure 9-3: Place the fingers of one hand under the infant, with the thumb on the abdomen. To palpate the kidneys, compress the fingers against the thumb;

the fingers support the flank while the thumb explores the area.[9]

The bladder can be percussed, or it can be palpated between the umbilicus and the symphysis pubis. A distended bladder may be palpated as a sub-umbilical fullness or mass. Because the bladder wall is thin, this organ may be difficult to palpate. Percussion may then be helpful to detect a full bladder over the symphysis pubis.[9]

MALE GENITALIA

Inspect the urogenital area with the male infant in the supine position. Figure 9-4 is a diagram of normal male genitalia. Gestational age has a great impact on the appearance of the external genitalia. Figure 9-5 illustrates the changes in external genitalia with advancing

FIGURE 9-4 ▲ Normal newborn genitalia (male).

FIGURE 9-4 ▲ Normal newborn genitalia (male).

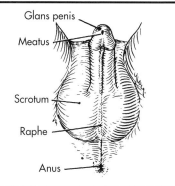

Glans penis
Meatus
Scrotum
Raphe
Anus

From: Grumbach MM, and Conte FA. 1992. Disorders of sexual differentiation. In *William's Textbook of Endocrinology,* 8th ed., Wilson JD, and Foster DW, eds. Philadelphia: Saunders, 331. Reprinted by permission.

gestation. Rugae (wrinkles or creases) begin to form on the ventral surface of the scrotum at approximately 36 weeks gestation. At term, the scrotum is fully rugated and more deeply pigmented than the surrounding skin.

Palpate the scrotal sac and inguinal canal to locate the testes and to detect any masses. Prior to 28 weeks gestation, the testes are abdominal organs; at 28–30 weeks, they begin to descend into the inguinal canal. By term, the testes should be well situated in the scrotum.[1,5,10] When palpated, normal testes are firm and smooth and comparatively equal in size. They are ovoid in shape, usually mobile, and measure, on average, 1.4–1.6 cm in the term neonate.[5,11] Palmert and Dahms suggest the following technique for detecting testes in the inguinal area: (1) Place the infant supine. (2) Apply soap or oil to the infant's skin and examiner's fingers. (3) Using gentle to firm pressure, slide two or three fingers along the inguinal canal toward the scrotum. It may be necessary to repeat this maneuver numerous times before testes can be felt.[12]

Newborn males may have edema of the genitalia due to the effects of transplacentally acquired maternal hormones. Trauma may

FIGURE 9-5 ▲ Appearance of genitalia in (A) preterm, (B) term, and (C) postterm male neonates.

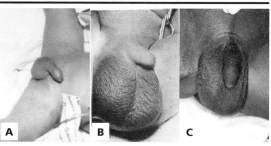

A   B   C

Term infant is from: Lepley CJ, Gardner SL, and Lubchenco LO. 1989. Initial nursery care. In *Handbook of Neonatal Intensive Care,* 2nd ed., Merenstein GB, and Gardner SL, eds. Philadelphia: Mosby, 88. Reprinted by permission.

occur during breech delivery (Figure 9-6) or in very large babies. Ecchymosis, edema, or even hematomas may be seen. These findings are transient and should begin to dissipate after a few days.

The prepuce, or foreskin, covers the entire head of the penis in an uncircumcised male neonate. Its function is to protect the urethral

FIGURE 9-6 ▲ Genital bruising with breech presentation.

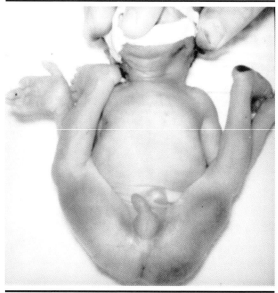

Courtesy of Dr. David A. Clark, Albany Medical Center and Wyeth-Ayerst Laboratories, Philadelphia, Pennsylvania.

FIGURE 9-7 ▲ **Technique for measuring penile length.**

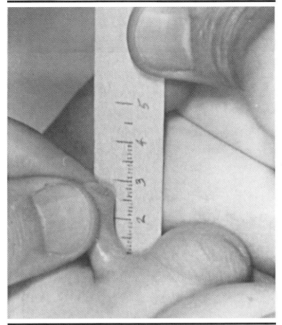

From: Palmert MR, and Dahms WT. 2006. Abnormalities of sexual differentiation. In _Fanaroff and Martin's Neonatal-Perinatal Medicine: Diseases of the Fetus and Infant,_ 8th ed., Martin RJ, Fanaroff AA, and Walsh MC, eds. Philadelphia: Mosby, 1559. Reprinted by permission.

FIGURE 9-8 ▲ **Normal newborn genitalia (female).**

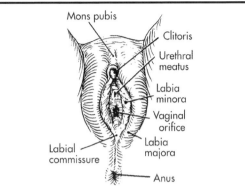

Adapted from: Grumbach MM, and Conte FA. 1992. Disorders of sexual differentiation. In _William's Textbook of Endocrinology,_ 8th ed., Wilson JD, and Foster DW, eds. Philadelphia: Saunders, 331. Reprinted by permission.

meatus from minor trauma.[11,13] Normally, the prepuce is tight, with a tiny orifice, but the opening is usually adequate to allow urination.[1] In newborns, the prepuce is adherent to the glans and cannot be retracted without disrupting its natural adherence to the surface of the glans. Therefore, forceful retraction should be avoided.[1,7] Physiologic phimosis, a nonretractable foreskin, is normal in young males and generally resolves in the first few years of life.[11,13,14]

Gentle traction is applied on the foreskin to visualize the urethral meatus at the central tip of the penis. The penis should be straight; erections are commonly seen in neonates. Observation and documentation of the force and direction of the urine stream while voiding are important. The urine stream should be forceful, straight, and continuous.[4,7]

Penile length and width should be assessed. The average stretched length of the penis in a term neonate is 3.5 cm, measured from the pubic bone to the tip of the glans (omitting excess foreskin).[5] Some neonates have a large deposit of adipose tissue overlying the pubic bone, giving the illusion of a small penis. In such cases, it is important to depress the fat pad while stretching the shaft for assessment of length. Comparative nomograms are available to document an abnormally sized penis.[12] There may be racial differences in the size of genitalia.[15,16] Male newborns with measurements that lie outside of the normal range should be compared to those of their racial background if such information is available. Figure 9-7 demonstrates a measurement technique for penile length. Penile width is measured midshaft on a stretched penis and should be 0.9–1.3 cm in a term neonate.[11]

If catheterization is necessary, a #5 French catheter or feeding tube should pass easily through the external meatus and urethra of either a preterm or a term male infant. By one year of age, the urethra should be able to accommodate a #8 French tube.[11,17]

FIGURE 9-9 ▲ Appearance of genitalia in (A) preterm and (B) term female neonates.

FIGURE 9-9 ▲ Appearance of genitalia in (A) preterm and (B) term female neonates.

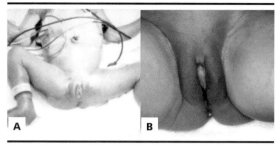

FIGURE 9-10 ▲ Hymenal tag in a neonate.

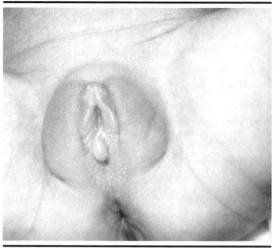

Female Genitalia

The female genitalia are also inspected with the newborn in the supine position. An illustration of the normal external female anatomy is provided in Figure 9-8. The labia majora are the outermost structures, extending from the mons pubis to the labial commissure. Medial to the labia majora are the labia minora, which join anteriorly to form the prepuce of the clitoris.[5]

For the first eight weeks of life, the term female neonate may have prominent labia, a large clitoris, and a urethral meatus that is difficult to visualize because of the influence of maternal estrogen. Maternal hormone exposure can stimulate a white, mucoid vaginal discharge and/or bleeding (pseudomenses). These findings may persist for up to ten days. The genitalia of breech-positioned and large babies may be edematous and ecchymotic for several days after delivery.[18]

Gestational age influences the appearance of the female genitalia (Figure 9-9). In preterm females, the labia minora and clitoris are very prominent, and the labia majora are small because of a lack of adipose tissue. The labia majora are larger in more mature neonates; in term females, they usually cover the clitoris and labia minora.

The labia and the inguinal and suprapubic areas are inspected and palpated to detect any masses, bulges, or swelling. The labia are then separated with gentle lateral and downward traction of the examiner's fingers. The clitoris is the uppermost structure, located at the junction of the labia minora. Normal values for clitoral measurements in the newborn have been published.[5]

Directly below the clitoris and above the vaginal opening is the urethral meatus. The perineum is the area between the vaginal opening and the anus; it should be smooth, without dimpling or fistulas. Normally, in the term female, the perineum is as wide as a fingertip. Abnormal length of the perineum with abnormal spacing between the vaginal, urethral, and anal orifices is occasionally associated with GU anomalies.[12] The vaginal orifice measures 1.5 cm in the average term female.[19] The hymen is a thickened avascular membrane with a central orifice. A hymenal tag (Figure 9-10) is a common neonatal variation that usually disappears in a few weeks.

Abnormal Findings on Abdominal Examination

Abdominal Distention

Abdominal distention is a frequent finding in the neonate because of poorly developed abdominal musculature. Masses or, less commonly, ascites can be causes of abdominal distention. Most palpable abdominal masses in newborns are of renal origin.[7,9] The most common renal causes of abdominal masses in neonates are hydronephrosis and multicystic dysplastic kidneys.[1] Dilated, enlarged ureters caused by urinary tract obstruction can also present as abdominal masses.

Because the urinary bladder is higher in the abdomen in the neonate than in the older infant, bladder distention is a frequent cause of abdominal distention and the most common midline abdominal mass. Persistent bladder distention might signify structural urethral defects, bladder obstruction, or neuromuscular disease. An abdominal mass is a cause for concern and warrants further investigation.

Ascites is an intra-abdominal collection of fluid. Percussion reveals its presence. Lower urinary tract obstruction, particularly posterior urethral valves, can be a cause of ascites. In these cases, ascitic fluid is composed of urine that has either escaped through a frank rupture in the collecting system or leaked through a renal calyx into the peritoneal cavity.[1]

ABDOMINAL WALL DEFECTS

Triad syndrome or *prune belly syndrome (PBS),* a congenital deficiency of the abdominal musculature, is readily apparent at birth (see Figure 8-1). The incidence of PBS is approximately 1 per 50,000 births.[20] Its characteristics are a large, flaccid, wrinkled abdominal wall, undescended testes, and various genitourinary malformations, such as hydroureter, hydronephrosis, and renal dysplasia. Occasionally, imperforate anus, intestinal malrotation, rib cage anomalies, cardiovascular abnormalities, and lower limb defects are also present. This syndrome is seen almost exclusively in males; reports of affected females are rare.[21]

Exstrophy of the bladder is a part of a spectrum of malformations involving defects of the urinary and genital tracts, musculoskeletal

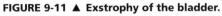

FIGURE 9-11 ▲ Exstrophy of the bladder.

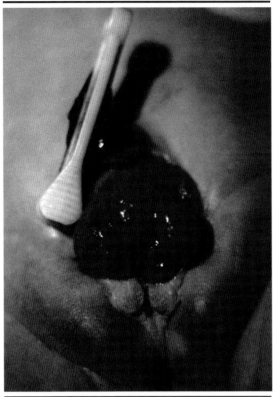

From: Clark DA. 2000. *Atlas of Neonatology,* Philadelphia: Saunders, 201. Reprinted by permission.

system, and sometimes the intestinal tract.[20] It is a rare condition, occurring in approximately 1 per 24,000–40,000 births, and is more common in males. Variants of this condition include epispadias and cloacal exstrophy.[2] As the result of an embryologic defect, there is an absence of muscle and connective tissue in the anterior abdominal wall over the bladder. This presents as eversion and protrusion of the bladder through the abdominal wall defect (Figure 9-11). The ureteral orifices may be identified on the exposed bladder surface. Complete exstrophy of the bladder is associated with epispadias in some male infants (Figure 9-12).

In cloacal exstrophy, the defect is more extensive and may include an omphalocele containing intestines, liver, and spleen (Figure 9-13). Loops of cecum and terminal ileum

FIGURE 9-12 ▲ Exstrophy of the bladder with epispadias.

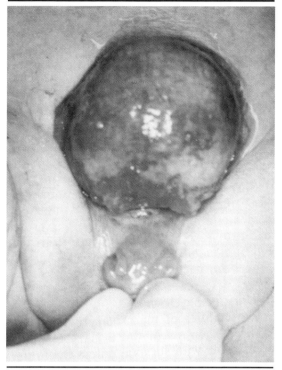

From: Kaplan GW, and McAleer IM. 2005. Structural abnormalities of the genitourinaty tract. In *Neonatology: Pathophysiology and Management of the Newborn,* 6th ed., MacDonald MG, Mullett MD, and Seshia MMK, eds. Philadelphia: Lippincott Williams & Wilkins, 1077. Reprinted by permission.

FIGURE 9-13 ▲ Newborn male with cloacal exstrophy.

Note separate bladder components (**B**), associated omphalocele (**O**), terminal ileum (**I**), cecum (**C**), and bifid penis (**arrows**).

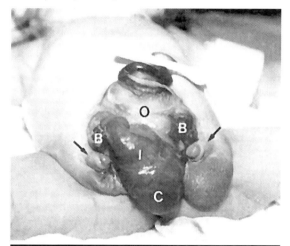

From: Zaontz MR, and Packer MG. 1997. Abnormalities of the external genitalia. *Pediatric Clinics of North America* 44(5): 1282. Reprinted by permission.

may be seen dividing the exposed bladder into two sections. In males, the penis is small and divided in half, whereas females may present with a bifid clitoris and uterus and a duplicate or exstrophic vagina.[22,23]

In bladder exstrophy and epispadias, the upper urinary tract is usually normal, but renal agenesis, horseshoe kidneys, hydronephrosis, and other renal anomalies have been reported. A wide array of abnormalities involving the cardiac, gastrointestinal, renal, musculoskeletal, and neurologic systems is associated with cloacal exstrophy.[22,23]

Umbilical Cord Anomalies

A single umbilical artery (SUA) is found in 0.3 percent of neonates. In an otherwise normal infant, further diagnostic workup is not indicated because SUA is associated with renal abnormalities in only 7 percent of cases.[24,25]

The urachus (see Figure 8-3) is an embryologic structure that connects the fetal bladder with the umbilicus. Postnatal patency of the urachal remnant can result in a clear discharge (urine) from an otherwise normal appearing umbilical cord. The discharge of urine may be intermittent or minimal. Obtaining the specific gravity of the discharge can confirm it to be urine. A large, edematous umbilical cord that does not separate in the normal amount of time may be the only sign of a patent urachus or of a urachal cyst.[7,26] Urinary drainage from a urachal remnant can lead to umbilical granuloma, redness, or swelling below the umbilicus. A sign of a persistent urachus is the retraction of the umbilical cord during urination. Evaluation for lower urinary tract obstruction should be considered in a neonate with a patent urachus.[5]

FIGURE 9-14 ▲ Distal hypospadias.

Note dorsal hooded foreskin, flattened glans, and distal shaft meatus.

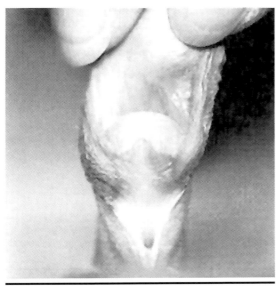

From: Zaontz MR, and Packer MG. 1997. Abnormalities of the external genitalia. *Pediatric Clinics of North America* 44(5): 1268. Reprinted by permission.

ABNORMALITIES OF THE MALE GENITALIA

THE PENIS

Aphallia (absence of a penis) and *diphallia* (duplicated penis) are rare conditions that require extensive reconstructive surgery. There are two types of duplications: bifid penis and true duplication. Bifid penis may occur in exstrophy-epispadias complex and is characterized by separation of the corporal body of the penis into two halves, with a single urethral meatus at the base of the shafts.[22,23] In true diphallia, there may be total duplication, with voiding and erectile function in individual shafts.[11]

Hypospadias is the abnormal location of the urethral meatus on the ventral surface of the penis. It is a common abnormality, occurring in approximately 8.2 per 1,000 births, and results from the incomplete development of the anterior urethra.[12] Failure of the urethra

FIGURE 9-15 ▲ Balanic (or glanular) hypospadias.

This is the most common form of hypospadias. The external urethral orifice is indicated by the arrow. There is a shallow pit at the usual site of the orifice. Note the moderate degree of chordee, causing the penis to curve ventrally.

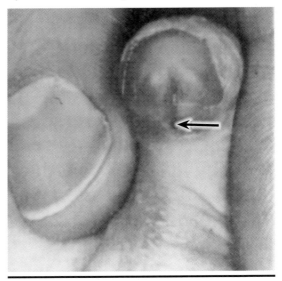

From: Jolly H. 1968. *Diseases of Children*, 2nd ed. Oxford: Blackwell Scientific Publications. Reprinted by permission.

to develop inhibits proper development of the prepuce. Most neonates with hypospadias also have a hooded or malformed prepuce (Figure 9-14).[12,27] It is important to locate the urethral meatus in a neonate with a malformed or hypoplastic prepuce and not simply to dismiss the malformation as a "natural circumcision."

Hypospadias can be classified into three categories based on meatal position. Balanic (glanular) hypospadias exists when the urethral opening is ventrally situated at the base of the glans (Figure 9-15). Penile hypospadias occurs when the meatus is found between the glans and the scrotum (Figure 9-16). Penoscrotal hypospadias (Figure 9-17) and perineal hypospadias are defined as the urethral opening at the penoscrotal junction and on the perineum, respectively.[1,5,28]

Isolated balanic (glanular) and penile hypospadias without other genital abnormalities or

FIGURE 9-16 ▲ Penile hypospadias.

The penis is short and curved (chordee). The external urethral orifice (arrow) is near the penoscrotal junction.

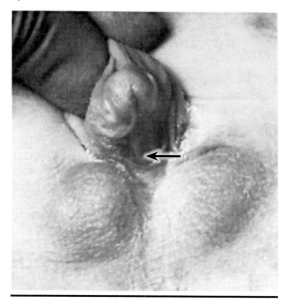

From: Moore KL, and Persaud TVN. 1998. *Before We Are Born: Essentials of Embryology and Birth Defects,* 5th ed. Philadelphia: Saunders, 320. Reprinted by permission.

FIGURE 9-17 ▲ Penoscrotal hypospadias.

The external urethral orifice (arrow) is located at the penoscrotal junction.

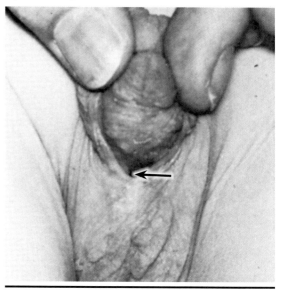

From: Moore KL, and Persaud TVN. 1998. *Before We Are Born: Essentials of Embryology and Birth Defects,* 5th ed. Philadelphia: Saunders, 320. Reprinted by permission.

dysmorphic features are rarely associated with chromosomal or endocrine disorders or with problems of sexual differentiation. Infants with penoscrotal or perineal hypospadias have a higher risk of these problems. Also, in infants with hypospadias and additional genital anomalies, such as cryptorchidism or micropenis (both discussed later in this chapter), the risk of endocrine imbalance or problems with sexual differentiation rises.[5,7,12,29] Further investigation is warranted in these cases.

Chordee is a bend in the shaft of the penis. It is an aspect of penile development that occurs between the 16th and the 20th week of gestation and may be seen in some normal premature infants. In these infants, it may resolve spontaneously within the first few months of life.[17] However, it is more common for chordee to be caused by fibrous tissue growth in an area of failed urethral development or by

skin traction from skin deficiency as seen in hypospadias or epispadias.[5,12,30] Chordee may not be evident without the presence of an erection.[11,22] Ventral chordee frequently, but not always, accompanies hypospadias (see Figure 9-15).

A variant of hypospadias that may be identified only after circumcision is called mega-meatus with intact prepuce. In this type, there is a well-formed, complete foreskin; the hypospadias is hidden by the prepuce, and there is no chordee.[14,31]

Epispadias, the location of the urethral meatus on the dorsal aspect of the penis, varies in severity from a glanular defect (Figure 9-18) to the complete version seen in exstrophy of the bladder (see Figure 9-12). All forms of epispadias are associated with differing degrees of dorsal chordee.[30]

Circumcision should not be performed on neonates with hypospadias or epispadias

FIGURE 9-18 ▲ Epispadias.

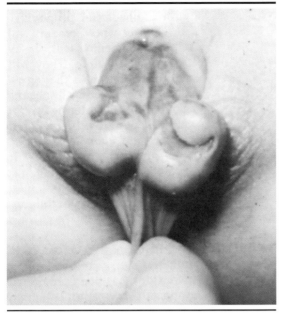

From: Kaplan GW, and McAleer IM. 2005. Structural abnormalities of the genitourinaty tract. In *Neonatology: Pathophysiology and Management of the Newborn,* 6th ed., MacDonald MG, Mullett MD, and Seshia MMK, eds. Philadelphia: Lippincott Williams & Wilkins, 1087. Reprinted by permission.

because the foreskin may be used in the repair of these defects. Parents should be notified that reconstructive surgery by a pediatric urologist might be required. Repair is generally performed after six months of age.[1]

Hypospadias or epispadias can cause abnormalities in voiding.[30,32] A weak urine stream, especially in the presence of a distended bladder, suggests the possibility of lower urinary tract obstruction (commonly, posterior urethral valves). The neonate with a spinal cord abnormality such as a sacral tumor, spinal cord tethering, caudal regression syndrome, or myelomeningocele may also have abnormalities in voiding as the result of a neurogenic bladder. In these newborns, lesions of the nervous system interrupt the conduction of impulses from the brain to the bladder, preventing normal micturition.

FIGURE 9-19 ▲ Webbed penis.

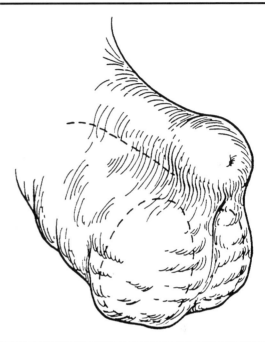

From: Rozanski TA, and Bloom DA. 1997. Male genital tract. In *Surgery of Infants and Children: Scientific Principles and Practice,* Oldham KT, Colombani PM, and Foglia RP, eds. Philadelphia: Lippincott-Raven, 1547. Reprinted by permission.

A *micropenis* is an abnormally short or thin penis that is more than two standard deviations below the mean of length and width for age using standard charts. The evaluation and management of a newborn with a true micropenis frequently requires an endocrinologist and a geneticist.[1,11,31] (See **Abnormal Sexual Differentiation/Ambiguous Genitalia** later in this chapter.)

Priapism is a persistent, seemingly painless penile erection that usually resolves spontaneously. Factors that may contribute to its development are polycythemia and birth trauma; many cases of priapism are idiopathic.[32] The neonate with a *webbed penis* (Figure 9-19) has a normal urethra and scrotum. However, the scrotal skin extends onto the ventral surface of the shaft, obscuring the penoscrotal angle and making the penis appear short.[5,7,31,32]

FIGURE 9-20 ▲ Hydrocele.

A. Large hydrocele that resulted from an unobliterated portion of the precessus vaginalis. **B.** Hydrocele of the testis and spermatic cord resulting from peritoneal fluid passing into an unclosed processus vaginalis.

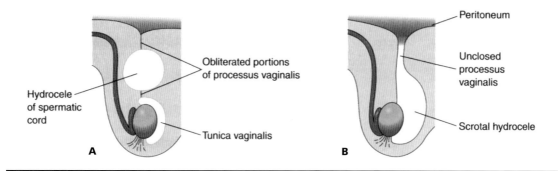

From: Moore KL, and Persaud TVN. 2008. *The Developing Human: Clinically Oriented Embryology,* 8th ed. Philadelphia: Saunders, 282. Reprinted by permission.

THE SCROTUM

Cryptorchidism—literally, hidden testis— refers to a testis or testes that assume an extrascrotal location.[11,12,27] The condition occurs when one or both testes fail to descend completely into the scrotum. It is detected by the inability to palpate one or both testes in the scrotal sac. Cryptorchidism is seen in approximately 3.7 percent of term males and in 21 percent of all premature neonates, with an incidence of nearly 100 percent in extremely preterm neonates.[12] A unilateral, undescended testis is more commonly seen than is bilateral cryptorchidism. Bilateral cryptorchidism presents as an empty, hypoplastic scrotal sac.

A truly undescended testis is one that is interrupted in its usual path of descent, whereas an ectopic testis pursues an abnormal course of descent and may be found in a superficial inguinal pouch.[12,33,34] Anorchia is the absence of testicular tissue.[11] A retractile testis is a normally descended organ that recedes into the inguinal canal because of activity of the cremasteric muscle. Because this muscle is

FIGURE 9-21 ▲ Inguinal hernia.

A. Incomplete congenital inguinal hernia resulting from persistence of the proximal part of the processus vaginalis. **B.** Complete congenital inguinal hernia into the scrotum resulting from persistence of the processus vaginalis. Cryptorchidism, a commonly associated anomaly, is also illustrated.

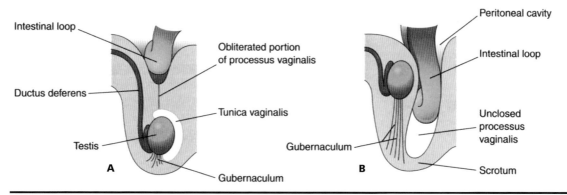

From: Moore KL, and Persaud TVN. 2008. *The Developing Human: Clinically Oriented Embryology,* 8th ed. Philadelphia: Saunders, 282. Reprinted by permission.

FIGURE 9-22 ▲ Transillumination of a scrotal hydrocele.

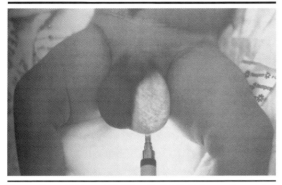

From: Coen RW, and Koffler H. 1987. *Primary Care of the Newborn.* Boston: Little, Brown, 33. Reprinted by permission.

FIGURE 9-23 ▲ Hydrometrocolpos.

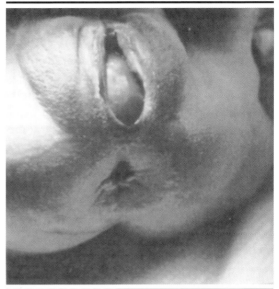

From: Coen RW, and Koffler H. 1987. *Primary Care of the Newborn.* Boston: Little, Brown, 90. Reprinted by permission.

inactive in newborns, retractile testes do not occur in this age group.[33] Thus, an empty or a hypoplastic scrotal sac in a neonate, when detected by observation and palpation, indicates truly undescended testes, ectopic testes (outside the external inguinal ring), or anorchia (absent testes).[1,7,20]

Most undescended testes will descend by three months of age. Spontaneous descent rarely occurs after nine months of age.[12,32] Diagnosis of true cryptorchidism and subsequent surgical intervention, called orchiopexy, is important because of an associated risk of infertility and malignancy in the cryptorchid testis.[12,20,27] Retractile testes usually grow and develop normally.[12]

Cryptorchidism may be an isolated defect or a coincidental finding in many malformations and syndromes. Neonates with undescended testes and other abnormal features, such as micropenis, bifid scrotum, and hypospadias, should be evaluated for endocrine problems and gender ambiguity.[12,27,29,34]

Hernias and hydroceles commonly present as bulges or swellings in the groin or scrotum.[5,25] Both are the result of a patent processus vaginalis; however, they differ in several ways.[2,26] A *hydrocele* (Figure 9-20) is a nontender, fluid-filled scrotal mass overlying the testis and spermatic cord. It presents as a scrotal swelling and is caused by the passage of peritoneal fluid through the patent processus vaginalis into the scrotum or by the persistence of peritoneal fluid that has not been reabsorbed.[5,26,27] Neonates commonly (57.9 percent of all newborn males) present with hydroceles.[5] Upon examination, the entire circumference of the testis can be palpated.[25,35]

An actual or a potential indirect *inguinal hernia* may be associated with a hydrocele. Loops of intestine can herniate through the persistent processus vaginalis into the scrotum (Figure 9-21). The incidence of hernias is inversely proportional to gestational age and birth weight.[2] Prematurity increases the incidence of inguinal hernia in both males and females, although they are seen more often in males.[2,5] Other conditions associated with the development of inguinal hernias are family history, hydrops fetalis, meconium peritonitis, urinary and chylous ascites, ambiguous genitalia, hypospadias and epispadias, cryptorchidism,

FIGURE 9-24 ▲ Inguinal hernias (A) before and (B) after reduction.

Inguinal hernias occur more frequently in extremely premature females than in those born closer to term. The uterus, fallopian tubes, and ovaries, as well as the bowel, may herniate. A hymenal tag is apparent after reduction in **B**.

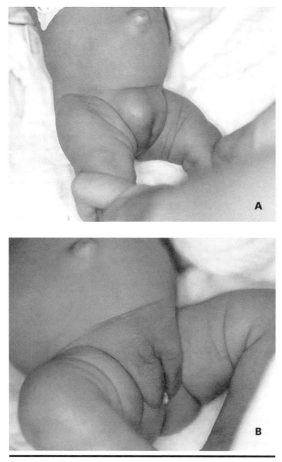

From: Fletcher M. 1998. *Physical Diagnosis in Neonatology.* Philadelphia: Lippincott-Raven, 388. Reprinted by permission.

cystic fibrosis, ventriculoperitoneal shunts, congenital hypothyroidism, and Beckwith-Wiedemann syndrome.[9,36]

The presence of intestine in the scrotal sac renders the entire circumference of the testis impalpable.[18,37] A scrotal mass or swelling from a hydrocele may be further distinguished from that caused by a hernia in that a hydrocele appears translucent on transillumination (Figure 9-22). This may not be a universal finding,

however. Hernias may also transilluminate because the bowel contains air.[36] Hernias are reducible and hydroceles are not.

To reduce a hernia, the examiner should grasp the most distal portion of the scrotum on the affected side with the fingers of one hand and apply firm, steady, upward pressure in the direction of the internal ring.[38] The scrotal sac will decrease in size as the intestines return to the abdomen through the internal ring.

Bowel incarceration and strangulation and ischemic injury to the testis are potential complications of inguinal hernias. Incarceration is the inability to easily reduce the hernia; in strangulation, the loop of bowel becomes trapped, leading to ischemia and ultimate necrosis.[2,35] Redness, pain, symptoms of intestinal obstruction, and difficulty in reduction are evidence of incarceration.[27]

Hernia repair can be deferred if the hernia is easily reducible and there are no signs of incarceration, but surgery should be scheduled as soon as possible. Most hydroceles resolve in the first year of life.[2] Communicating hydroceles are, in reality, indirect inguinal hernias; therefore, repair is recommended if they persist after two years of age.[39]

Testicular torsion, or twisting of the testis on its spermatic cord, may occur prenatally and is usually unilateral. The neonate presents with a hard, swollen scrotum that is red to bluish red in color and does not transilluminate. This condition compromises blood supply to the testis; therefore, it requires urgent evaluation and possibly emergency management.[2,27,31] Ischemia of more than 12 hours duration usually results in irreversible damage and loss of the gonad.[27] With prenatal torsion, the duration of the torsion is unknown; by birth, irreversible ischemic damage to the testis may have occurred. Testicular torsion is painful in older children, but pain is not a universal finding in neonates.[12,27,38] Therefore, one should

FIGURE 9-25 ▲ **Newborn male infant (46,XY) with ambiguous genitalia.**

Note penoscrotal hypospadias (arrow). Testes are palpable in the scrotum.

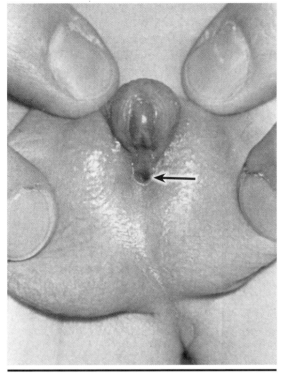

From: Palmert MR, and Dahms WT. 2006. Abnormalities of sexual differentiation. In *Fanaroff and Martin's Neonatal-Perinatal Medicine: Diseases of the Fetus and Infant,* 8th ed., Martin RJ, Fanaroff AA, and Walsh MC, eds. Philadelphia: Mosby, 1565. Reprinted by permission.

not be misled into discounting the possibility of testicular torsion in the case of a newborn male with a red, swollen scrotum that is not tender.

ABNORMALITIES OF THE FEMALE GENITALIA

Hydrocolpos (distention of the vagina) and *hydrometrocolpos* (distention of the vagina and the uterus) (Figure 9-23) are the result of either incomplete canalization of the vagina during gestation or an imperforate hymen.[5,17] These conditions present in the newborn as lower abdominal masses and frequently as urinary

FIGURE 9-26 ▲ **Newborn female with ambiguous genitalia: clitoral enlargement and fusion of labia majora.**

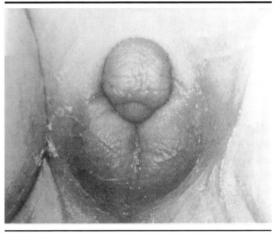

From: Moore KL, and Persaud TVN. 1998. *Before We Are Born: Essentials of Embryology and Birth Defects,* 5th ed. Philadelphia: Saunders, 307. Reprinted by permission.

tract obstructions. Urine retention may occur secondary to mass effect.[40] When the hymen is imperforate, it may bulge secondary to accumulation of vaginal secretions, creating the appearance of a shiny, cystic mass between the labia.[17]

The urethral meatus should be just ventral to the vaginal opening. Deviation from this position may indicate a urogenital sinus or ambiguous genitalia.[40]

Inguinal hernias occur less frequently in females than in males.[36] When they do occur, they may present as a reducible swelling of the labia (Figure 9-24). Occasionally, a gonad may be palpated in the suprapubic area. The question may arise as to whether the infant is a female with a prolapsed ovary or a genotypic male with ambiguous genitalia. This is due to the fact that ovaries usually do not descend.[41]

Clitoromegaly has been defined as an eight- to tenfold increase in clitoral index (defined as width times length). Causes of clitoromegaly in the newborn include endocrine abnormalities (congenital adrenal hyperplasia), maternal factors (increased androgen production, drugs), and syndromes (Beckwith-Wiedemann, true hermaphroditism).[5]

ABNORMAL SEXUAL DIFFERENTIATION/ AMBIGUOUS GENITALIA

Ambiguous genitalia (Figures 9-25 and 9-26) may be defined as the presence of a phallic structure that is not discretely male or female, an abnormally located urethral meatus, and the inability to palpate one or both gonads in males.[4] One should suspect problems of sexual differentiation in phenotypic males with bilateral impalpable testes, perineal hypospadias, or unilateral undescended testis with hypospadias. Similarly, phenotypic females with clitoral hypertrophy, a palpable gonad, inseparably fused labia, or abnormal openings or dimpling on the perineum should be evaluated.[1,12,42]

The association of ambiguous genitalia with serious underlying endocrine disorders and the understandable distress of the parents mandate rapid identification and evaluation of these newborns. It is imperative that an endocrinologist, a genetic specialist, a urologist, and a psychologist/social worker be included on the evaluation team. The infant should be referred to simply as "baby" until the appropriate sex of rearing is determined.

SUMMARY

Evaluation of the GU tract in the newborn is important to ensure rapid detection and treatment of abnormalities. Too frequently, this examination is cursory, and abnormalities, both major and minor, go unnoticed. Identification of problems in the neonatal period may preserve organ function and prevent mortality and morbidity in the future.

REFERENCES

1. Vogt BA, Dell KM, and Davis ID. 2006. The kidney and urinary tract. In *Neonatal-Perinatal Medicine: Diseases of the Fetus and Infant,* 8th ed., Martin RJ, Fanaroff AA, and Walsh MC, eds. Philadelphia: Mosby, 1659–1683.

2. Parker L. 2007. Genitourinary system. In *Comprehensive Neonatal Care: An Interidisciplinary Approach,* 4th ed., Kenner C, and Lott J, eds. Philadelphia: Saunders, 175–202.

3. Friedlich PS, Evans JR, and Seri I. 2005. Clinical evaluation of renal and urinary tract disease. In *Avery's Diseases of the Newborn,* 8th ed., Taeusch HW, Ballard RA, and Gleason CA, eds. Philadelphia: Saunders, 1267–1271.

4. Ritchey ML. 2007. Renal anomalies. In *The Kelalis-King-Belman Textbook of Clinical Pediatric Urology,* 5th ed., Docimo SG, Canning DA, and Khoury AK, eds. New York: Informa Healthcare, 293–312.

5. Fletcher M. 1998. *Physical Diagnosis in Neonatology.* Philadelphia: Lippincott Williams & Wilkins, 368–383.

6. Barratt TM, and Niaudet P. 2003. Clinical evaluation. In *Pediatric Nephrology,* 5th ed., Avner ED, Harmon WE, and Niaudet P, eds. Philadelphia: Lippincott Williams & Wilkins, 387–398.

7. Vogt BA, Davis ID, and Avner ED. 2002. The kidney. In *Care of the High-Risk Neonate,* 5th ed., Klaus MH, and Fanaroff AA, eds. Philadelphia: Saunders, 425–446.

8. Arant BS. 2007. Fetal and neonatal renal function. In *The Kelalis-King-Belman Textbook of Clinical Pediatric Urology,* 5th ed., Docimo SG, Canning DA, and Khoury AK, eds. New York: Informa Healthcare, 313–325.

9. Thigpen J. 2007. Gastrointestinal system. In *Comprehensive Neonatal Care: An Interidisciplinary Approach,* 4th ed., Kenner C, and Lott J, eds. Philadelphia: Saunders, 92–133.

10. Kolon TF, Patel RP, and Huff DS. 2004. Cryptorchidism: Diagnosis, treatment, and long-term prognosis. *Urologic Clinics of North America* 31(3): 469–480.

11. Rozanski TA, and Bloom D. 1997. Male genital tract. In *Surgery of Infants and Children: Scientific Principles and Practice,* Oldham KT, Colombani PM, and Foglia RP, eds. Philadelphia: Lippincott Williams & Wilkins, 1543–1558.

12. Palmert MR and Dahms WT. 2006. Abnormalities of sexual differentiation. In *Neonatal-Perinatal Medicine: Diseases of the Fetus and Infant,* 8th ed., Martin RJ, Fanaroff AA, and Walsh MC, eds. Philadelphia: Mosby, 1550–1596.

13. Cartwright PC, Masterson TA, and Snow B. 2007. Office pediatric urology. In *The Kelalis-King-Belman Textbook of Clinical Pediatric Urology,* 5th ed., Docimo SG, Canning DA, and Khoury AK, eds. New York: Informa Healthcare, 194–214.

14. Elder JS. 2007. Abnormalities of the penis and urethra. In *Nelson Textbook of Pediatrics,* 18th ed., Kleigman RM, et al., eds. Philadelphia: Saunders, 2253–2260.

15. Phillip M, et al. 1996. Clitoral and penile sizes of full term newborns in two different ethnic groups. *Journal of Pediatric Endocrinology & Metabolism* 9(2): 175–179.

16. Lian WB, Lee WR, and Ho LY. 2000. Penile length of newborns in Singapore, *Journal of Pediatric Endocrinology & Metabolism* 13(1): 55–62.

17. Brown MR, Cartwright PC, and Snow BW. 1997. Common office problems in pediatric urology and gynecology. *Pediatric Clinics of North America* 44(5): 1091–1115.

18. Sansoucie DA, and Cavaliere TA. 2007. Assessment of the newborn and infant. In *Comprehensive Neonatal Care: An Interdisciplinary Approach,* 4th ed., Kenner C, and Lott J, eds. Philadelphia: Saunders, 677–718.

19. Adkins EA. 1997. The female genital tract. In *Surgery of Infants and Children: Scientific Principles and Practice,* Oldham KT, Colombani PM, and Foglia RP, eds. Philadelphia: Lippincott Williams & Wilkins, 1559–1575.

20. Mesrobian HG, Balcom AH, and Durkee CT. 2004. Urologic problems of the neonate. *Pediatric Clinics of North America* 51(4): 1051–1062.

21. Hudson RG, and Skoog SJ. 2007. Prune belly syndrome. In *The Kelalis-King-Belman Textbook of Clinical Pediatric Urology,* 5th ed., Docimo SG, Canning DA, and Khoury AK, eds. New York: Informa Healthcare, 1081–1114.

22. Martin T. 2007. Cloacal exstrophy: A case study. *Neonatal Network* 26(1): 21–30.

23. Hyun SJ. 2006. Cloacal exstrophy. *Neonatal Network* 25(2): 101–115.

24. Rennie JM. 2005. Examination of the newborn. In *Roberton's Textbook of Neonatology,* 4th ed., Rennie JM, and Roberton NRC, eds. Philadelphia: Churchill Livingstone, 249–266.

25. Lissauer T. 2006. Physical examination of the newborn. In *Neonatal-Perinatal Medicine: Diseases of the Fetus and Infant,* 8th ed., Martin RJ, Fanaroff AA, and Walsh MC, eds. Philadelphia: Mosby, 513–528.

26. Moore KL, and Persaud TVN. 2008. *The Developing Human: Clinically Oriented Embryology,* 8th ed. Philadelphia: Saunders, 243–284.

27. Zderic SA. 2005. Developmental abnormalities of the genitourinary system. In *Avery's Diseases of the Newborn,* 8th ed., Taeusch HW, Ballard RA, and Gleason CA, eds. Philadelphia: Saunders, 1287–1297.

28. Pinkstaff D, and Noseworthy J. 2005. Hypospadias. In *Principles and Practice of Pediatric Surgery*, 2nd ed., Oldham KT, et al., eds. Philadelphia: Lippincott Williams & Wilkins, 1611–1619.

29. Reddy PP, DeFoor WR, and Sheldon CA. 2005. Intersex status. In *Principles and Practice of Pediatric Surgery,* 2nd ed., Oldham KT, et al., eds. Philadelphia: Lippincott Williams & Wilkins, 1637–1679.

30. Zaontz MR, and Packer MG. 1997. Abnormalities of the external genitalia. *Pediatric Clinics of North America* 44(5): 1267–1297.

31. Kennedy AP, and Figueroa TE. 2005. Common urologic problems in the fetus and neonate. In *Intensive Care of the Fetus and Neonate,* 2nd ed., Spitzer AR, ed. Philadelphia: Mosby, 1369–1384.

32. Barthold JS, and Kass EJ. 2007. Prune belly syndrome. In *The Kelalis-King-Belman Textbook of Clinical Pediatric Urology,* 5th ed., Docimo SG, Canning DA, and Khoury AK, eds. New York: Informa Healthcare, 1239–1270.

33. Elder JS. 2007. Disorders and anomalies of the scrotal contents. In *Nelson Textbook of Pediatrics,* 18th ed., Kliegman RM, et al., eds. Philadelphia: Saunders, 2260–2265.

34. Husman DA. 2002. Cryptorchidism. In *Clinical Pediatric Urology,* 4th ed., Belman AB, King LR, and Kramer SA, eds. London: Martin Dunitz, 1295–1308.

35. Benjamin K. 2002. Scrotal and inguinal masses in the newborn period. *Advances in Neonatal Care* 2(3): 140–148.

36. Skoog SJ, and Colin MJ. 1995. Pediatric hernias and hydroceles: The urologist's perspective. *Urologic Clinics of North America* 22(1): 119–130.

37. Jarvis C. 2000. *Physical Examination and Health Assessment,* 3rd ed. Philadelphia: Saunders, 778.

38. Skoog SJ. 1997. Benign and malignant pediatric scrotal masses. *Pediatric Clinics of North America* 44(5): 1229–1250.

39. Berseth CL, and Poenaru, D. 2005. Abdominal wall problems. In *Avery's Diseases of the Newborn,* 8th ed., Taeusch HW, Ballard RA, and Gleason CA, eds. Philadelphia: Saunders, 1113–1122.

40. Merguerian PA, and McLorie GA. 1992. Disorders of the female genitalia. In *Clinical Pediatric Urology,* 3rd ed., Kelalis PP, King LR, and Belman AB, eds. Philadelphia: Saunders, 1084–1105.

41. Hyun G, and Kolon TF. 2004. A practical approach to intersex in the newborn period. *Urologic Clinics of North America* 31(3): 435–443.

42. His-Yang W, and Snyder HM. 2007. Intersex. In *The Kelalis-King-Belman Textbook of Clinical Pediatric Urology,* 5th ed., Docimo SG, Canning DA, and Khoury AK, eds. New York: Informa Healthcare, 1147–1160.

NOTES

NOTES

10 Musculoskeletal System Assessment

Ellen P. Tappero, DNP, RN, NNP-BC

Careful scrutiny of the musculoskeletal system during the newborn's physical examination is imperative because (1) it is vital to the confirmation of musculoskeletal abnormalities detected on prenatal ultrasound such as spinal malformations, limb length discrepancies, and clubfoot deformities and (2) the information recorded during the first exam forms the database for all future examinations. The musculoskeletal system provides stability and mobility for all physical activity. It consists of the body's bones (Figure 10-1), joints, and their supporting and connecting tissues. In addition to allowing movement and providing structure, the musculoskeletal system protects vital organs (brain, spinal cord), stores minerals (calcium, phosphorus), and produces red and white blood cells.

The bones of the newborn are soft because they are composed mostly of cartilage, which contains only a small amount of calcium. The process of ossification occurs rapidly during the first year of life. Compared with the skeleton of an adult or a child, the newborn's skeleton is flexible, and the joints are elastic. This elasticity is necessary to enable the infant to pass through the birth canal. Unlike the bones of the skeletal system, the muscular system is almost completely formed at birth. Growth in

FIGURE 10-1 ▲ Infant's skeletal structure.

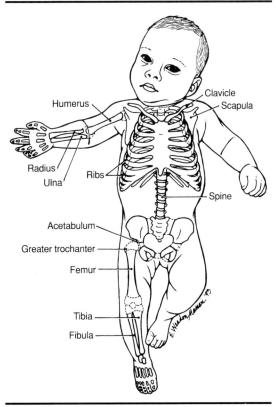

the size of the muscle is caused by hypertrophy, rather than by hyperplasia of the cells.[1]

A thorough evaluation of the musculoskeletal system involves the techniques of inspection, palpation, and, on some occasions, listening. It includes an appraisal of (1) posture, position, and gross anomalies; (2) discomfort from bone or joint movement; (3) range of joint motion; (4) muscle size, symmetry, and strength; and (5) the configuration and motility of the back. Normal variations in shape, size, contour, or movement may be the result of position *in utero* or genetic factors. These normal variations should be distinguished from congenital anomalies and birth trauma. Early diagnosis of musculoskeletal disorders and early intervention often preempt the need for complex medical treatment and lead to more favorable outcomes.[2]

Disorders that affect the musculoskeletal system may also originate from the neurologic system. An asymmetric Moro reflex, for example, may be caused by pain from a broken bone or a muscle injury, or it may be the result of a neurologic defect. Because there is some overlap between the musculoskeletal and neurologic examinations, assessment of muscle strength and motor activity are discussed with other neurologic assessments in Chapter 11.

PRENATAL HISTORY

Obtaining a comprehensive prenatal history is vital to the musculoskeletal assessment because a normal uterine environment is essential to the development of the fetus. Any event or condition that changes the intrauterine environment can alter fetal growth, movement, or position. Such prenatal factors as oligohydramnios, maternal uterine malformations, abnormal growth patterns, exposure to teratogenic agents, and breech presentation may adversely affect the development and maturation of the musculoskeletal system *in utero*. The perinatal history should be reviewed for possible birth trauma or neurologic insult. The practitioner must note such factors as duration of labor, signs of fetal distress, and the type of delivery

(vaginal or cesarean). These factors may have a bearing on conditions such as cerebral palsy, brachial palsy, and torticollis. In multiple gestation, the birth order is also worth noting because there is a higher incidence of developmental dysplasia of the hip (DDH) in firstborn children.[3] An accurate gestational age assessment or estimated date of confinement from the obstetric record is necessary for accurate assessment of the infant's posture and muscle tone.

GENERAL SURVEY

Ideally, a thorough physical examination should be done within the first 24 hours after delivery. Because it is difficult to find a totally motionless, cooperative newborn, much of the musculoskeletal examination must be done while watching the newborn or while examining other systems. Nondisturbing maneuvers should be performed early in the examination and potentially distressing maneuvers near the end. For example, the head and neck should be palpated early and the hips examined near the end. The practitioner must compile all the information produced by the exam and record all findings concerning the musculoskeletal system in a systematic manner.

For examination, the newborn should be completely undressed and positioned initially on the back. The examination area should be well lit, warm, and free of drafts. A radiant warmer or other heat source is necessary to prevent loss of body heat. The practitioner should develop a routine for examining the newborn so that no part of the musculoskeletal system is overlooked. The examination routine varies from practitioner to practitioner. Most proceed from head to toe.

Examination of the bony structures is important in a newborn examination because it is one of the first opportunities to assess intrauterine development. Deviations from normal may be the first indicator of a genetic abnormality or disease.[4]

The best instrument for measuring an infant's length, head circumference, and chest circumference is a narrow steel measuring tape. However, most nurseries provide paper tapes, which may be less accurate. Folding the paper tape in half lengthwise may add strength as well as decrease slippage when measuring rounded contours such as the head.[5]

MEASUREMENTS

Measurement of growth as reflected in increased body weight and length along expected pathways and within certain limits is one of the most important indicators of health in an infant.[4] Measurements taken soon after birth demand careful attention to detail because they will act as a baseline for subsequent assessments of growth and development. All measurements are plotted on a growth chart and correlated with gestational age (Chapter 3).

Weight

Infants should be weighed without clothing or diaper and at approximately the same time each day. Using an infant scale, put a protective cloth or paper liner in place, and then place the infant on the scale.[6,7] Weigh newborns in both pounds and ounces and in grams. Newborn weight varies with gestational age as well as race. Average weight for a term newborn is between 2,700 and 4,000 g (6 to 9 lb).[7] African American, Asian, Hawaiian, and Filipino infants generally weigh less than Caucasian newborns. Birth weights of Native American newborns vary a great deal; there can be as much as 350 g separating the mean birth weights of different tribes.[6] All newborns initially lose weight, with a loss of 10 percent or less considered acceptable. Birth weight should be regained within the first two weeks. In general, infants double their birth weight by four to five months of age.

Length

The infant's recumbent length is measured from the heel to the crown (top of the head). The infant should be placed supine, with legs extended and the head flat. Make a mark on the bed to indicate the crown and a mark at the heel of the infant. Measure the distance between those two marks. Direct measurement of the infant is difficult because of head molding and incomplete extension of the knees. An alternate method for measuring length, although less accurate, is to hold the zero point of the tape at the heel and to run the tape along the surface of the bed to the top of the head. Mark the spot on the tape with a finger, remove the tape, and read the measurement.[8] The length of term newborns at birth varies between 48 and 53 cm (19 to 21 inches).[1] Specialized devices to measure length may be available in some facilities.

Head Circumference

The head should be measured over the occipital, parietal, and frontal prominence, avoiding the ears. The average findings in a term newborn are 33 to 35 cm (13 to 14 inches), with normal variations of 32.5 to 37.5 cm (12.5 to 14.5 inches).[7,8] As a general rule, the head circumference in centimeters is equal to one-half the length in centimeters plus 10.[9]

Chest Circumference

Measurement of chest circumference is no longer a routine part of newborn physical examination in many hospitals. It can, however, be a useful measurement when compared with the head circumference if one suspects a problem in the head or chest size. If it is measured, the chest circumference should be assessed at the nipple line during expiration. In term infants, the average chest circumference is approximately 2 cm smaller than the head circumference, with the average being 30.5 to 33 cm (12 to 13 inches).[1,8] The head and chest circumferences may be about the same for the

FIGURE 10-2 ▲ Posture of a term newborn.

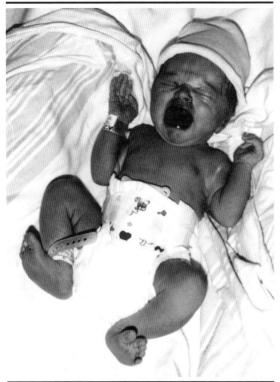

FIGURE 10-3 ▲ Posture of the preterm infant.

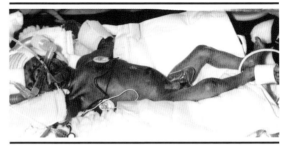

Dorsiflexion: flexion toward the back, as in flexion of the foot so that the forefoot is higher than the ankle

Plantar flexion: extension of the foot so that the forefoot is lower than the ankle

Rotation (neck): as in turning the face to the side

Valgus: bent outward or twisted away from the midline of the body

Varus: turned inward

Everted: turning out and away from the midline of the body

Inverted: turning inward toward the midline of the body

first five months of life. The more immature the newborn, the greater the difference is between the head and chest circumferences at birth.[6]

TERMINOLOGY

The following terms are used to accurately and consistently describe skeletal positions and muscle movements observed during examination:

Flexion: bending a limb at a joint

Extension: straightening a limb at a joint

Abduction: moving a limb away from the midline of the body

Adduction: moving a limb toward or past the midline of the body

Pronation: turning the face down

Supination: turning the face up

GENERAL INSPECTION

Inspection should proceed from the general to the specific. General inspection includes observation for symmetry of movement, as well as size, shape, general alignment, position, and symmetry of different parts of the body. Soft tissues and muscles should be observed for swelling, muscle wasting, and symmetry.

In the extremities, no asymmetry of length or circumference, constrictive bands, or length deformities should be noted. Unequal length or circumference has been associated with skeletal anomalies, tumors, and intra-abdominal neoplasms.[6,10]

The ratio of extremity length to body length is also observed. If a discrepancy is seen, measurements of thoracic length and extremities should be recorded. The gestational age of the

FIGURE 10-4 ▲ Breech presentation showing flexed, abducted hips and extended knees.

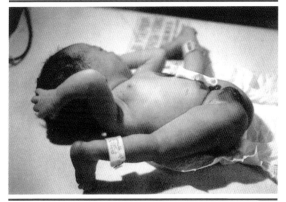

From: Clark DA. 2000. *Atlas of Neonatology.* Philadelphia: Saunders, 9. Reprinted by permission.

FIGURE 10-5 ▲ Breech presentation showing flexed, abducted hips and extended knees.

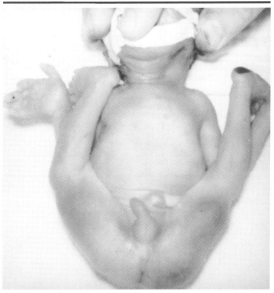

Courtesy of Dr. David A. Clark, Albany Medical Center and Wyeth-Ayerst Laboratories, Philadelphia, Pennsylvania.

newborn determines the normal values for these measurements. In the term newborn, the ratio of upper body length to the length of the lower body segment should not exceed 1.7:1.[9,11] This ratio is most useful in determining whether a small newborn is proportionate or has congenitally shortened lower extremities, as in achondroplasia.[12]

Term newborns lie in a symmetric position with the limbs flexed, the legs partially abducted at the hips so that the soles of the feet may nearly touch each other (Figure 10-2). The head is slightly flexed and positioned in the midline or turned to one side. The resting position of the newborn is often that of the tonic neck reflex (see Figure 11-5). Spontaneous motor activity of flexion and extension, alternating between the arms and legs, is random and uncoordinated. The fingers are usually flexed in a fist, with the thumb under the fingers. Slight tremors may be seen in the arms and legs with vigorous crying during the first 48 hours of life. Any tremors noted after four days of age while the infant is at rest are considered abnormal and signal a neurologic problem.[4] The resting posture of the preterm infant is one of extension (Figure 10-3) and is discussed in Chapter 11.

The position and appearance of the extremities at birth can reflect intrauterine position. Because the lower extremities of the fetus have been folded on the abdomen, the newborn's lower extremities often appear externally rotated and bowed, with everted feet. The infant delivered in a breech presentation often has flexed, abducted hips and extended knees (Figures 10-4 and 10-5). These positional deformities can usually be corrected by passive joint manipulation and should not be confused with congenital malformations.

PALPATION

Palpation is the next important technique used in the examination of the newborn's musculoskeletal system. This technique, along with observation, is used on each extremity to identify component parts (for example, the two bones in the forearm), function, and normal range of motion. Some aspects of this assessment are shared with the gestational age

TABLE 10-1 ▲ Normal Neonatal Range of Motion in the Upper Extremities

Joint or Bony Unit	Flexion	Extension	External Abduction	Internal Rotation	Rotation
Shoulder	Close to 180°	≥25°	Close to 180°	≥45°	≥80°
Elbow	145°	165°–170°			
Forearm				Supination* ≥80°	Pronation* ≥80°
Wrist	75°–80°	65°–75°			
Digits	Able to clench	Full extension			
Metacarpal-phalangeal		0°			
Interphalangeal		0° → 5°–15°			

*These maneuvers are done while the humerus is held immobile and the elbow is at 90 degrees.

From: Scanlon JW, et al. 1979. *A System of Newborn Physical Examination.* Baltimore: University Park Press, 40. Reprinted by permission of the author.

assessment. Muscular contour in the term infant is smooth, and despite lack of strength, the infant's muscles should feel firm and slightly resist pressure. If an infant feels limp, the condition should never be mistaken for a mere characteristic of immaturity. Further assessment is necessary to rule out a neurologic defect. When testing range of motion, note any asymmetry, tightness, or contractures. Range of motion of all joints is greatest in infancy, gradually lessening as the infant matures. As with posture and muscle tone, the range of joint motion varies with gestational age. It is not necessary to assess the exact number of degrees of range of motion, but only whether the range of movement is less than normal or significantly beyond normal findings. Never use excessive force to assess range of motion.

NECK

The neck is passively examined for rotation and for anterior and lateral flexion and extension. Rotation of 80 degrees and lateral flexion of 40 degrees to both the right and left sides are considered normal. In anterior flexion, the chin should touch or almost touch the chest, and on extension, the occipital part of the head should touch or almost touch the back of the neck. When there is asymmetric rotation or lat-

eral flexion or when range of motion is limited, x-rays of the neck should be taken.

UPPER EXTREMITIES

Examination of the upper extremities includes the bones of the shoulder girdle (the clavicle and scapula) as well as the humerus, elbow, forearm, and hand. Normal ranges for joint movements of the upper extremities are listed in Table 10-1. Asymmetry in range of motion may indicate weakness, paralysis, fractures, or infection. Failure to move an extremity can indicate spinal cord injury or brachial plexus palsy.

Clavicles

The clavicles are inspected and palpated for size, contour, and crepitus (grating that can be felt or heard on movement of ends of a broken bone). A fractured clavicle should be suspected when there is a history of a difficult delivery, irregularity in contour, shortening, tenderness, or crepitus on palpation. An asymmetric Moro reflex (Chapter 11) may also be seen. A broken clavicle is one of the most common birth injuries in newborns.[2,13]

Humerus

Length and contour of each humerus should also be noted. A fractured humerus should be suspected if there is a history of difficult

FIGURE 10-6 ▲ **Single palmar crease (simian crease).**

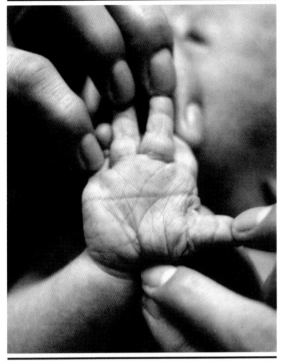

From: Clark DA. 2000. *Atlas of Neonatology.* Philadelphia: Saunders, 31. Reprinted by permission.

FIGURE 10-7 ▲ **Landmarks used in measuring palm and finger length.**

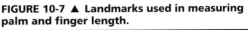

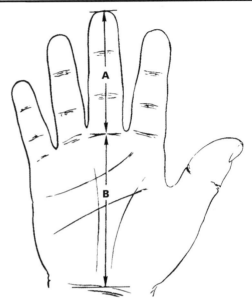

From: Feingold M. 1994. Congenital malformations. In *Neonatology: Pathophysiology and Management of the Newborn,* 4th ed. Avery GB, Fletcher MA, and MacDonald MG, eds. Philadelphia: Lippincott Williams & Wilkins, 761. Reprinted by permission.

delivery, one feels a mass caused by hematoma formation, or there are signs of pain during palpation. After the clavicle, the humerus is the bone most often fractured during the birth process.[2,13]

Elbow, Forearm, and Wrist

The elbow, forearm, and wrist are examined for size, shape, and number of bones, as well as for range of joint motion. It is sometimes difficult to evaluate the elbow in infants because the normal neonate has a mild flexion contracture that does not disappear until a few weeks after birth. Wrist flexion varies with the infant's gestational age, with greater wrist flexion seen in the term than in the preterm infant.

Hand

The hand should be examined for shape, size, and posture while the fingers are examined for number, shape, and length. Inspection of palm creases should also be included. Although a single crease across the palm (Figure 10-6) is usually associated with Down syndrome, it is often found in normal infants. It can be found in 4 percent of the population and is seen bilaterally in 1 percent.[14] However, a combination of short fingers, an incurved little finger, a low-set thumb, and a single palmar (simian) crease should lead the examiner to investigate the possibility of Down syndrome. In term infants, the distance from the tip of the middle finger to the base of the palm is 6.75 ± 1.25 cm. Middle finger length to total hand length is usually 0.38 to 0.48:1 (Figure 10-7).[9] Macrodactyly, an enlarged finger or toe, may be normal, or it may be a sign of neurofibromatosis (Figure 10-8).[15] Flexed fingers with the index finger overlapping the third finger (Figure 10-9) should lead one to investigate the possibility of trisomy 18.[16]

FIGURE 10-8 ▲ **Macrodactyly.**

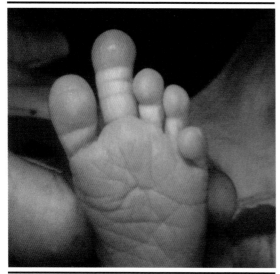

From: Clark DA. 2000. *Atlas of Neonatology.* Philadelphia: Saunders, 225. Reprinted by permission.

Examine the nails for size and shape. The nails are usually smooth and soft and extend to the fingertips. They may be long in postterm infants or may be absent or spoon shaped in the presence of some syndromes. Nails may appear hypoplastic if the infant's hands are edematous. A detailed discussion of nail examination is found in Chapter 4.

SPINE

The back is examined with the newborn lying prone or held suspended with the examiner's hand under the chest. First inspect the spine from the base of the skull to the coccyx, noting any skin disruption, tufts of hair, soft or cystic masses, hemangiomas, a pilonidal dimple (Figure 10-10), cysts, or sinus tracts. Such pathologic conditions may be signs of a congenital spinal or neurologic anomaly. The position of the scapula should also be noted while the infant is in the prone position to rule out Sprengel's deformity, a winged or elevated scapula.

The entire length of the spine should be palpated to determine the presence of dorsal spinal

FIGURE 10-9 ▲ **Finger position in an infant with trisomy 18.**

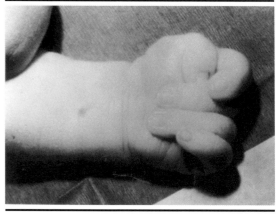

Courtesy of Eva Sujansky, MD, Associate Professor of Pediatrics, University of Colorado Health Sciences Center.

processes and any abnormal curvatures. Gross abnormalities such as scoliosis (Figure 10-11), lordosis, and kyphosis are easily observed. A lateral curvature, however, is usually secondary to *in utero* position. A convex curvature of the thoracic and lumbar spine will be apparent

FIGURE 10-10 ▲ **Pilonidal dimple.**

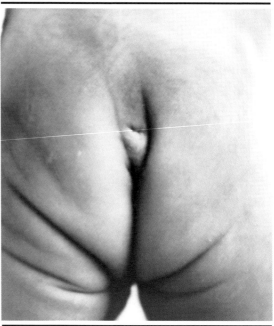

Courtesy of Dr. David A. Clark, Albany Medical Center.

FIGURE 10-11 ▲ Scoliosis.

Scoliosis denotes spinal curvature convex to the right or left. Scoliosis in the newborn is rare, but when it occurs, it is usually associated with a structural anomaly of the vertebral column. Infants with scoliosis are usually female, and the condition may be familial. **A.** Inspection of the infant in the supine position may lead to equivocal signs. But when the baby is lifted by the armpits (**B**), the scoliosis becomes obvious.

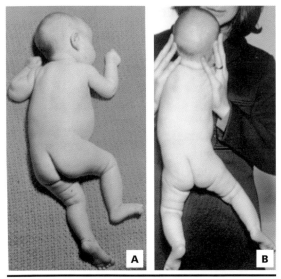

From: Milner RDG, and Herber SM. 1984. *Color Atlas of the Newborn.* Oradell, New Jersey: Medical Economics, 88. Reprinted by permission of Blackwell Science.

FIGURE 10-12 ▲ Convex curvature of the thoracic and lumbar spine.

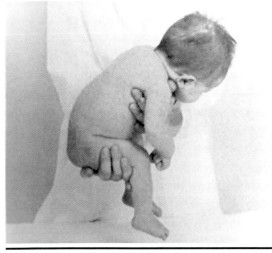

From: Jarvis C. 1992. *Physical Examination and Health Assessment.* Philadelphia: Saunders, 705. Reprinted by permission.

FIGURE 10-13 ▲ Spinal curves of the adult (left) and infant (right).

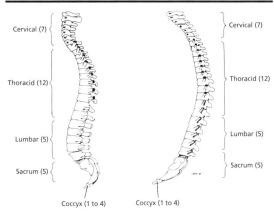

Cervical (7)

Thoracid (12)

Lumbar (5)

Sacrum (5)

Cervical (7)

Thoracid (12)

Lumbar (5)

Sacrum (5)

Coccyx (1 to 4)   Coccyx (1 to 4)

From: Alexander MM, and Brown MS. 1979. *Pediatric History Taking and Physical Diagnosis for Nurses,* 2nd ed. Philadelphia: Mosby, 292. Reprinted by permission of the authors.

when the infant is in a sitting position (Figure 10-12). The lumbar and sacral curves that are seen in adults develop later, when the infant sits up and begins to stand (Figure 10-13).[8] Extension and lateral bending of the spine can be noted by passive flexion. Flexion and extension should be smooth and rhythmic, without muscle spasm. A neurologic evaluation is necessary to complete the examination of the spine. Techniques are explained in Chapter 11.

LOWER EXTREMITIES

Examination of the lower extremities includes the hip, femur, tibia, fibula, knee, ankle, and foot. Normal ranges for joint movement in the lower extremities are listed in Table 10-2.

Hips

The hips of a newborn generally have a flexion contracture. When the pelvis is stabilized and the lumbar spine is flattened out by extending one leg flat and flexing the other leg with the knee to the chest, a flexion contracture of the hip can be detected in the extended leg. The degree of flexion contracture on the extended leg is the angle that is measured

TABLE 10-2 ▲ Normal Neonatal Range of Motion in the Lower Extremities

Joint or Extremity	Flexion	Extension	Abduction	Adduction	Internal Rotation	Rotation
Hip	145°		90°	10°–20°	40°	80°
Knee	120°–145°	90°				
Ankle	Dorsiflexion: above resting position Plantar flexion: >10° from resting position					
Forefoot			≥10°–15°	≥10°–15°		
Hindfoot			Valgus ≥10°	Varus ≥5°		

From: Scanlon JW, et al. 1979. *A System of Newborn Physical Examination.* Baltimore: University Park Press, 42. Reprinted by permission of the author.

between the thigh and the horizontal plane of the bed or examining table.[6] Normal newborns have an approximately 30 degree flexion contracture that usually resolves by one year of age.[17] The stability of the hip must also be evaluated to rule out DDH. Asymmetry of skin folds in the gluteal and femoral regions is a sensitive but nonspecific indicator that suggests that the hip is abnormal (Figure 10-14).

FIGURE 10-14 ▲ Asymmetric gluteal folds.

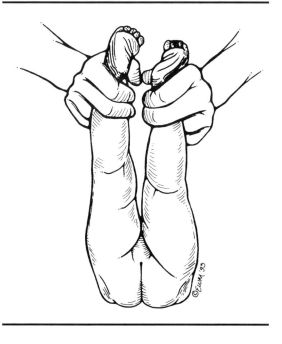

The Ortolani and Barlow maneuvers are the most reliable screening tests for evaluating hip stability (Figure 10-15 A and B). Although they arsracy of the examination.

The Ortolani maneuver is a test of hip reduction. It produces the reduction of the dislocated femoral head into the acetabulum by abduction. A helpful tip is to remember that the "O" in Ortolani means that the hip is "out." The maneuver is used to place the hip back into a normal position. With the infant positioned supine, the practitioner flexes the infant's knee and hip, then grasps the thigh with the thumb positioned along the inner thigh and the third or fourth finger placed over the greater trochanter laterally. While the practitioner abducts the hip, the practitioner's finger on the greater trochanter presses up against the head of the femur, and the hand presses the shaft of the femur toward the mattress. A positive Ortolani test is produced when a palpable "clunk" is noted, indicating that the femoral head has slipped from a dislocated position into the acetabulum. Higher-pitched clicks and snaps can be heard and felt but are not associated with hip pathology; they usually result from movement of tendons, ligaments, or fluid in the hip joint.[14,15,19]

The Barlow maneuver determines whether the femoral head can be dislocated from the acetabulum and is the opposite of the Ortolani

TABLE 10-2 ▲ Normal Neonatal Range of Motion in the Lower Extremities

Joint or Extremity	Flexion	Extension	Abduction	Adduction	Internal Rotation	Rotation
Hip	145°		90°	10°–20°	40°	80°
Knee	120°–145°	90°				
Ankle	Dorsiflexion: above resting position Plantar flexion: >10° from resting position					
Forefoot			≥10°–15°	≥10°–15°		
Hindfoot			Valgus ≥10°	Varus ≥5°		

From: Scanlon JW, et al. 1979. *A System of Newborn Physical Examination.* Baltimore: University Park Press, 42. Reprinted by permission of the author.

between the thigh and the horizontal plane of the bed or examining table. Normal newborns have an approximately 30 degree flexion contracture that usually resolves by one year of age.[17] The stability of the hip must also be evaluated to rule out DDH. Asymmetry of skin folds in the gluteal and femoral regions is a sensitive but nonspecific indicator that suggests that the hip is abnormal (Figure 10-14).

FIGURE 10-14 ▲ Asymmetric gluteal folds.

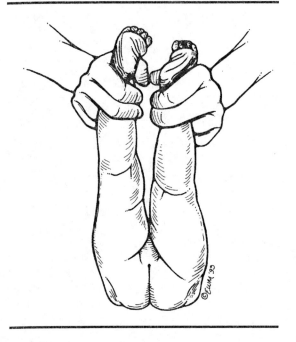

The Ortolani and Barlow maneuvers are the most reliable screening tests for evaluating hip stability (Figure 10-15 A and B). Although they are described as separate tests, in clinical practice, both maneuvers are done in a sequence, not as separate examinations. The infant must be in a supine position and on a relatively firm surface. These are not forceful examinations; a forceful exam only makes the infant cry and yields unreliable results. A crying, kicking infant can generate enough muscle strength by tightening the adductors and hamstrings to create a false result.[18] The cooperation of the infant and the patience of the practitioner affect the accuracy of the examination.

The Ortolani maneuver is a test of hip reduction. It produces the reduction of the dislocated femoral head into the acetabulum by abduction. A helpful tip is to remember that the "O" in Ortolani means that the hip is "out." The maneuver is used to place the hip back into a normal position. With the infant positioned supine, the practitioner flexes the infant's knee and hip, then grasps the thigh with the thumb positioned along the inner thigh and the third or fourth finger placed over the greater trochanter laterally. While the practitioner abducts the hip, the practitioner's finger on the greater trochanter presses up against the head of the femur, and the hand presses the shaft of the femur toward the mattress.

FIGURE 10-15 ▲ Ortolani and Barlow maneuvers.

A. Ortolani: The fingers are on the trochanter and thumb grips the femur as shown. The femur is lifted forward as the thighs are abducted. If the femur head was dislocated, it can be felt to reduce. **B.** Barlow: The thighs are adducted, and if the femur head dislocates, it will be both felt and seen as it suddenly jerks over the acetabulum.

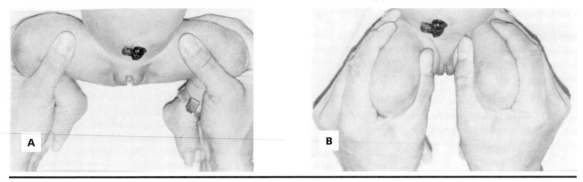

From: Robertson WW. 2005. Orthopedics. In *Neonatology: Pathophysiology and Management of the Newborn,* 6th ed. MacDonald MG, Seshia MMK, and Mullett MD, eds., Philadelphia: Lippincott Williams & Wilkins, 1429. Reprinted by permission.

maneuver. The practitioner's hand position is the same as for the Ortolani maneuver, with the infant's hip and leg flexed. As the knee is brought to the center (adducted) from the abducted position, the practitioner's thumb pushes laterally on the upper inner thigh. A "clunk" indicates that the femoral head has slipped over the lateral edge of the acetabulum and demonstrates an unstable hip joint that is dislocatable. The amount of force needed to push the femoral head out of or into the acetabulum is minimal.

A variation of the Barlow maneuver is to stabilize the pelvis with one hand while using the other hand to try to move the thigh anteriorly and posteriorly (upward and downward) without flexing the hip. This maneuver enables the practitioner to determine if the femoral head can be displaced posteriorly out of the acetabulum.

Legs

Palpate the legs to confirm the presence of the femur, tibia, and fibula. Fractures should be suspected when there is a history of difficult delivery or when palpation reveals irregularities in contour, crepitation, or masses resulting from hematoma formation. Although birth trauma

rarely causes a fracture of the femur, avulsion of the femoral epiphysis can occur and should be suspected if there is pain on passive movement or little spontaneous movement of the leg.[13] Femoral length can be observed by testing for the Galeazzi (or Allis's) sign. Keeping the feet flat on the bed and the femurs aligned, flex both of the infant's knees. With the tips of the big toes in the same horizontal plane, face the feet and observe the height of the knees.[6] It will be apparent if one knee is higher than the other, a positive sign. A discrepancy in knee height should also lead one to investigate for DDH (Figure 10-16).[15] Twenty-four percent of patients with congenital constricting bands have leg length discrepancy.[10]

The lower extremities are examined for length and shape. Congenital limb deficiencies are easy to identify, and an x-ray will confirm the deficiency (Figures 10-17 and 10-18). The lower extremities of newborns frequently have mild bowing and internal rotation of the lower leg because of intrauterine environmental conditions and fetal positioning. The bowed appearance is usually a combined rotational deformity caused by external rotation of the hip and internal tibial torsion from

FIGURE 10-16 ▲ Allis's sign.

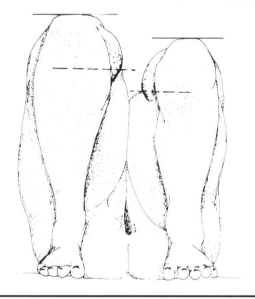

From: Alexander MM, and Brown MS. 1979. *Pediatric History Taking and Physical Diagnosis for Nurses,* 2nd ed. St. Louis: Mosby-Year Book, 301. Reprinted by permission of the authors.

FIGURE 10-17 ▲ Infant with congenital limb deficiency of the leg.

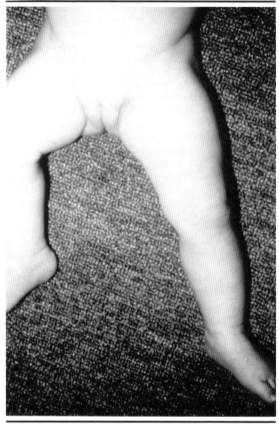

Courtesy of Mark Erickson, MD, The Children's Hospital, Denver, Colorado.

in utero positioning.[15,18,20] With the infant supine, draw an imaginary line connecting the anterior-superior iliac spine with the mid-patella, and continue down to the foot. If the line falls medial to the big toe, external tibial torsion is present. If the line falls lateral to the second toe, internal tibial torsion (a slight varus curvature) is present (Figure 10-19). Internal tibial torsion is a common physiologic feature of almost all newborns and is the usual cause of in-toeing in children from birth to two years of age. Because this is a physiologic rather than a pathologic condition, spontaneous recovery can be anticipated with normal growth and development.[15,20] Although lateral tibial bowing without a significant shortening of the extremity is considered normal in the newborn, anterior bowing is an abnormal finding, and an orthopedic consultation should be sought.

Ankles and Feet

Examination of the ankles and feet includes observation of the resting position and stimulation for active motion. To stimulate for motion, stroke the sole as well as the dorsal, medial, and lateral sides of the foot. Passive motion of the ankle in dorsiflexion and plantar flexion varies, depending on the infant's position *in utero.* For example, ankle and forefoot adduction, a positional deformity, can be differentiated from congenital equinovarus (clubfoot) malformation by passively positioning the foot in the midline and dorsiflexing it. A clubfoot or other structurally abnormal foot and ankle will not have a full range of motion and will resist dorsiflexion.

FIGURE 10-18 ▲ X-ray of congenital limb deficiency.

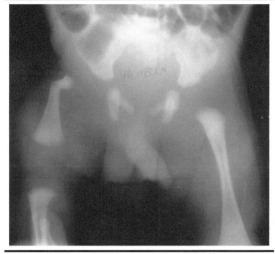

Courtesy of Mark Erickson, MD, The Children's Hospital, Denver, Colorado.

FIGURE 10-19 ▲ Examination for tibial torsion.

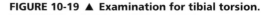

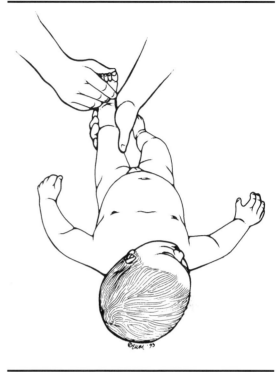

The toes should be examined for number, position, and spacing between them. Overlapping toes in infancy is usually a hereditary condition; correction may involve only stretching or stabilizing the toe by taping it in the correct position.[21] The soles of the feet should be inspected as part of the gestational age assessment. Most newborns are flat-footed as the result of a plantar fat pad (a pad of fat in the longitudinal arch of the foot), which gradually disappears during the first year of life.

MUSCULOSKELETAL ANOMALIES

Congenital anomalies of the musculoskeletal system may be evident as the absence of a part, extra parts, or malformed or malfunctioning tissue. Congenital anomalies usually affect the infant's movement, muscle tone, or posture. It is not within the scope of this chapter to discuss all the musculoskeletal anomalies the practitioner may encounter. However, many of the common problems and other special conditions seen in neonates are included in this section.

ANOMALIES OF THE NECK

Klippel-Feil Syndrome

Klippel-Feil syndrome is a defect of the cervical vertebrae in which there is both a decrease in the number of vertebrae and a fusion of two or more vertebrae. The cause is unknown, although current theories involve generalized fetal insult, *in utero* vascular insult, or neural tube abnormalities.[15] In some instances, the syndrome is familial, indicating a genetic transmission.[22] On physical examination, the neonate's neck usually appears shorter than normal, and motion is limited in all directions. There may be asymmetry in both rotation and lateral flexion. The classic signs on physical examination of short neck, low posterior hairline, and limitation of neck motion are seen in less than 50 percent of neonates with this syndrome.[3,15] The asymmetric motion may be confused with torticollis (see following

FIGURE 10-20 ▲ Torticollis.

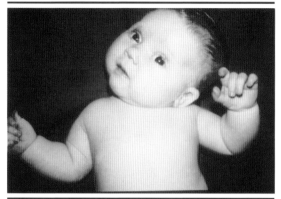

Courtesy of Mark Erickson, MD, The Children's
Hospital, Denver, Colorado.

section), but an x-ray of the neck will confirm the presence of the Klippel-Feil deformity. Other bony abnormalities, such as Sprengel's deformity and congenital scoliosis, are associated with Klippel-Feil deformity.[3,22]

Torticollis

Congenital torticollis, or wry neck, is "a spasmodic, unilateral contraction of the neck muscles."[9] It is thought to be the result of birth trauma, intrauterine malposition, muscle fibrosis, or venous abnormality in the muscle.[3,15,18] This anomaly is not usually seen in the immediate newborn period, but a hematoma may sometimes be palpated, or soft tissue swelling may be noted over the involved sternocleidomastoid muscle shortly after birth. Torticollis usually appears as a firm, fibrous mass or tightness in the sternocleidomastoid muscle at approximately two weeks of age. The mass is 1 to 2 cm in diameter, hard, immobile, and felt in the midportion of the sternocleidomastoid muscle.[3,15] In infants with this condition, the head is tilted laterally toward the involved side, with the chin rotated away from the affected shoulder (Figure 10-20).[3,15,22] Infants with this anomaly should be further evaluated for associated conditions such as metatarsus adductus and hip dysplasia. If the mass is detected early, most neonates with congenital muscular

torticollis can be treated with stretching exercises performed by the parents.[15,22] If the mass goes unnoticed, however, the torticollis may not be detected until there is plagiocephaly or asymmetry of the face and skull development. If the torticollis persists or goes untreated, there is a flattening of the occiput on the opposite side and a flattening of the frontal bones on the side of the lesion.[3,22]

Spinal Deformities

Congenital Scoliosis

Scoliosis in the neonate may range from undetectable to very severe. It is not chromosomal or inherited, but rather an embryonic defect. The structural basis for congenital scoliosis is a failure of vertebral formation, segmentation, or a variety of both. The failures can be in any area of the vertebral body (Figure 10-21). If the defect goes undetected, severe deformities can develop and affect neurologic function as well as cosmetic appearance. Upon diagnosis, the infant should also be evaluated for genitourinary tract anomalies (unilateral renal agenesis being the most common) because there is an increased incidence (20 to 30 percent) of these anomalies with congenital vertebral anomalies.[3,15,18] Klippel-Feil syndrome and Sprengel's deformity of the scapula are also seen with congenital scoliosis.[15,22,23]

Myelomeningocele

Myelomeningocele is a congenital neural tube defect that usually presents as a failure of closure at the caudal (tail) end of the vertebral column, permitting the meninges and sometimes the spinal cord to protrude into a saclike structure (Figure 10-22). Skin disruption is not always present, however, so any soft mass noted over the spine or just off the midline must be examined closely to rule out myelomeningocele. Because the functional deficit of the lower extremities is linked to the level of involvement of the myelomeningocele,

FIGURE 10-21 ▲ X-ray of congenital scoliosis.

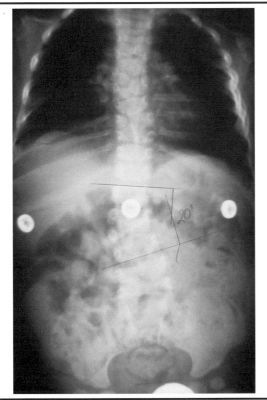

Courtesy of Mark Erickson, MD, The Children's Hospital, Denver, Colorado.

FIGURE 10-22 ▲ Myelomeningocele.

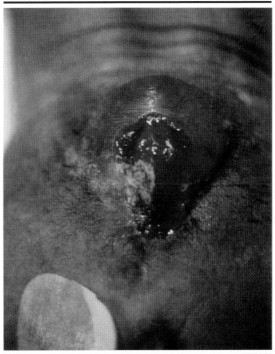

From: Clark DA. 2000. *Atlas of Neonatology.* Philadelphia: Saunders, 131. Reprinted by permission.

it is important to examine the muscle function of the lower extremities. This examination is discussed in Chapter 11.

UPPER EXTREMITY ANOMALIES

Sprengel's Deformity (Congenital Elevated Scapula)

Sprengel's deformity is one of the more common congenital anomalies of the shoulder girdle. It is characterized by an abnormally small, elevated scapula.[23,24] The elevation may be unilateral or, in 10 to 30 percent of cases, bilateral.[24] The asymmetry of the shoulder seen with unilateral involvement makes diagnosis relatively easy. On examination, the scapula is noted to be hypoplastic, elevated, and malrotated so that, when palpated, the vertebral border lies superiorly and more horizontal than

normal. The angle of the scapula may give the newborn the appearance of a webbed neck or a fullness at the base of the neck.[15,24] There is usually limitation of shoulder motion, particularly in abduction and forward flexion.[23,24] Internal and external shoulder rotation may be only slightly affected. Sprengel's deformity is frequently associated with congenital spinal problems, renal anomalies, and Klippel-Feil syndrome.[15,18,24]

Cleidocranial Dysostosis

Cleidocranial dysostosis is a defect in which there is the complete or partial absence of the clavicles (Figure 10-23). The incidence is estimated at 1 in 200,000. This skeletal dysplasia is inherited as an autosomal dominant trait, but approximately one-third of the cases are new mutations.[12,25] It is recognized by palpation and by the presence of excessive scapulothoracic motion where the newborn's

FIGURE 10-23 ▲ Cleidocranial dysostosis.

Infant showing marked adduction of the shoulders resulting from absence of the clavicles.

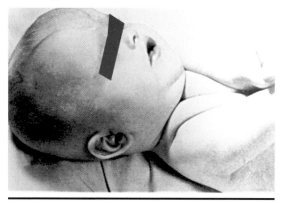

From: Swaiman KF, and Wright FS. 1982. *The Practice of Pediatric Neurology.* Philadelphia: Mosby, 441. Reprinted by permission.

FIGURE 10-24 ▲ Brachial plexus palsy.

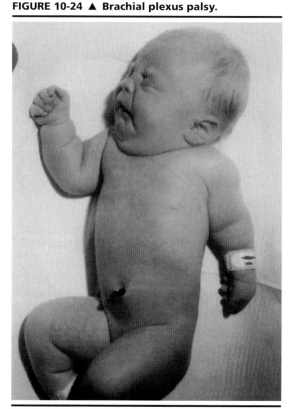

From: Clark DA. 2000. *Atlas of Neonatology.* Philadelphia: Saunders, 138. Reprinted by permission.

shoulders touch in midline. Bilateral absence of the clavicles is common, but there may also be segmental loss of the lateral or middle portion.[25] Complete absence of the clavicle is usually accompanied by defective ossification of the cranium, large fontanels, and delayed closure of the sutures.[6,12] Although the deformities may not be cosmetically pleasing, there is usually little functional disability, and therefore no treatment is required.

Brachial Plexus Palsy

Brachial plexus palsy is one of the more common birth injuries detected on the newborn examination, with an incidence of 0.7 to 4 per 1,000 live births.[11,14,26] Most cases are thought to be the result of prolonged and difficult labor involving traction and lateral flexion of the neck.[2,13,26] Brachial plexus injury has also been attributed to abnormal *in utero* forces on the posterior shoulder of the fetus as it passes over maternal bony prominences such as the sacral promontory. Increased *in utero* pressure and traction have also been proposed as the cause in an abnormal uterus such as a bicornuate or fibroid uterus.[13,26] Other perinatal risk factors include newborns who are large

for gestational age and those with a breech presentation.[3] Brachial plexus palsy is seen most often in large babies, who because of their size are vulnerable to stretching injuries to the components of the brachial plexus.[2,13,24,26] Shoulder dystocia in vertex deliveries and difficult arm or head extraction in breech deliveries increases the risk of brachial plexus injuries.[2,26]

There are three types of brachial plexus palsy, each with a different clinical presentation, depending on the site of injury and extent of neural injury The most common type of brachial plexus injury involves complete or partial paralysis of the shoulder muscles as a result of C5 and C6 neurologic injury. This type is known as Erb's palsy.[13,26] An infant with this type of upper arm paralysis holds the affected arm adducted and internally rotated, with extension at the elbow, pronation of the forearm, and flexion of the wrist (Figure 10-24). The grasp reflex remains intact, but the Moro reflex is absent on the affected side. A second type, Klumpke's palsy, involves C8 and T1 injury, with complete or partial paralysis of the forearm and hand muscles. This lower arm paralysis is rare. When the lower plexus is involved, the shoulder is in a relatively normal position with the wrist and hand flaccid, having little or no control. The third type of brachial plexus palsy, complete paralysis of the arm, involves injury to the plexus at all levels. It includes paralysis of the wrist and hand function in addition to shoulder and elbow dysfunction.[2,13,27] Because of the possibility of birth trauma as an etiology for the palsy, skeletal injury may coexist and should be ruled out radiographically.[3]

In cases of brachial plexus palsy where the nerve roots are not disrupted, infants regain neurologic function within several days as the hemorrhage and edema in the area resolve. Gentle handling and protection of the arm for the first few days should avoid additional injury to the plexus. Although most infants gain significant functional improvement by three months of age, close examination usually reveals tightness of the shoulder on internal rotation, difficulties in supination of the forearm, and abduction of the shoulder.[2,13] If the arm is flaccid at two to three months of age, surgery is recommended as soon as possible.[27] In newborns with peripheral nerve disruption or nerve root disruption, early intervention with microsurgery is recommended. Primary surgery is preferred at three to seven months for best results. Approximately 20 percent of brachial plexus injuries require surgery, and 90 percent of these patients achieve useful function of muscle groups above the elbow.[13,27]

FIGURE 10-25 ▲ Congenital absence of the radius.

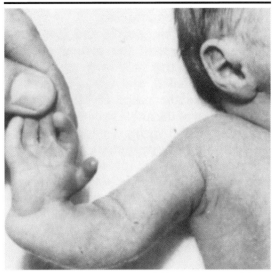

From: Robertson WW. 2005. Orthopedics. In *Neonatology: Pathophysiology and Management of the Newborn*, 6th ed., MacDonald MG, Seshia MMK, and Mullett MD, eds. Philadelphia: Lippincott Williams & Wilkins, 1432. Reprinted by permission.

Congenital Absence of the Radius (Radial Dysplasia)

This anomaly is the result of congenital absence or hypoplasia of the radial structures of the forearm and hand. It is sometimes referred to as radial dysplasia and is easy to recognize. In congenital absence of the radius, the hand and wrist are deviated 90 degrees or more (Figure 10-25). It occurs in between 1 in 30,000 and 1 in 100,000 live births.[15,24] It is seen in males more often than females.[23] Although radial hypoplasia alone may be inherited sporadically, infants presenting with this anomaly should be further evaluated for associations such as VACTERL (**v**ertebral anomalies, **a**nal atresia, **c**ardiac abnormalities, **t**racheo**e**sophageal abnormalities, **r**enal abnormalities, and **l**imb anomalies); Fanconi anemia; and Holt-Oram syndrome.[15,24,26] The clinical presentation is a shortened forearm with bowing of the ulna. The thumb is usually absent or hypoplastic. There is marked limited movement of the hand, wrist, and forearm. Treatment comprises

FIGURE 10-26 ▲ Pavlik harness.

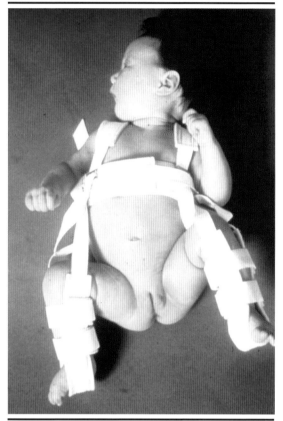

Courtesy of Mark Erickson, MD, The Children's
Hospital, Denver, Colorado.

both operative and nonoperative options and is recommended for cosmetic and functional reasons.[15,23,24] A consultation with a pediatric hand surgeon is required.

LOWER EXTREMITY ANOMALIES

Developmental Dysplasia of the Hip

DDH is one of the most significant deformities of the newborn period. It covers a spectrum of conditions that arise from abnormal development of the hip joint. These conditions range from minimal instability (in which the femoral head remains in the acetabulum) to irreducible dislocation (where the femoral head loses contact completely with the acetabular capsule and is displaced over the fibrocartilaginous rim).[19,28] DDH is thought to be caused

by lack of acetabular depth, ligamentous laxity, and/or abnormal intrauterine positioning, as in intrauterine breech position.

Approximately 16 to 25 percent of all DDH occurs in infants born after breech presentation.[18] About 2.5 to 6.5 infants per 1,000 live births develop hip dysplasia, but the true incidence of DDH can only be presumed because DDH is not always detectable at birth. The overall incidence of detectable dysplasia has been reported to be as high as 1 in 100 newborns with evidence of instability and 1 in 1,000 newborns with dislocation.[19,28] However, genetic and ethnic factors play a key role in the incidence of DDH, with incidence reported based on geography and ranging from 1.7 per 1,000 live births in Sweden to 188.5 per 1,000 in a district of Manitoba, Canada. African American and Asian infants are less likely than Native Americans or Eastern Europeans to display DDH. These differences may be caused by child rearing practices, such as swaddling, that keep the newborn's hips in adduction and extension rather than to genetic predisposition.[28] Females are more prone to the condition than males, and the left hip is more frequently affected than the right.[19,28,29] A family history revealing that a parent had a dislocated hip as a child or that an older sibling has hip dysplasia increases the risk for dislocated hip in the infant.[19,23,28] DDH is also more common in infants with other orthopedic conditions, such as torticollis, and in those with congenital foot deformities, such as clubfoot and metatarsus adductus.[23,28]

Early diagnosis and treatment appropriate to the specific anomaly are important for normal hip anatomy and function. When treatment is initiated early using simple devices such as the Pavlik harness (Figure 10-26) and the von Rosen splint, there is a 95 percent success rate.[28,29] The longer the dislocation remains untreated, the greater the chance of problems

FIGURE 10-27 ▲ Congenital absence of the fibula.

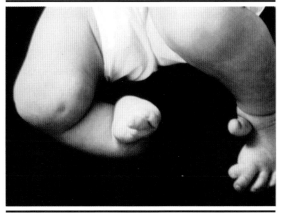

Courtesy of Mark Erickson, MD, The Children's
   Hospital, Denver, Colorado.

FIGURE 10-28 ▲ Genu recurvatum.

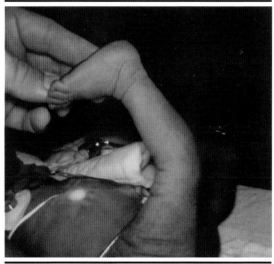

From: Clark DA. 2000. *Atlas of Neonatology.*
   Philadelphia: Saunders, 9. Reprinted by permission.

in returning the femoral head to its normal position and the less satisfactory the results.[28] Assessment techniques for and signs of DDH were discussed earlier in this chapter.

Congenital Absence of the Tibia or Fibula

Although congenital absence of a long bone is unusual, when it does occur, the deformity is easily recognized. Tibia or fibula absence may be partial or complete. When a portion of the bone is present, the deformity is likely to be less severe. In absence of the tibia, the clinical presentation is mild to marked shortening of the lower leg. The knee is unstable and has a flexion contracture. The foot may be normal or fixed in a mild to severe varus position.[2,30] In absence of the fibula, the clinical presentation is shortening of the involved leg, with bowing of the tibia anteriorly and medially (Figure 10-27). The foot deformity is often severe, with a valgus position.[28] Treatment depends upon the severity of the condition and focuses on the problems of foot deformity and leg length discrepancy. These deformities should be seen by an orthopedist early in the neonatal period. Many infants with congenital limb deficiencies frequently have other associated anomalies that represent an inherited syndrome. Because

of the high potential for genetic transmission of the disorder, the parents should be offered genetic counseling.[30]

Genu Recurvatum

Genu recurvatum, a rare anomaly with an estimated incidence of 1 per 100,000 live births, is a congenital dislocation or hyperextension of the knee (Figure 10-28). It is thought to result from a frank breech position *in utero* (41 percent of otherwise normal newborns exhibiting this anomaly were breech).[31] It may be a result of a prenatal developmental defect. It may be associated with oligohydramnios or fibrosis of the quadriceps muscle along with deficient hamstrings.[15,31] More common in females, genu recurvatum is usually seen bilaterally. Because early treatment prevents further deformity or interference with normal function, an orthopedic consultation should be initiated early.

Metatarsus Adductus

The most common congenital foot anomaly, metatarsus adductus is a deformity of the forefoot in which the metatarsal bones are deviated medially. The condition is probably the

FIGURE 10-29 ▲ Metatarsus adductus.

A. Structural metatarsus adductus. **B.** Structural metatarsus adductus. The forefoot does not abduct beyond neutral. **C.** Positional metatarsus adductus. The forefoot abducts beyond the midline.

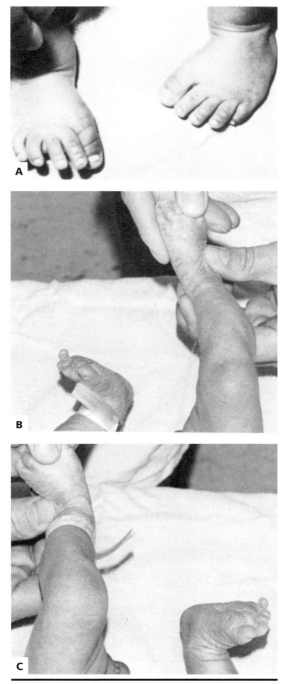

From: Robertson WW. 2005. Orthopedics. In *Neonatology: Pathophysiology and Management of the Newborn,* 6th ed., MacDonald MG, Seshia MMK, and Mullett MD, eds. Philadelphia: Lippincott Williams & Wilkins, 1434. Reprinted by permission.

result of intrauterine positioning. Multiple births and oligohydramnios, two conditions that decrease the room available for fetal movement, predispose the newborn to metatarsus adductus.[6,15] Other than the deviation, there are no pathologic changes in the structure of the foot. It occurs equally in both males and females and is seen bilaterally in approximately 50 percent of newborns who exhibit the anomaly.[15] Metatarsus adductus may be a positional (flexible) deformity with no bony abnormality involved or a structural (fixed) deformity (Figure 10-29). In a structural deformity, the arch appears to be greater than normal, and there may be a medial crease at its middle portion. The forefoot usually cannot be abducted beyond the midline (neutral position). In a positional deformity, the forefoot is very mobile and can be easily abducted. In infants with severe structural anomaly, the heel (hindfoot) is in a valgus position. In a positional metatarsus adductus, the heel is likely to be in a neutral position. Approximately 85 percent of neonatal metatarsus adductus deformities resolve by three years of age and develop normal foot position and function without treatment.[3,15] A positional deformity of the involved foot will correct spontaneously or may be treated with stretching exercises. Because there is an association between metatarsus adductus and DDH, the hip should be examined carefully when this anomaly is noted on physical examination.[31] In a rigid foot, an orthopedic consultation is necessary for early treatment because manipulative stretching exercises and casting may be required. Surgery is indicated only when casting is unable to produce a flexible foot.[15]

Clubfoot (Talipes Equinovarus)

Clubfoot (Figure 10-30) is a complex foot deformity that is readily apparent at birth. It is one of the most common congenital anomalies, whose incidence varies with race

FIGURE 10-30 ▲ Clubfoot.

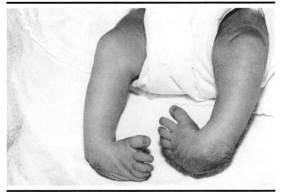

Courtesy of Carol Trotter, St. John's Mercy Medical
Center, St. Louis, Missouri.

and sex. In Caucasians, the birth frequency is approximately 1 per 1,000 live births, with males affected twice as often as females.[15,21,32] The highest incidence is seen in Polynesians at a rate of 6.8 per 1,000 births. Asian infants are the least likely to present with clubfoot, with it occurring at a rate of 0.6 per 1,000 live births.[21,32] The cause of congenital clubfoot is unknown, but it is likely a combination of genetic and environmental factors. Within affected families, the probability is approximately 3 percent for siblings and 20–30 percent for the offspring of affected parents.[21,32]

Clinical presentation of the deformity is characterized by three primary components: (1) adduction of the forefoot (points medially), (2) pronounced varus of the heel, and (3) downward pointing of the foot and toes (equinus positioning). Clubfoot may be unilateral, but involvement is bilateral in about 50 percent of the cases.[15,21] There are variations in the severity of clubfoot. Some are relatively flexible and correctable with conservative measures such as exercises and serial casting. Surgical correction is necessary when conservative measures fail.[21] Treatment can often be started in the nursery. An orthopedic consultation should be initiated on the day of birth.

Conditions Affecting Upper and/or Lower Extremities

Congenital Constricting Bands (Streeter Dysplasia)

Presenting as a band encircling the arms, legs, fingers, or toes, Streeter dysplasia can vary from mild, shallow indentations of the soft tissue to severe constrictions causing partial or complete amputation (Figures 10-31 through 10-34). Occasionally, craniofacial structures are affected. This deformity is estimated to occur in 1 per 15,000 births, with the upper extremities more frequently involved than the lower extremities.[15,24] It is associated with other musculoskeletal deformations in 50 percent of cases, with the most common being clubfoot. There may be cleft lip and facial deformities as a result of the amniotic bands.[24] The etiology is unknown, but the majority of evidence suggests that there is an abnormal attachment of the amnion to the fetus, because the amnion has either lost its integrity or ruptured and adhered to a fetal body part, causing compression or amputation.[14] Treatment depends on the severity of the condition. Severe bands may need to be treated as an emergency, especially if there is evidence of vascular or lymphatic obstruction. A surgical consultation is needed for these cases.

Syndactyly

Congenital webbing of the fingers or toes—syndactyly—is one of the most common congenital anomalies (Figure 10-35). Syndactyly is frequently a familial tendency.[2] The severity of involvement varies from minimal "bridging" between adjacent fingers/toes to complete webbing of the hand/foot. The more severe the syndactyly, the greater the likelihood of bony abnormalities as well. Syndactyly of the toes does not interfere with function, but may be unacceptable cosmetically. Although surgical treatment is not required, it may be requested by the parents. Treatment for syndactyly of the

FIGURE 10-31 ▲ Congenital constricting bands (amniotic bands).

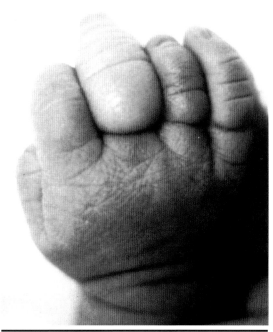

From: Clark DA. 2000. *Atlas of Neonatology.*
   Philadelphia: Saunders, 23. Reprinted by permission.

FIGURE 10-33 ▲ Congenital constricting bands (amniotic bands).

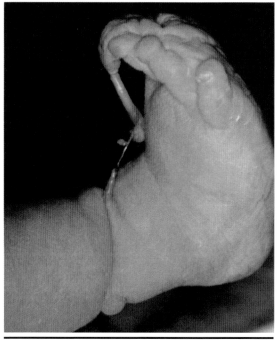

From: Clark DA. 2000. *Atlas of Neonatology.*
   Philadelphia: Saunders, 24. Reprinted by permission.

fingers depends on the severity of the webbing and the presence or absence of bony abnormalities. When multiple fingers are involved, function may deteriorate as the fingers grow. Early

FIGURE 10-34 ▲ Amniotic bands resulting in finger amputation.

FIGURE 10-32 ▲ Congenital constricting bands (amniotic bands).

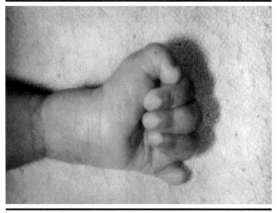

Courtesy of Dr. David A. Clark, Albany Medical Center
   and Wyeth-Ayerst Laboratories, Philadelphia,
   Pennsylvania.

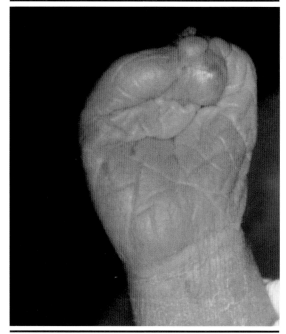

From: Clark DA. 2000. *Atlas of Neonatology.*
   Philadelphia: Saunders, 23. Reprinted by permission.

FIGURE 10-35 ▲ Two variations of syndactyly of the fingers.

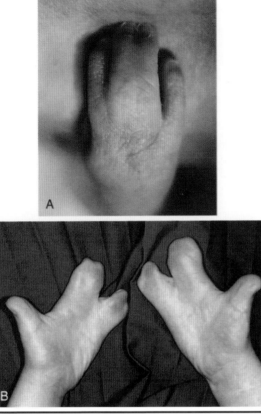

From: Clark DA. 2000. *Atlas of Neonatology.* Philadelphia: Saunders, 222. Reprinted by permission.

correction should therefore be considered. An orthopedic consultation is needed.

Polydactyly

Extra digits—polydactyly—are common abnormalities affecting both the hands and the feet (Figures 10-36 and 10-37), with an incidence of approximately 2 per 1,000 live births.[15] Polydactyly is seen more commonly in African American infants, with an incidence of 1 in 300 live births. The incidence in Caucasian infants is 1 in 3,000 live births. It occurs more frequently in infants who have a positive family history.[15,32] The most common type of polydactyly is a floppy digit or skin tag on either the radial or the ulnar side of the

FIGURE 10-36 ▲ Polydactyly of the toes.

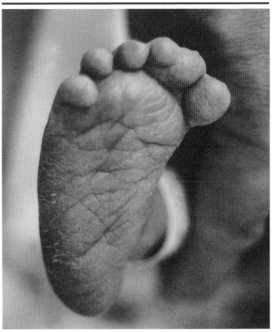

From: Clark DA. 2000. *Atlas of Neonatology.* Philadelphia: Saunders, 225. Reprinted by permission.

hand. Polydactyly may, however, involve the duplication of a normal-looking digit, giving the infant a functional six-fingered hand or a

FIGURE 10-37 ▲ Polydactyly of the fingers.

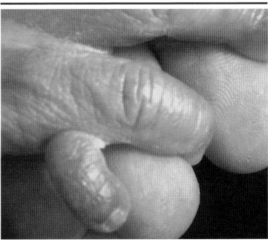

From: Clark DA. 2000. *Atlas of Neonatology.* Philadelphia: Saunders, 222. Reprinted by permission.

foot with six toes. Treatment depends on the extent of the anomaly. Consultation is required so that therapeutic decisions can be based on functional as well as cosmetic considerations.

SUMMARY

The examination of the musculoskeletal system provides a wealth of information about the overall development of the infant *in utero,* as well as the newborn's potential for normal development and function. Many of the common congenital anomalies of infancy are found in the musculoskeletal system. Although these abnormalities may not interfere with vital functions (as do those of the respiratory, cardiovascular, or other systems), they are a frequent cause of parental anxiety. The more accomplished the examiner becomes at performing the musculoskeletal examination, the easier it is to recognize deviations from normal, potential problems, and the necessity to initiate early interventions.

REFERENCES

1. Wheeler B, and Wilson D. 2007. Health promotion of the newborn and family. In *Wong's Nursing Care of Infants and Children,* 8th ed., Hockenberry MJ, and Wilson D, eds., Philadelphia: Mosby, 267–272.

2. Robertson WW. 2005. Orthopedics. In *Avery's Neonatology: Pathophysiology and Management of the Newborn,* 6th ed., MacDonald MG, Mullett MD, and Seshia MMK, eds. Philadelphia: Lippincott Williams & Wilkins, 1428–1443.

3. Sponseller PD. 2006. Bone, joint, and muscle problems. In *Oski's Pediatrics: Principles and Practice,* 4th ed., McMillan JA, et al., eds. Philadelphia: Lippincott Williams & Wilkins, 2470–2473, 2481–2493.

4. Szilagyi PG. 2007. Assessing children: Infancy through adolescence. In *Bates' Guide to Physical Examination and History Taking,* 9th ed., Bickley LS, and Szilagyi PG, eds. Philadelphia: Lippincott Williams & Wilkins, 685, 690–696, 705–706, 727–730.

5. Lawrence RA. 1984. Physical examination. In *Assessment of the Newborn: A Guide for the Practitioner,* Ziai M, Clark T, and Merritt TA, eds. Boston: Little, Brown, 99–101.

6. Seidel HM, et al. 2006. *Mosby's Guide to Physical Examination,* 6th ed. Philadelphia: Mosby, 62, 117–124, 734–738, 753–754.

7. Hockenberry MJ, and Barrera P. 2007. Communication and physical and developmental assessment of the child: Growth measurements. In *Wong's Nursing Care of Infants and Children,* 8th ed., Hockenberry MJ, and Wilson D, eds. Philadelphia: Mosby, 166–169, 197–198.

8. Jarvis C. 2004. General survey, measurement, and vital signs. In *Physical Examination and Health Assessment,* 4th ed., Jarvis C, ed. Philadelphia: Saunders, 190–193.

9. Scanlon JW, et al. 1979. *A System of Newborn Physical Examination.* Baltimore: University Park Press, 39–43.

10. Moseley C. 2006. Leg-length discrepancy. In *Lovell and Winter's Pediatric Orthopedics,* 6th ed., Morrissy RT, and Weinstein SL, eds. Philadelphia: Lippincott Williams & Wilkins, 1214–1227.

11. Fletcher MA. 1998. *Physical Diagnosis in Neonatology.* Philadelphia: Lippincott-Raven, 405–418, 441–453.

12. Sponseller PD, and Ain ML. 2006. The skeletal dysplasias. In *Lovell and Winter's Pediatric Orthopedics,* 6th ed., Morrissy RT, and Weinstein SL, eds. Philadelphia: Lippincott Williams & Wilkins, 205–250.

13. Mangurten HH. 2006. Birth injuries. In *Neonatal-Perinatal Medicine: Diseases of the Fetus and Infant,* 8th ed., Martin RJ, Fanaroff AA, and Walsh MC, eds. Philadelphia: Mosby, 529–559.

14. Brozanski BS, and Bogen DL. 2007. Neonatology. In *Atlas of Pediatric Physical Diagnosis,* 5th ed., Zitelli BJ, and Davis HW, eds. Philadelphia: Mosby, 33–47.

15. Cooperman DR, and Thompson GH. 2006. Neonatal orthopedics. In *Neonatal-Perinatal Medicine: Diseases of the Fetus and Infant,* 8th ed., Martin RJ, Fanaroff AA, and Walsh MC, eds. Philadelphia: Mosby, 1755–1786.

16. Jones KL. 2005. *Smith's Recognizable Patterns of Human Malformation,* 6th ed. Philadelphia: Saunders, 13.

17. Beebe AC, and Kerpsack JM. 2005. Pediatric musculoskeletal examination. In *Pediatric Orthopaedics: Core Knowledge in Orthopaedics,* Dorman JP, ed. Philadelphia: Mosby, 16–27.

18. Tolo VT, and Wood B. 1993. *Pediatric Orthopaedics in Primary Care.* Philadelphia: Lippincott Williams & Wilkins, 16–21, 30–33, 92–93, 143–154.

19. American Academy of Pediatrics. 2000. Clinical practice guidelines: Early detection of developmental dysplasia of the hip. *Pediatrics* 105(4 part 1): 896–905.

20. Halpern KV, Erol B, and Dorman JP. 2004. Common musculoskeletal conditions related to intrauterine compression and effects of mechanics on endochondral ossification. In *Fetal and Neonatal Physiology,* 3rd ed, Polin RA, Fox WW, and Abman SH, eds. Philadelphia: Saunders, 1838–1844.

21. Kasser JR. 2006. The foot. In *Lovell and Winter's Pediatric Orthopedics,* 6th ed., Morrissy RT, and Weinstein SL, eds. Philadelphia: Lippincott Williams & Wilkins, 1262–1280, 1307–1308.

22. Loder R. 2006. The cervical spine. In *Lovell and Winter's Pediatric Orthopedics,* 6th ed., Morrissy RT, and Weinstein SL, eds. Philadelphia: Lippincott Williams & Wilkins, 886–891.

23. Deeney VF, et al. 2007. Orthopedics. In *Atlas of Pediatric Physical Diagnosis.* 5th ed, Zitelli BJ, and Davis HW, eds. Philadelphia: Mosby, 781–865.

24. Waters PM. 2006. The upper limb. In *Lovell and Winter's Pediatric Orthopedics,* 6th ed., Morrissy RT, and Weinstein SL, eds. Philadelphia: Lippincott Williams & Wilkins, 926–930, 942–946, 977–978.

25. Van Heest AE. 1996. Congenital disorders of the hand and upper extremity. *Pediatric Clinics of North America* 43(5): 1113–1133.

26. Chang B, and Kozin SH. 2005. Upper extremity disorders. In *Pediatric Orthopaedics: Core Knowledge in Orthopaedics,* Dorman JP, ed. Philadelphia: Mosby, 181–196.

27. Storment M. 2001. Guidelines for therapists: Treating children with brachial plexus injuries. Kent, Ohio: United Brachial Plexus Network. Retrieved July 18, 2007, from www.ubpn.org/awareness/A2002storment.html.

28. Erol B, and Dormans JP. 2005. Hip disorders. In *Pediatric Orthopaedics: Core Knowledge in Orthopaedics,* Dorman JP, ed. Philadelphia: Mosby, 224–264.

29. Weinstein SL. 2006. Developmental hip dysplasia and dislocation. In *Lovell and Winter's Pediatric Orthopedics,* 6th ed., Morrissy RT, and Weinstein SL, eds. Philadelphia: Lippincott Williams & Wilkins, 987–1037.

30. Morrissy RT, Giavedoni BJ, and Coulter-O'Berry C. 2006. The limb-deficient child. In *Lovell and Winter's Pediatric Orthopedics*, 6th ed., Morrissy RT, and Weinstein SL, eds. Philadelphia: Lippincott Williams & Wilkins, 1339–1349.

31. Schoenecker PL, and Rich MM. 2006. The lower extremity. In *Lovell and Winter's Pediatric Orthopedics,* 6th ed., Morrissy RT, and Weinstein SL, eds. Philadelphia: Lippincott Williams & Wilkins, 1157–1211.

32. Wallach DM, and Davidson RS. 2005. Pediatric lower limb disorders. In *Pediatric Orthopaedics: Core Knowledge in Orthopaedics,* Dorman JP, ed. Philadelphia: Mosby, 206–211.

BIBLIOGRAPHY

- Barkauskas VH, et al. 1994. *Health and Physical Assessment.* Philadelphia: Mosby, 801–805.
- Furdon SA, and Donlon CR. 2002. Examination of the newborn foot: Positional and structural abnormalities. *Advances in Neonatal Care* 2(5): 248–258.
- Furdon SA, and Benjamin K. 2004. Physical assessment. In *Core Curriculum for Neonatal Intensive Care Nursing,* 3rd ed., Verklan MT, and Walden M, eds. Philadelphia: Saunders, 165–166.
- Milner RDG, and Herber SM. 1984. *Color Atlas of the Newborn.* Oradell, New Jersey: Medical Economics.
- Swaiman KF, and Wright FS. 1982. *The Practice of Pediatric Neurology,* 2nd ed. Philadelphia: Mosby, 441.
- Witt C. 2003. Detecting developmental dysplasia of the hip. *Advances in Neonatal Care* 3(2): 65–75.

NOTES

Notes

11 Neurologic Assessment

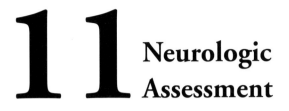

Pamela Dillon Heaberlin, RN, MS, NNP-BC

The neurologic evaluation is a critical part of neonatal assessment. A single examination may verify the presence of normal or abnormal neurologic responses and status. Serial follow-up of the abnormal neurologic examination is necessary to validate anomalies identified on the first examination and to document their changes or disappearance over time. Steady improvement in responses and disappearance of abnormal responses during the neonatal period offer a better prognosis than static abnormal responses.

A common approach to assessment of neurologic status is through the systematic testing of specific functions of the nervous system, including the motor system, reflexes, sensory system, and cranial nerves. This approach is followed here. More formal neurologic assessments, designed as clinical and research tools, are available. The neurologic evaluation developed by Amiel-Tison is designed to evaluate neonates at term or corrected term age during the first year of life and emphasizes neuromotor function.[1] Prechtl has also developed and validated a neurologic examination for the term neonate.[2] Another comprehensive neurologic examination has been designed by Lilly and Victor Dubowitz and is applicable to both term and preterm neonates.[3] The Dubowitz exam places heavy

emphasis on evaluation of movement and tone. It also includes some behavioral items that are evaluated on the Brazelton assessment, further discussed in Appendix B.

MATERNAL AND FAMILY HISTORY

The neurologic examination should be preceded by a thorough review of the history for genetic or neurologic problems of the family, maternal medical difficulties, as well as the use of medications, alcohol, or illicit drugs. Any test results of chromosome analysis, prenatal ultrasounds, and fetal well-being maturity should be noted. The intrapartum course is reviewed for abnormal presentation, prolonged labor, precipitous delivery, fetal distress, and difficult or operative extraction. Anesthetic agents and medications administered around the time of delivery may also affect the neurologic examination and should be noted. The history is also surveyed for Apgar scores, the cord blood pH and for the presence of perinatal depression, difficulties in transition, and feeding ability. The gestational age is noted. An accurate assessment of gestational age (Chapter 3) is essential for appropriate interpretation of posture, tone, and reflexes. Neurologic response varies predictably at different stages of maturity.

FIGURE 11-1 ▲ Posture and passive tone. Increase of tone with maturity showing the ascending direction of tone.

Gestational age	28 wk	30 wk	32 wk	34 wk	36 wk	38 wk	40 wk
Posture	Completely hypotonic	Beginning of flexion of the thigh at the hip	Stronger flexion	Froglike attitude	Flexion of the 4 limbs	Hypertonic	Very hypertonic
Heel to ear maneuver							
Popliteal angle	150°	130°	110°	100°	100°	90°	80°
Dorsiflexion angle of the foot			40–50°		20–30°		Premature reached 40 weeks 40° / Full term
Scarf sign	Scarf sign complete with no resistance		Scarf sign more limited		Elbow slightly passes the midline		Elbow does not reach the midline
Return to flexion of forearm	Absent (upper limbs very hypotonic lying in extension)			Absent (flexion of forearms begins to appear when awake)	Present but weak, inhibited	Present, brisk, inhibited	Present, very strong, not inhibited

From: Amiel-Tison C. 1991. Newborn neurologic examination. In *Rudolph's Pediatrics,* 19th ed., Rudolph AM, and Hoffman J, eds. Stamford, Connecticut: Appleton & Lange, 178. Reprinted by permission.

OBSERVATION

Observation before disturbing the neonate is necessary to evaluate for the presence of dysmorphic features, evidence of birth trauma, skin lesions, posture, and activity.

Evidence of *birth trauma* may include cephalhematoma, a depressed area of the skull, forceps marks, lacerations, abrasions, bruising, petechiae, and localized swelling. If evidence of trauma is found on the face or limbs, spontaneous movement and symmetry of movement should be evaluated to identify possible underlying damage to the nerves.

Certain types of *skin lesions* may be significant in the assessment of neurologic abnormalities. Café au lait spots of 1.5 cm or larger or more than three in number may indicate the presence of neurofibromatosis, one of the more common autosomal dominant genetic disorders. In this disease, dysplastic tumors occur along nerves and sometimes in the eyes and/or meninges as well as at other sites in the body and on the skin.[4]

Port wine nevi involving both eyelids, with bilateral distribution, or those that are unilateral but involve all three branches of the trigeminal nerve are associated with a significantly higher incidence of eye and central nervous system abnormalities.[5] They may indicate the presence of Sturge-Weber syndrome with underlying

FIGURE 11-2 ▲ Increase in active tone with maturity is illustrated. Note the ascending direction of tone.

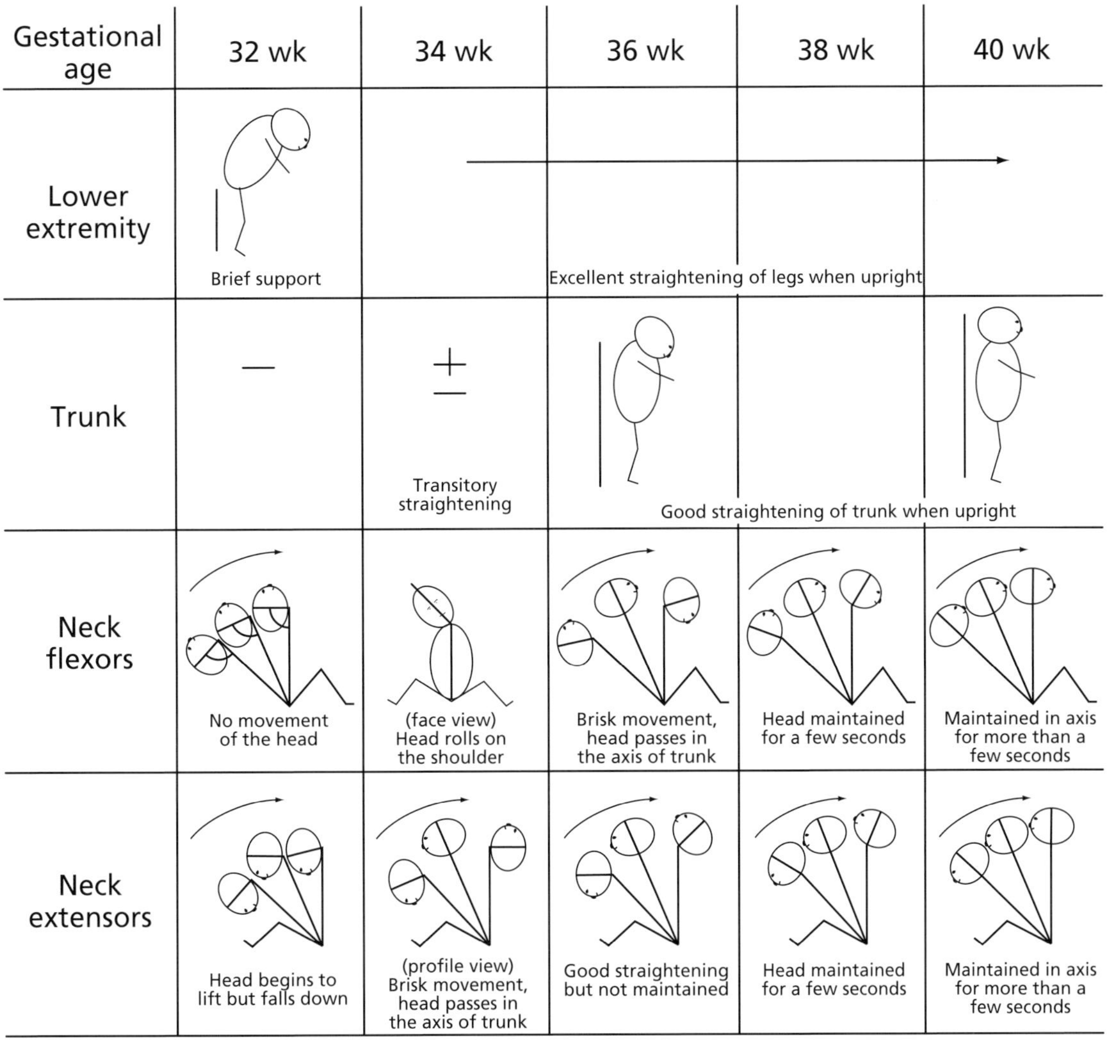

Gestational age	32 wk	34 wk	36 wk	38 wk	40 wk
Lower extremity	Brief support		Excellent straightening of legs when upright		
Trunk	—	± Transitory straightening	Good straightening of trunk when upright		
Neck flexors	No movement of the head	(face view) Head rolls on the shoulder	Brisk movement, head passes in the axis of trunk	Head maintained for a few seconds	Maintained in axis for more than a few seconds
Neck extensors	Head begins to lift but falls down	(profile view) Brisk movement, head passes in the axis of trunk	Good straightening but not maintained	Head maintained for a few seconds	Maintained in axis for more than a few seconds

From: Amiel-Tison C. 1991. Newborn neurologic examination. In *Rudolph's Pediatrics,* 19th ed., Rudolph AM, and Hoffman J, eds. Stamford, Connecticut: Appleton & Lange, 179. Reprinted by permission.

arteriovenous malformations. Glaucoma and leptomeningeal vessels in the brain that can lead to seizures are other abnormalities.

Areas of skin depigmentation can be significant because they can indicate the earliest manifestation of tuberous sclerosis, a progressive degenerative neurologic disease in which collections of abnormal neurons and glia occur in the subependymal and cortical areas of the brain. The skin lesion is white, macular, and has irregular leaflike borders. One or several lesions may be present.

If the neonate is awake and crying, attention should be paid to the *quality of the cry, symmetry of movement,* and *facial expression.* A loud, lusty cry is usual in the term neonate. A weaker cry may be heard in the premature, depressed, or ill neonate. A high-pitched cry may be heard in infants with neurologic disturbances, metabolic abnormalities, and drug withdrawal. Neonates with high-pitched, incessant crying and who are also hyperirritable should raise the concern of possible drug withdrawal, excessive nicotine exposure, or exposure to selective serotonin reuptake inhibitors.[6,7] A catlike cry may be heard with cri du chat syndrome, which results from deletion of the short arm of the fifth chromosome. Stridor should raise the concern of partial vocal cord paralysis related to cervical nerve damage or to partial webs, stenosis, or malacia of the airway. Lack of movement of an extremity may indicate trauma and nerve damage. Lack of movement of one arm may indicate brachial plexus injury: Erb's palsy (damage to the upper spinal roots C-5 and C-6), Klumpke's palsy (damage to the lower spinal roots C-8 and T-1), or involvement of all the roots that make up the plexus. If respiratory distress or sustained tachypnea is present in the neonate with a brachial plexus injury, the possibility of phrenic nerve damage and resultant diaphragm paralysis should be considered. According to Volpe, approximately 5 percent of brachial plexus injuries have phrenic nerve injury.[8] Facial asymmetry or unilateral lack of expression is most commonly seen as an isolated finding in infants with facial weakness due to Bell's palsy. The etiology may be intrauterine positioning with pressure on the fetal facial nerve from the maternal sacral prominence or secondary to direct trauma from a difficult extraction or forceps delivery. Bruising is often present.[8]

Another, more serious cause of facial asymmetry is congenital hypoplasia of the depressor anguli oris muscle. This condition is characterized by an asymmetric facial appearance and is most evident when the neonate is crying. The essential finding is a failure of one corner of the mouth to move down and out. Other functions of the facial muscles are normal. The clinical significance of this disorder is its association with other abnormalities—commonly,

congenital cardiovascular anomalies and, rarely, neuroblastoma.[8]

Bilateral facial weakness is also seen in neuromuscular disorders characterized by generalized hypotonia and weakness at the level of the muscle, such as congenital myotonic or muscular dystrophy. The clinical presentation includes a tentlike appearance of the upper lip, a partly open mouth, and generalized hypotonia. Congenital facial diplegia syndrome (Möbius syndrome) is a condition in which severe bilateral facial weakness is also seen. The upper face is more affected than the lower, the face is expressionless, and the eyes remain partially open. Neuromuscular junction disorders, such as myasthenia gravis and infantile botulism, are other conditions associated with generalized hypotonia, including the face. Other etiologies for generalized facial weakness include posterior fossa hematoma, cerebral contusion, and hypoxic-ischemic encephalopathy.[8]

The neonate's resting *posture* should be noted and its appropriateness for gestational age gauged. The normal term neonate lies with hips abducted and partially flexed and with knees flexed. The arms are usually adducted and flexed at the elbow (Figures 11-1 and 11-2). The hand is normally loosely fisted, and the thumb may lie in the palm or adjacent to the fingers. At 28 weeks gestational age, the newborn's arms and legs are extended, with little tone. From 28 to 40 weeks gestational age, tone increases in a caudocephalic direction, with increased tone in flexion observed first in the legs (around 32 to 34 weeks) and later in the arms (around 34 to 36 weeks). In the premature neonate, the adductor muscles are hypotonic; although flexion is seen as gestational age increases, the limbs are often flat against the bed surface. In this posture, the legs are abducted, and the lateral thigh rests against the surface of the bed. This position, often referred to as the "frog leg" position, is abnormal in neonates of more than 36 weeks gestation. Neonates of 32 weeks gestation or more who lie with their extremities completely extended are demonstrating abnormal postural tone. Depressed postural tone in the arms is suggested by flaccid extension of the arms or by some degree of flexion at the elbow but with open palmar surfaces facing up at 36 weeks or greater. In addition, cortical thumb—a persistent tightly fisted hand in which the thumb is firmly enclosed by the fingers—may indicate neurologic abnormality. When observation identifies any postural abnormality, it should be reconfirmed during the examination of tone and reflexes.

The *quality of movements* should also be evaluated in the active neonate. Term neonates move their limbs smoothly. In the preterm neonate, tremors and jitteriness may be present normally. Jitteriness can often be benign in term neonates and is sometimes seen with vigorous crying. It may also be a sign of disorders such as hypoglycemia, hypocalcemia, drug withdrawal, and hypoxic-ischemic encephalopathy. Jitteriness must be distinguished from seizure activity (Table 11-1). Although the distinction can be subtle in the neonatal period, jitteriness is characterized by rapid alternating movements of equal amplitude in both directions. In contrast, the clonic movements seen during true seizures have a fast and slow component and are not as rapid. Noise, touch, or other environmental stimuli can elicit jitteriness, which can be stopped by flexing or holding the involved extremity. Seizures are generally not initiated by stimulation, nor can they be eliminated by flexing or holding. In addition, jitteriness is not associated with any subtle signs of seizure activity, such as abnormal eye movements.

TABLE 11-1 ▲ Distinguishing Seizure Activity from Jitteriness

Clinical finding	Seizure	Jitteriness
Abnormal gaze or eye movements	Yes	No
Stimulus sensitive	No	Yes
Ceases with passive flexion	No	Yes
Autonomic changes	Yes	No
Predominant movement	Clonic jerking	Tremor

Adapted from: Volpe JJ. 2008. *Neurology of the Newborn*, 5th ed. Philadelphia: Saunders, 214. Reprinted by permission.

The neonate's *state* should be noted both before and during the examination, which optimally is performed with the neonate in the quiet alert state. Timing the examination for 30 minutes to one hour before a feeding may increase the chances of the neonate being in this state. Prior to 28 weeks gestation, it is difficult to identify periods of wakefulness. Stimulation (such as a gentle shake) may result in eye opening and apparent alerting for short periods. At approximately 28 weeks gestation, there is an increase in the level of alertness, and both stimulated and spontaneous alerting can be seen. The premature neonate has longer sleep cycles than the term neonate. Sleep-wake cycles are more apparent by 32 weeks gestation, and stimulation is usually not necessary to arouse and alert the neonate. By 37 weeks, increased alertness can be readily observed.

EXAMINATION OF THE HEAD

The status of the fontanels and sutures should be evaluated initially by gentle palpation in the noncrying neonate (Chapter 5). The examiner forms a general impression as to whether the fontanels are soft and flat or full or bulging. The size of the fontanels and sutures is next determined by palpation. A full or bulging fontanel with widened sutures may indicate increased intracranial pressure and hydrocephalus. Widening of the sutures alone, with a normal anterior fontanel, may be caused by abnormal ossification seen with intrauterine growth restriction. The head is palpated for other abnormalities, such as cephalhematoma and nondisplaceable sutures.

Head circumference is measured, plotted on a growth chart, and the percentile determined based on gestational age. A neonate with a head circumference greater than the 90th percentile for gestational age and weight and height below the 90th percentile may have hydrocephaly, macrocephaly, or hydranencephaly. The skull configuration in hydrocephalus is frequently globular. Posterior ballooning of the skull is seen with hydrocephalus caused by Dandy-Walker syndrome, which consists of congenital agenesis of the foramen of Magendie and Luschka with dilation of the fourth ventricle. Abnormalities in skull configuration are also seen in some neonates with craniosynostosis. When a large head circumference and percentile for gestational age are identified, transillumination of the skull can be helpful. In a dark room and after the examiner's eyes have adapted to the reduced light, a rubber-cuffed flashlight or other transillumination device is applied firmly to the skull (see Figure 5-1). A glow of more than 2 cm around the rubber cuff of the flashlight is abnormal and reflects fluid accumulation.

Neonates with small head circumferences (less than the tenth percentile for gestational age) may have microcephaly caused by a chromosomal abnormality, intrauterine infection, or maternal drug and alcohol intake. Marked molding of the head following birth may give the erroneous impression of microcephaly, especially when the shape of the head is conical.

Although not a routine part of the newborn physical examination, auscultation of the skull for bruits may be of value when arteriovenous malformation or aneurysm is suspected. Flow disturbances resulting from interference with the normal laminar flow through vessels may cause vessel wall vibrations heard as systolic murmurs and referred to as bruits. Bruits may be heard in Sturge-Weber syndrome, usually accompanied by facial hemangioma; it is therefore important to listen for bruits in neonates with this skin lesion. Arteriovenous malformations may lead to unexplained high-output cardiac failure in neonates, and an examination for bruits may assist in making the diagnosis. Auscultation is carried out with the bell of the stethoscope placed over the temporal, frontal, and occipital areas.

MOTOR EXAMINATION

Evaluation of muscle tone involves examination of resting posture, passive tone, and active tone of the major muscle groups. Tone can also be categorized as phasic, which correlates with passive tone and deep tendon reflexes, and postural, which correlates with active tone. Phasic tone is a brief, forceful contraction in response to a short-duration, high-amplitude stretch. Postural tone is a long-duration, low-amplitude stretch in response to gravity. The two tone types are tested separately and can vary independently.

PHASIC TONE

Phasic tone is evaluated by testing the resistance of the upper and lower extremities to movement and by the activity of the deep tendon reflexes. Resistance of the extremities to passive movements can be evaluated by the scarf sign (Chapter 3) and by arm and leg recoil. Minimal resistance is normal at 28 weeks; resistance increases with maturity. Tendon reflexes are elicited by sharp percussion with the examiner's finger or a small reflex hammer over the tendon. The biceps reflex and the patellar (or knee jerk) reflex are basic reflexes that can be tested in the neonate. These are most active in the first two days after birth and when the neonate is alert. Of all the tendon reflexes, the

FIGURE 11-3 ▲ Normal traction response seen in the term neonate.

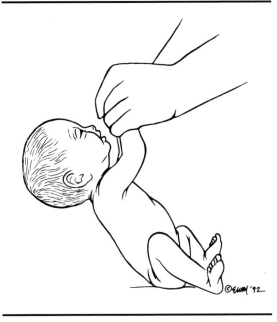

FIGURE 11-4 ▲ Traction response indicating hypotonia.

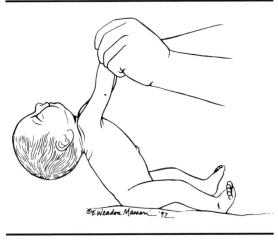

patellar is the most frequently demonstrated after birth. Innervation for the knee jerk is at the second through fourth lumbar segments. It is tested by tapping the patellar tendon just below the patella while the examiner's hand supports the neonate's knee in a flexed position. The normal response is extension at the knee and visible contraction of the quadriceps. The biceps reflex is innervated at the fifth and sixth cervical nerve roots and is tested by holding the neonate's arm with the elbow in flexion and the examiner's thumb over the insertion of the biceps tendon. The examiner's thumb is tapped with a reflex hammer, and flexion of the biceps occurs.

Weak or absent reflexes may be seen in neonates less than 28 weeks gestational age, in those depressed from birth asphyxia or sepsis, and in those with dysfunction of the motor unit (i.e., the motor neuron, peripheral nerve, muscle and neuromuscular junction). Neonates with acute encephalopathy are frequently areflexic initially. As they improve,

reflexes return, but they may be depressed initially and later become increased or exaggerated. Exaggerated deep-tendon reflexes are also seen in neonates with drug withdrawal syndrome. Asymmetric deep-tendon reflexes may reflect either central or peripheral nervous system impairment. Clonus is rapid movement of a particular joint brought about by sudden stretching of a tendon. Ankle clonus can be evaluated by holding the anterior portion of the neonate's foot with the hip and knee in flexion and dorsiflexing the forefoot. The response usually consists of several repetitive jerks (beats) of the foot or no movement at all. Sustained clonus (with more than eight to ten beats occurring) may indicate cerebral irritation.

POSTURAL TONE

Postural tone is best tested by the traction response (or pull-to-sit maneuver), which tests the ability to resist the pull of gravity. The traction response is tested by grasping the neonate's hands and pulling him slowly from the supine to a sitting position. The normal term neonate reinforces this maneuver by contracting the shoulder and arm muscles, followed by

TABLE 11-2 ▲ Patterns of Abnormal Muscle Tone in the Neonate

Abnormality	Significance
Generalized increased or decreased tone	CNS insult or systemic illness
Increased arm flexor tone with increased leg extensor tone	Normal in crying neonate
	CNS irritability (e.g., hypoxic-ischemic injury, hemorrhage, increased intracranial pressure)
Increased neck extensor tone more than neck flexor tone	Seen in crying neonates
	Hypoxic-ischemic injury
	Meningitis
	Increased intracranial pressure
Tight popliteal angle, increased as compared to leg tone	Intracranial hemorrhage
Asymmetric popliteal angles beyond 40 weeks	Hypertonia, hemiplegia

CNS: central nervous system

From: Hill A. 1998. Development of tone and reflexes in the fetus and newborn. In *Fetal and Neonatal Physiology,* 2nd ed., Polin RA, and Fox WW, eds. Philadelphia: Saunders, 2169. Reprinted by permission.

flexion of the neck. As the neonate is pulled to sit, his head leaves the bed almost immediately, lagging only minimally behind the body (Figure 11-3). When the infant reaches the sitting position, the head remains erect momentarily and then falls forward. During traction, flexion occurs in the elbows, knees, and ankles. In the term neonate, more than minimal head lag is abnormal and may indicate postural hypotonia (Figure 11-4). Neck flexion in response to traction is absent in preterm neonates under 33 weeks. Because normal postural tone requires the integrated functions of the entire central nervous system, hypotonia (indicating depressed postural tone) may result from disturbances in the central nervous system, the peripheral nervous system, or the skeletal muscles. As with the other components of the neurologic examination, postural tone should be tested with the neonate in an awake alert state. When a large subgaleal hemorrhage or an extremely large caput is present, there may be more difficulty with the performance of the neck righting in the pull-to-sit maneuver. It may be difficult to determine whether the poor performance represents a mechanical problem caused by the extra weight of the head or a neurologic problem related to birth trauma. Normal findings on the evaluation of other reflexes, tone, and activity are reassuring. The infant should be retested prior to discharge.

Testing muscle strength is imprecise in the neonate because differentiating between hypotonia and muscle weakness is difficult. The strength of the upper extremities is gauged by using the pull-to-sit maneuver described previously and the grasp reflex. The strength of the lower extremities is evaluated by observing the stepping reflex, readily elicited by 37 weeks gestational age, and gauging the neonate's ability to support his weight when his feet are against a flat surface.

Movement should be evaluated and the presence of abnormal involuntary movements, such as jerking or jitteriness, noted. At 28 to 32 weeks gestational age, slow twisting movements of the trunk as well as rapid, wide-amplitude movements of the limbs are seen. By 32 weeks gestational age, movements are more flexor and tend to occur in unison. At 36 weeks gestational age, active flexor movements of the lower extremities often occur in an alternating rather than a bilateral symmetric pattern. The term neonate's upper and lower extremities move in an alternating pattern. Typical of the neonatal period are mass movements that occur in response to environmental stimuli and discomfort. During the first few weeks of life, coarse tremors or brief trembling of the chin may occur normally, as may occasional uncoordinated movements.

ABNORMALITIES OF TONE

The motor examination may detect hypotonia or hypertonia. *Hypotonia* is the more common abnormality observed in the neonatal neurologic examination. A focal injury to the cerebrum can result in contralateral hemiparesis involving the face and upper extremities more than the lower extremities. Injury to the parasagittal cerebral region (which may be caused by cerebral perfusion abnormalities) results in weakness of the upper limbs more than the lower limbs. If spinal cord injury occurs, it is frequently in the cervical region and can result in flaccid weakness of the extremities; the face and cranial nerves are usually not affected. Neuromuscular junction diseases, such as myasthenia gravis and infantile botulism, cause generalized weakness and hypotonia. Disorders of the lower motor neurons (such as Werdnig-Hoffmann disease) cause flaccid weakness of the extremities with initial sparing of the face and cranial nerves. Fasciculation (spontaneous contraction of a group of fibers in a motor unit) can also be seen in Werdnig-Hoffmann disease and is best observed in the tongue. Inspection of the tongue reveals continuous and rapid twitching movements. Damage to nerve roots results in discrete patterns of focal weakness, the location of which depends on the root involved. One example is the unilateral loss of movement seen in the arm of a neonate with brachial plexus palsy.

Hypertonia is a less common finding in the neonatal period. If it is present, passive manipulation of the limbs often increases the tone. Opisthotonus (marked extensor hypertonia with arching of the back) is sometimes seen with bacterial meningitis, severe hypoxic-ischemic brain damage, massive intraventricular hemorrhage, and tetanus. Table 11-2 lists patterns of abnormal muscle tone and their possible significance.

TABLE 11-3 ▲ Neonatal Reflexes

Reflex	Age (Weeks of Gestation; Months Postnatal)		
	Onset (Weeks)	Well-Established (Weeks)	Disappearance (Months)
Suck	28	32–34	12
Rooting	28	32–34	3–4
Palmar grasp	28–32	32	2
Tonic neck	35	4	7
Moro	28–32	37	6
Stepping	35–36	37	3–4
Truncal incurvation	28	40	3–4
Babinski	34–36	38	12

Adapted from: Volpe JJ. 2008. *Neurology of the Newborn*, 5th ed. Philadelphia: Saunders, 121–147; and Barness LA. 1991. *Manual of Pediatric Physical Diagnosis*. Philadelphia: Mosby, 17.

ASSESSMENT OF DEVELOPMENTAL REFLEXES

Developmental reflexes are sometimes referred to as primary or primitive reflexes because they do not require functional brain above the diencephalon. Although there are many developmental reflexes, it is usual to test only those commonly present in most newborns. The normal timing of appearance and disappearance of the developmental reflexes is presented in Table 11-3. Development of reflexes with maturation from 28 to 40 weeks is shown in Table 11-4.

SUCKING REFLEX

The sucking reflex is normally present at birth, even in the premature neonate, although it is weaker with decreasing gestational age. The stimulus consists of touching or gently stroking the lips. In response, the neonate's mouth opens, and sucking movements are initiated. The examiner's gloved finger can be introduced into the mouth to evaluate strength and coordination of the suck.

TABLE 11-4 ▲ Development of Reflexes with Maturity from 28 to 40 Weeks Gestation

Gestational Age (weeks)	28	30	32	34	36	38	40
Sucking	Weak and not really synchronized with deglutition		Stronger and better synchronized with deglutition		Perfect		
Grasp	Present but weak			Stronger		Excellent	
Response to traction	Absent		Begins to appear	Strong enough to lift part of the body weight		Strong enough to lift all of the body weight	
Moro reflex	Weak, obtained just once, incomplete		Complete reflex ⟶	⟶	⟶		
Crossed extension	Flexion and extension in a random pattern, purposeless reaction		Good extension but no tendency to adduction		Tendency to adduction but imperfect	Complete response with Extension Adduction Fanning of the toes	
Automatic walking	—	—	Begins tiptoeing with good support on the sole and a righting reaction of the legs for a few seconds				
				Pretty good; very fast tiptoeing		• A premature newborn who has reached 40 weeks. Walks in a toe-heel progression or tiptoes. • A term newborn of 40 weeks gestation. Walks in a heel-toe progression on the whole sole of the foot.	

Adapted from: Amiel-Tison C. 1991. Newborn neurologic examination. In *Rudolph's Pediatrics,* 19th ed., Rudolph AM, and Hoffman J, eds. Stamford, Connecticut: Appleton & Lange, 178. Reprinted by permission.

ROOTING REFLEX

To evaluate the rooting reflex, stroke the cheek and corner of the neonate's mouth. The infant's head should turn toward the stimulus, and the mouth should open.

PALMAR GRASP

Stimulating the palmar surface of the neonate's hand with a finger should cause him to grasp the finger. Attempts to withdraw the finger should lead to a tightened grasp. When the palmar grasp is tested with both hands, the term neonate can be lifted off the bed for a few seconds. If palmar grasp is weak or absent in a term neonate, cerebral, local nerve, or muscle injury may be present.

TONIC NECK REFLEX

To elicit the tonic neck reflex, place the neonate in a supine position and turn his head to one side. The neonate should extend the upper extremity on the side toward which the head is turned and flex the upper extremity on the opposite side (Figure 11-5). This is sometimes called the fencing position. If the response cannot be obtained or if even slight turning of the head consistently produces a marked tonic neck reflex, these can be important indicators of abnormality.

MORO REFLEX

The Moro reflex is a response to the sensation of loss of support. The most effective and reproducible method of stimulating it is to hold the neonate in a supine position with

FIGURE 11-5 ▲ The tonic neck reflex.

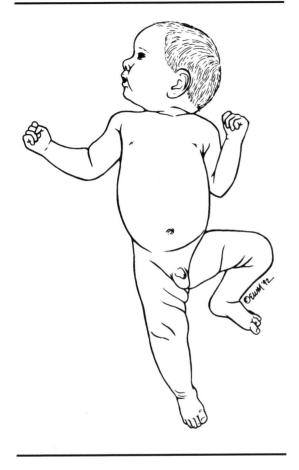

FIGURE 11-6 ▲ The Moro reflex.

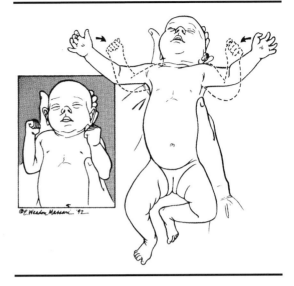

may occur in depressed neonates. Asymmetry of movements may indicate a localized neurologic defect, such as brachial plexus injury or fractured clavicle.

A loud noise or bumping the side of the incubator or crib often produces a Moro-like response. This is usually a startle reflex—consisting of flexion of the extremities and palmar grasping—but not a complete Moro.

STEPPING REFLEX

When the neonate is held upright and the soles of the feet are allowed to touch a flat surface, alternating stepping movements can be observed. The stepping is more active 72 hours after birth.

TRUNCAL INCURVATION (GALANT) REFLEX

The truncal incurvation reflex is tested with the neonate in ventral suspension, with his anterior chest wall in the palm of the examiner's hand. Firm pressure with the thumb or a cotton swab is applied parallel to the spine in the thoracic area. A positive response is flexion of the pelvis toward the side of the stimulus.

his head several centimeters off the bed. Then withdraw the hand supporting the head, and the infant's head falls back into the examiner's hand or against the surface of the bed. The infant's first response is a spreading movement in which the arms are extended and abducted and the hands are opened (Figure 11-6). That response is followed by inward movement and some flexion of the arms, with closing of the fists. An audible cry may accompany this reflex in neonates greater than 32 weeks gestational age. Premature neonates have incomplete responses, with abduction of the arms but without flexion, adduction, or cry. Complete absence of the reflex is abnormal and

TABLE 11-5 ▲ Testing Cranial Nerve Function of Infants

Cranial Nerve	Function
I	Smell
II, III, IV, VI	Optical blink reflex—shine light in open eyes, note rapid closure Regards face or close object Eyes follow movement
V	Rooting reflex, sucking reflex
VII	Facial movements (e.g., wrinkling forehead and nasolabial folds) symmetric when crying or smiling
VIII	Loud noise yields Moro reflex (until 4 months) Acoustic blink reflex—infant blinks in response to a loud hand clap 30 cm (12 in) from head (Avoid making air current.) Eyes follow direction of sound
IX, X	Swallowing, gag reflex
XI	Head turns normally from side to side, shoulder height is equal
XII	Coordinated sucking and swallowing Pinch nose, infant's mouth will open and tongue rise in midline

Adapted from: Jarvis C. 1992. *Physical Examination and Health Assessment*. Philadelphia: Saunders, 765. Reprinted by permission.

Babinski Reflex

The response to stimulation of the sole of the foot is usually plantar flexion. In the neonatal period, the Babinski reflex is positive if extension or flexion of the toes occurs. Consistent absence of any response is abnormal and may indicate central depression or abnormal spinal nerve innervation. In children older than 18 months, an abnormal response is extension or fanning of the toes; either response indicates upper motor neuron abnormalities.

Assessment of Sensory Function

The peripheral sensory system functions include touch and pain. The withdrawal reflex is stimulated to evaluate peripheral sensory function. Touching the sole of the foot with a pin provokes flexion of the stimulated limb and extension of the contralateral limb. Response is present in most neonates of 28 weeks gestational age and above. In neonates, extension of the contralateral limb varies, and sometimes flexion of both limbs is seen. This assessment is rarely performed as part of a routine neurologic examination but may be performed in cases of myelomeningocele or suspected spinal cord transection to delineate the level of abnormality.

Evaluation of the Cranial Nerves (Table 11-5)

Olfactory-Cranial Nerve (I)

The neonate's sense of smell is rarely tested because disturbances in olfaction are rarely a feature of neurologic disease in the neonate. The sense of smell is present in neonates, and those of nursing mothers are able to discriminate between their mother's breast pad and that of another woman.[8] Gross evaluation can be done using strong-smelling substances such as anise, peppermint, or clove oil and evaluating for grimacing, sniffing, or startle responses.

Optic-Cranial Nerve (II)

Visual acuity, visual fields, and a funduscopic examination provide information on the function of the optic-cranial nerve. The ability of the neonate's eyes to fix on an object and follow it over a 60-degree arc is evaluated. The object may be the examiner's face, simple black-and-white pictures depicting facial features, or a ball held 10 to 12 inches from the neonate's eyes and moved from side to side. During the examination, occasional nystagmus (an involuntary rapid movement of the eyeball) may be seen in the neonate. Wandering or persistent nystagmus is abnormal and may indicate loss of vision. When a light is introduced into the periphery of the neonate's visual field, his head should turn toward it. Pupillary size and constriction in response to light are also evaluated. Funduscopic examination is performed, and the character of veins and arteries, the macula, and the optic disc is evaluated. A thorough examination of the optic disc requires pupillary dilation. Pupillary abnormalities and possible etiologies are shown in Table 11-6.

Oculomotor (III), Trochlear (IV), and Abducens-Cranial (VI) Nerves

These nerves supply the pupil and the extraocular muscles. Pupillary response to light is tested and should be present at 28 to 30 weeks gestational age. Spontaneous movements of the eyes, their size, and their symmetry are evaluated. The presence of ptosis, proptosis, sustained nystagmus, or strabismus is noted.

Movement of the eyes as the position of the head is turned is evaluated. The "doll's eye" maneuver consists of gently rotating the head from side to side and evaluating for deviation of the eyes away from the direction of rotation—for example, in a normal response, when the head is turned to the right, the eyes deviate to the left (Figure 11-7). If the eyes remain in a fixed position regardless of head rotation, brainstem dysfunction may be present. If the eyes move in the same direction as the head is rotated, brainstem or oculomotor nerve dysfunction may be present. When it is not possible to rotate the neonate's head, the semicircular canals can be stimulated by introducing cold water into the ear canal. In this maneuver, the eyes should deviate to the side of the cold water. This response is lost when the pontine centers are compromised.

Trigeminal-Cranial Nerve (V)

The trigeminal-cranial nerve supplies the jaw muscles and is responsible for the sensory innervation of the face. The three divisions of this nerve are mandibular, maxillary, and ophthalmic. If unilateral facial paralysis is present,

TABLE 11-6 ▲ Pupillary Abnormalities in the Neonatal Period

Etiology	Pupillary Reactivity
Bilateral increase in size	
Hypoxic-ischemic encephalopathy	Reactive early in course Unreactive later in course
Intraventricular hemorrhage	Unreactive
Local anesthetic intoxication	Unreactive
Bilateral decrease in size	
Hypoxic-ischemic encephalopathy	Reactive
Unilateral decrease in size	
Horner syndrome	Reactive
Unilateral increase in size	
Subdural hematoma	Unreactive
Unilateral mass	Unreactive
Third nerve palsy	± Unreactive
Hypoxic-ischemic encephalopathy	± Unreactive

Modified from: Volpe JJ. 2008. *Neurology of the Newborn,* 5th ed. Philadelphia: Saunders, 137. Reprinted by permission.

damage to the motor component of this nerve may cause the jaw to deviate to the paralyzed side when the mouth is open. Strength of the masseter muscle is judged by placing a gloved

FIGURE 11-7 ▲ The "doll's eye" maneuver.

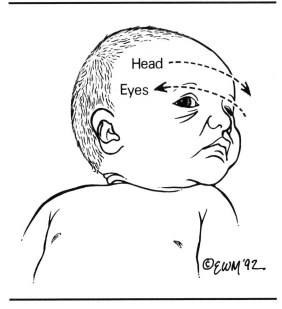

TABLE 11-7 ▲ Causes of Facial Weakness in the Neonatal Period

Cerebral
  Hypoxic-ischemic encephalopathy
  Cerebral contusion

Nerve
  Traumatic nerve damage
  Hematoma in posterior fossa

Neuromuscular junction
  Myasthenia gravis
  Infantile botulism

Nuclear injury
  Möbius syndrome
  Hypoxic-ischemic encephalopathy

Muscle
  Myotonic dystrophy
  Muscular dystrophy
  Facioscapulohumeral dystrophy
  Myopathy
  Mitochondrial disorder
  Muscle hypoplasia

Modified from: Volpe JJ. 2008. *Neurology of the Newborn,* 5th ed. Philadelphia: Saunders, 140. Reprinted by permission.

finger in the neonate's mouth and evaluating the strength of the biting portion of the suck. The sensory component of this nerve can be estimated by response to touch (as in the rooting reflex) or by the response to gentle touching of the eyelashes with a piece of cotton. The corneal reflex can be tested by blowing air into the neonate's eye to elicit a blink or by gently touching the cornea with a small piece of cotton.

FACIAL-CRANIAL NERVE (VII)

The facial-cranial nerve controls facial expression. Facial symmetry is evaluated in the noncrying, undisturbed neonate and in the crying neonate. Severe injury to the facial nerve may result in marked facial weakness. If the entire nerve on one side of the face is damaged, the neonate will be unable to wrinkle his brow or close his eyes well with crying, and his mouth will appear to draw to the normal side. Nasolabial creases will also be asym-

metric. Causes of facial weakness are listed in Table 11-7.

AUDITORY-CRANIAL NERVE (VIII)

The auditory component of the auditory-cranial nerve can be grossly tested in the neonate by assessing response to a loud noise. The response may be a blink or a startle. Noting whether the infant responds to your voice by turning his head toward you during the examination can also be used to estimate hearing. If he fails to respond to stimuli on repeat examinations, more accurate hearing tests (such as auditory evoked potentials) should be performed. The vestibular component is tested by rotating the neonate from side to side and eliciting the "doll's eye" movement.

GLOSSOPHARYNGEAL-CRANIAL NERVE (IX)

The glossopharyngeal-cranial nerve controls tongue movement. It can be evaluated by inspecting tongue movement, eliciting a gag reflex, and noting the position of the uvula. If weakness of the nerve is present, the uvula deviates to one side.

VAGUS-CRANIAL NERVE (X)

The motor portion of the vagus-cranial nerve supplies the soft palate, pharynx, and larynx. Bilateral lesions of this nerve impair swallowing. Nerve function is evaluated by listening to the cry for abnormalities such as hoarseness, stridor, or aphonia. The ability to swallow indicates a functioning nerve.

ACCESSORY-CRANIAL NERVE (XI)

Control of the sternocleidomastoid and the trapezius muscles is under the accessory-cranial nerve. Evaluation of the neonate's head position when the head is turned from one side to the other should be made. Paralysis of the sternocleidomastoid muscle is suggested by difficulty in turning the head to the affected side. Observations of shoulder height are made to

TABLE 11-8 ▲ Causes of Impaired Suck and Swallow in the Neonatal Period

Cerebral
  Encephalopathy with bilateral cerebral involvement

Nuclear
  Traumatic facial nerve damage
  Hypoxic-ischemic encephalopathy
  Möbius syndrome
  Werdnig-Hoffmann disease
  Arnold-Chiari malformation

Nerve
  Hypoxic-ischemic encephalopathy
  Bilateral laryngeal paralysis
  Posterior fossa hematoma or mass

Neuromuscular junction
  Myasthenia gravis
  Infantile botulism

Muscle
  Myotonic dystrophy
  Muscular dystrophy
  Myopathies
  Facioscapulohumeral muscular dystrophy

Modified from: Volpe JJ. 2008. *Neurology of the Newborn*, 5th ed. Philadelphia: Saunders, 143. Reprinted by permission.

evaluate the trapezius muscle function. When the upper fibers of the trapezius are paralyzed, the corresponding shoulder will be lower than the unaffected one.

HYPOGLOSSAL-CRANIAL NERVE (XII)

The hypoglossal-cranial nerve supplies the muscles of the tongue. Atrophy or abnormal movements of the tongue are assessed, as well as the gag, suck, and swallow reflexes. A weak suck and delayed swallowing are present with damage to the nerve. Other causes of impaired suck and swallow are listed in Table 11-8.

ASSESSMENT OF THE AUTONOMIC NERVOUS SYSTEM

The function of the segmental and peripheral centers of the autonomic nervous system is well established in the term neonate. This system has priority in maturation because it controls the activity of systems and organs essential for life. Vital signs, skin, and sphincters are areas

that can be assessed. Observations of trends in temperature, blood flow, heart rate, blood pressure, respiratory rate, and pupillary response to light are made. The anal sphincter is observed to see if the opening is normal or patulous (distended). The anocutaneous reflex, or "anal wink," is tested by evaluating the response to cutaneous stimulation of the perianal skin. The normal response is contraction of the external sphincter. Bladder sphincter function is more difficult to assess. Constant dribbling of urine or bladder distention and the need to credé the bladder may indicate a neurogenic bladder. A normal variant demonstrating autonomic vasomotor instability in the neonate is the harlequin sign (Chapter 4). When the neonate is lying on his side, the dependent area becomes red, and the upper area appears pale in contrast.

ABNORMALITIES

PERINATAL ASPHYXIA

Neurologic examination plays a role in the assessment of the asphyxiated newborn. Perinatal asphyxia is an insult to the fetus and newborn resulting from lack of oxygen and perfusion. It is associated with tissue hypoxia and acidosis. The biochemical definition of asphyxia is acidosis, hypoxia, and hypercapnia. Hypoxic-ischemic encephalopathy—a result of asphyxia—is a syndrome characterized by recognizable clinical, biochemical, and pathologic features. The spectrum of hypoxic-ischemic encephalopathy can be divided into categories. *Mild encephalopathy* is associated with irritability, jitteriness, and hyperalertness. *Moderate encephalopathy* is characterized by lethargy, hypotonia, a decrease in spontaneous movements, and seizures. *Severe encephalopathy* is characterized by coma, flaccidity, disturbed brainstem function, and seizures. Infants at risk for encephalopathy include those with a low cord pH, Apgar score of less than 5, and

TABLE 11-9 ▲ Maternal Drug Use and Fetal Central Nervous System Abnormality

Drug	Abnormality
Isotretinoin (Accutane)	Microcephaly, absence of the cerebellar vermis, hydrocephalus, Arnold-Chiari malformation, Dandy-Walker syndrome
Antiepileptic drugs	Microencephaly, anencephaly, myelomeningocele, hydrocephalus
Primidone (Mysoline)	Microcephaly, hydrocephalus, spina bifida, anencephaly
Cocaine	Microcephaly, cerebral infarction, encephalocele
Narcotics	Microcephaly, strabismus
Warfarin (Coumadin)	Microcephaly, hydrocephalus, brain atrophy, Dandy-Walker syndrome
Ethanol	Microcephaly

Adapted from: Dodson WE. 1989. Deleterious effects of drugs on the developing nervous system. *Clinics in Perinatology* 16(2): 340–343, 348–353.

those who need resuscitation. Early recognition of the infant at risk for encephalopathy, a complete and early neurologic examination, and the use of the amplitude integrated electroencephalogram at the bedside are important because these infants may qualify for specific brain-oriented interventions. The window for these interventions is narrow, however, so early and complete neurologic evaluation of the infant at risk is vital.[9]

The evolution of severe encephalopathy has been studied and is somewhat predictable.[8] From birth to 12 hours, the neonate with severe encephalopathy usually demonstrates stupor or coma, periodic breathing, minimal movement, and seizures. Pupillary and oculomotor responses are intact. By 12 to 24 hours, the neonate's level of consciousness appears to improve, but this apparent improvement is accompanied by apneic spells, weakness, jitteriness, and severe seizures. Between 24 and 72 hours, the neonate's level of consciousness deteriorates, and stupor and coma may be associated with respiratory arrest. The pupils

become fixed and dilated, and the doll's eye response is lost. Those neonates who survive 72 hours or longer usually demonstrate improvement, over days to weeks, in the level of consciousness, but hypotonia and weakness are common. Disturbances in suck, swallow, gag, and tongue movements may impair the ability to feed.

Specific patterns of limb weakness reflect the area of brain injury resulting from asphyxia. In term neonates, injury occurs predominantly to the parasagittal areas, zones between the cerebral arteries that are most affected by changes in blood flow and oxygenation. Weakness of the shoulder girdle and proximal upper extremities results from injury to this area of the brain. Focal ischemic injury in the area of the middle cerebral artery also presents frequently in the term neonate and is demonstrated by hemiparesis. In the premature neonate, decreased arterial blood flow affects the periventricular area and results in periventricular leukomalacia. Damage to the periventricular area results in weakness in the lower extremities.[8]

MATERNAL DRUG USE

Drug use during pregnancy may affect the fetus and the newborn by producing malformations and withdrawal. A group of drugs known as selective serotonin reuptake inhibitors is now being implicated in a number of neurobehavioral abnormalities in the term newborn. The signs most often seen include tremors, shaking, agitation, spasms, hyper- or hypotonia, irritability, and sleep disturbances. Medical interventions include supportive care and ventilatory support.[6] Nicotine can also cause neurobehavioral disturbances in the term newborn. Infants exposed to tobacco have increased signs of stress, hypertonicity, and excitability.[7] Other specific drugs and their relationship to central nervous system malformations and abnormal neurologic signs are listed in Tables 11-9 and 11-10.

Neuromuscular Disorders

Components of the central and peripheral nervous systems are responsible for the control of movement and tone. Originating in the cerebral cortex and terminating in the muscle itself, these components compose what is known as the motor system. Generally, evidence of a central encephalopathy as the cause of abnormalities of the motor system is absent. The main clinical findings in affected neonates are hypotonia and weakness, often with an alert appearance. Examination is directed toward evaluation of the muscle size, tone, tendon reflexes, muscle fasciculation, and fatiguing. Arthrogryposis, characterized by fixed position and limitation of limb movement, may be a major presenting feature of neuromuscular disease in the neonate. Atrophic muscles and decreased tendon reflexes are usually present. Limitation of fetal movement from any condition can lead to arthrogryposis. It may result from conditions affecting the brain, anterior horn cell, nerve, neuromuscular junction, or muscle. Neurogenic causes are the most common and include brain malformations, chromosomal defects, genetic syndromes, and destructive lesions of the central nervous system.[10]

Spinal Cord Injuries

Injuries to the spinal cord are usually seen following deliveries that overstretch the vertebral axis or overrotate the body in relation to the head. These injuries may occur with cephalic or breech presentations. Occasionally, a loud pop or snap is heard during the delivery. Clinical manifestations depend upon the level and severity of the injury. Transection injuries are irreversible; partial or complete recovery is possible with injuries caused by compression or ischemia. Following spinal cord injury, a state of shock and difficulty initiating respiration are common. Lesions above C3 or C4 paralyze the diaphragm. Lower cervical and upper

TABLE 11-10 ▲ Maternal Drug Use and Neonatal Neurologic Abnormality

Drug	Abnormality
Isotretinoin (Accutane)	Hypotonicity, decreased reflexes, feeding problems, facial nerve paralysis, lack of visual responsiveness, seizures
Narcotics	Withdrawal symptoms; increased activity, tone, and arousal to stimulation
Phencyclidine	Hypertonicity, decreased reflexes, bursts of agitation, rapid changes in level of consciousness
Cocaine	Depressed interactive behavior, poor organizational responses to environmental stimuli

Adapted from: Dodson WE. 1989. Deleterious effects of drugs on the developing nervous system. *Clinics in Perinatology* 16(2): 340–343, 350–352.

thoracic cord lesions result in flaccidity of the legs and portions of the arms. Lack of perceptible response to pinprick can be demonstrated below the level of spinal injury.[11,12]

Defects in Closure of the Anterior Neural Tube

Anencephaly

Anencephaly is the result of defective closure of the anterior neural tube. The defect in the skull begins at the vertex and may extend to the foramen magnum. Dermal covering is absent; hemorrhagic and fibrotic cerebral tissue lies exposed to view. The cranium is underdeveloped, resulting in shallow orbits and protruding eyes. The most common variety of anencephaly involves the forebrain and variable amounts of the upper brainstem. Associated abnormalities (such as adrenal hypoplasia and lung defects) are frequently seen.

Encephalocele

Encephalocele is a restricted disorder of neural development involving closure of the anterior neural tube. There is a protrusion of meninges and sometimes cerebral tissue, which is covered by skin. The defect in the

FIGURE 11-8 ▲ Types of spina bifida and the commonly associated malformations of the nervous system.

Diagrammatic sketches illustrating various types of spina bifida and the commonly associated anomalies of the vertebral arch, spinal cord, and meninges. **A.** Spina bifida occulta. Observe the unfused vertebral arch. **B.** Spina bifida with meningocele. **C.** Spina bifida with myelomeningocele. **D.** Spina bifida with myeloschisis. The types illustrated in B to D are referred to collectively as spina bifida cystica because of the cystlike sac associate with them.

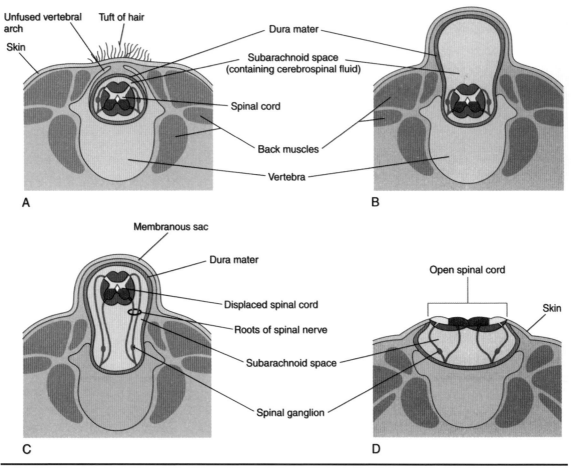

From: Moore KL, and Persaud TVN. 2008. *The Developing Human: Clinically Oriented Embryology,* 8th ed. Philadelphia: Saunders, 391. Reprinted by permission.

skull that allows protrusion is referred to as a bifid cranium.

Occasionally, cranium bifidum may be present without protrusion of meninges or fluid and instead appears as a small, tissue-covered opening on the skull. Noticeable tufts of normal hair may surround the defect. Encephaloceles most commonly occur in the midline of the occipital bone, but they may also occur in the parietal area, temporal area, or a frontal nasopharyngeal area. Occasionally,

they appear to be protruding from the eye socket.

The severity of the clinical findings is related to the location, size, and contents of the sac. Encephaloceles may vary from tiny protrusions to massive protrusions the size of the skull. The sac may contain cerebrospinal fluid, meninges, and cerebral tissue. Severe deficits occur if brain tissue and part of the ventricular system are trapped in the defect. Microcephaly, spasticity, seizures, and cortical

TABLE 11-11 ▲ Myelomeningocele and Sensory, Motor, Sphincter, and Reflex Function

Lesion	Innervation	Cutaneous Sensation	Motor Function	Working Muscles	Sphincter	Reflex
Cervical/ thoracic	Variable	Variable	None	None	None	—
Thora- columbar	T12	lower abdomen	None	None	None	—
	L1	Groin	Weak hip flexion	iliopsoas	None	—
	L2	Anterior upper thigh	Strong hip flexion	Iliopsoas and sartorius	None	—
Lumbar	L3	Anterior distal knee and thigh	Knee extension	Quadriceps	None	Patellar
	L4	Medial leg	Knee flexion, hip adduction	Medial hamstrings	None	Patellar
Lumbosacral	L5	Lateral leg, medial knee and foot	Foot dorsiflexion and eversion	Anterior tibial	None	Ankle jerk
	S1	Sole of foot	Foot plantar flexion	Gastrocnemius, soleus, posterior tibial	None	Ankle jerk
Sacral	S2	Posterior leg and thigh	Toe flexion	Flexor hallucis	Bladder and rectum	Anal wink
	S3	Middle of buttock	Toe flexion	Flexor hallucis	Bladder and rectum	Anal wink
	S4	Medial buttock	Toe flexion	Flexor hallucis	Bladder and rectum	Anal wink

Note: To assess the degree of dysfunction and level of lesion, evaluate the neonate with myelomeningocele for the presence of cutaneous sensation, motor function, working muscles, sphincter control, and reflexes.

Adapted from: Volpe JJ. 2008. *Neurology of the Newborn,* 5th ed. Philadelphia: Saunders, 10; and Noetzel M. 1989. Myelomeningocele: Current concepts of management. *Clinics in Perinatology* 16(2): 318. Reprinted by permission.

blindness are associated with structural defects of the occipital lobe. Skull x-rays are valuable in identifying the defect in the skull (the bifid cranium). Transillumination and ultrasound can be useful in identifying the extent of brain tissue in the sac.

DEFECTS IN CLOSURE OF THE POSTERIOR NEURAL TUBE

Spina bifida, meningocele, and myelomeningocele are defects arising from abnormal closure of the posterior neural tube (Figure 11-8).

Spina Bifida Occulta

A malformation arising from lack of closure or incomplete closure of the posterior portion of the vertebrae, spina bifida is the mildest form of all neural tube defects. It occurs most commonly in the lower lumbar and lumbosacral area and is covered with skin. The meninges and spinal cord are normal. The presence of tufts of hair, lipomas, or other abnormalities along the spine may indicate the presence of serious underlying defects. A dimple on the spine should be differentiated from a sinus. A dimple is a common finding and rarely indicates an underlying problem. It is usually located just superior to the anal opening. A dermal sinus can occur anywhere along the midline of the back, but is most frequently seen in the lumbar region. Although dimples generally have no clinical significance, sinuses may terminate in subcutaneous tissue, a cyst, or a fibrous band or may be associated with spina bifida and extend into an open spinal cord.

FIGURE 11-9 ▲ The brain and its coverings.

A. Schematic illustration of a coronal section through the brain and coverings. **B.** Enlargement of the area at the top of A.

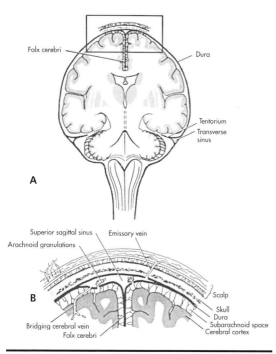

From: deGroot J, and Chusid JG. 1988. *Correlative Neuroanatomy*, 12th ed. Stamford, Connecticut: Appleton & Lange, 211. Reprinted by permission.

To inspect the dimple or sinus, try to visualize the skin covering the end of the site. This may be difficult with deep sinuses. Probing the site with instruments is contraindicated; in the case of an open spine, direct trauma to spinal elements as well as possible introduction of bacteria into the defect could occur. With skin lesions other than dimples, evaluation is indicated. X-ray or ultrasound of the involved area is helpful in identifying the vertebral abnormalities and the relationship of the defect to the meninges and cord.

Meningocele

Lesions associated with spina bifida, meningoceles usually involve more than one vertebra. The meninges, covered by a thin atrophic skin, protrude through the bony defect. The spinal roots and nerves are normal, and neurologic deficits are unusual.

Myelomeningocele

Myelomeningoceles are lesions associated with spina bifida in which there is often bilateral broadening of the vertebrae or absence of the vertebral arches. In this type of lesion, the meninges, spinal roots, and nerves protrude. Remnants of the spinal cord are fused, and the neural tube is exposed on the dorsal portion of the mass. Most of these lesions occur in the lumbar spine. Generally, the higher the defect is on the spine, the greater the degree of paralysis. Thoracic-level defects may be associated with marked abnormalities in spinal curvature and defects of the hips and lower extremities. Abnormalities in neurologic function depend on the level of the lesion (Table 11-11). Attention should be paid to examination of the motor, sensory, and sphincter functions and the reflexes. Hydrocephalus is a frequent finding associated with myelomeningocele. The status of head size and its percentile for gestational age, fontanel pressure, and width of sutures should be determined initially and periodically. Transillumination of the head following admission can be useful; serial brain ultrasounds are indicated.

The hydrocephalus seen with myelomeningocele is frequently associated with the Arnold-Chiari malformation (inferior displacement of the medulla and fourth ventricle into the upper cervical canal and elongation and thinning of the upper medulla and lower pons). Inferior displacement of the lower cerebellum through the foramen magnum into the lower cervical canal is also a feature. Hydrocephalus is thought to result from aqueductal stenosis and blockage of the cerebrospinal fluid outflow from the fourth ventricle. Neurologic, neurosurgical, urologic, and orthopedic consultations are commonly required for these patients.

INTRACRANIAL HEMORRHAGE

PRIMARY SUBARACHNOID HEMORRHAGE

A common type of neonatal intracranial hemorrhage, primary subarachnoid hemorrhage may occur in both the term and the preterm neonate, but is more common in the former. Bleeding occurs from vessels within the subarachnoid space, and the blood (hemorrhage) is usually most prominently located over the surface of the cerebral hemispheres (Figure 11-9). The etiology is thought to be trauma or hypoxia. Complications are rare.

Minor hemorrhages may go undetected because the neonate will generally be asymptomatic. Moderate degrees of hemorrhage may result in seizure activity in a neonate who otherwise appears well. One or more seizures can occur, but the neonate is stable between them.

Rarely, a massive subarachnoid hemorrhage may occur followed by rapid clinical deterioration and death. In those neonates surviving a major hemorrhage in the subarachnoid area, the development of hydrocephalus is possible. These neonates usually have histories of severe perinatal asphyxia and some degree of trauma. Hydrocephalus occurs with major hemorrhages due to decreased spinal fluid absorption by the inflamed arachnoid villi, resulting in adhesions in the subarachnoid space. Adhesions may also occur around the outflow of the fourth ventricle, leading to obstruction and hydrocephalus.

SUBDURAL HEMORRHAGE

The least common type of intracranial hemorrhage, subdural hemorrhage is most often caused by trauma. It is seen more frequently in the term than the preterm neonate. These hemorrhages are caused by (1) rupture of the tentorium, (2) occipital diastasis, (3) falx lacerations, and (4) rupture of superficial cerebral veins.[8]

FIGURE 11-10 ▲ Major cranial veins and dural sinuses.

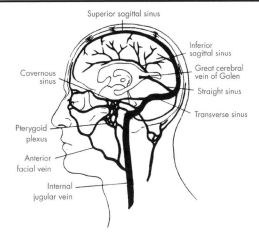

From: Volpe JJ. 2008. *Neurology of the Newborn,* 5th ed. Philadelphia: Saunders, 486. Reprinted by permission.

The dura is a fibrous tissue with two layers: an outer periosteal layer and an inner meningeal layer. These layers separate in areas to form sinuses into which major veins drain. One of the layers of separation is called the falx. The falx divides the cerebral hemispheres. The superior and inferior sagittal sinus and the vein of Galen lie close to the falx. Another area of the dura called the tentorium separates the cerebral hemispheres from the cerebellum. The straight sinus, vein of Galen, and transverse sinus lie in close proximity to the tentorium.

Tentorial laceration may result in rupture of the vein of Galen, straight sinus, or transverse sinus (Figure 11-10). A tentorial tear/laceration is usually caused by trauma associated with a difficult delivery and the need for forceps instrumentation/extraction. Clots extend into the posterior fossa and, if large, cause compression of the brain. When the neonate has a large hemorrhage in this area, neurologic disturbances will be present from birth, with signs of midbrain–upper pons compression such as stupor, coma, lateral deviation of the eyes that does not change with the doll's eye maneuver, and unequal pupils with abnormal response to light. Opisthotonos may also be present. When bradycardia is seen, it generally indicates severe compression from a massive hemorrhage. As the size of the clot increases, stupor becomes coma, pupils become fixed and dilated, and the signs of lower brainstem compression such as abnormal eye movements and apnea occur.

Occipital diastasis is a traumatic injury that results in separation of the cartilaginous joint between the squamous and lateral portions of the occipital bone. This can lead to tearing of the dura and the occipital sinuses with massive bleeding below the tentorium. The same clinical features as described for tentorial laceration occur. Smaller degrees of hemorrhage and hematoma formation in the posterior fossa lead to a different clinical evolution of signs. Initially, the neonate may have no abnormal neurologic signs. These signs begin to develop over hours or days as continued seepage of blood and gradual enlargement of the hematoma occur. Clinical signs of increased intracranial pressure ensue, followed by signs of disturbance of the brainstem, including respiratory depression, apnea, oculomotor abnormalities, and facial paresis. Seizures are also commonly seen.

When *falx laceration* has occurred with bleeding from the superior sagittal sinus, hematoma development in the cerebral fissure occurs. Marked neurologic signs develop only when the clot has extended infratentorially, and then the clinical signs are those described for tentorial laceration.

Rupture of the superficial cerebral veins results in blood collecting over the cerebral convexities. Three neurologic presentations have been associated with hemorrhage in this area. The first and most common that occurs with minor hemorrhages is either hyperirritability and a hyperalert appearance or no clinical signs at all. The second presentation includes signs of focal cerebral disturbances. Seizures are common; hemiparesis with eye deviation to the side opposite the hemiparesis can occur. The doll's eye maneuver remains normal because this is a cerebral lesion, not a brainstem lesion. Dysfunction of the third cranial nerve, the oculomotor, on the side of the hematoma, results in a poorly reactive or nonreactive pupil on the side of the lesion. The third presentation is secondary to chronic subdural effusion. The neonate has few or no clinical signs in the neonatal period, but presents months later with an enlarging head.

PERIVENTRICULAR-INTRAVENTRICULAR HEMORRHAGE

Periventricular-intraventricular hemorrhage (PV-IVH) is the most common cause of intracranial hemorrhage seen in the premature neonate. The incidence of IVH increases with decreasing gestational age. The correlation with gestational age is related to the site of bleeding, the subependymal germinal matrix. In this area of the brain, there is a matrix of poorly supported, thin-walled capillaries. It is located near the caudate nucleus at or slightly posterior to the foramen of Monro. At 28 weeks gestational age, the vessels in this area begin to involute, and involution continues so that the subependymal germinal matrix is no longer present by term.

Hemorrhage that starts in the periventricular germinal matrix can be localized in this area, or it may rupture into the ventricular system and, if large enough, cause distention of the lateral ventricles. Adjacent cerebral tissue can also be damaged as a result of hemorrhage in the germinal matrix, resulting in a parenchymal clot or infarction.

Large intraventricular hemorrhages have a high incidence of associated hydrocephalus. Most commonly, hydrocephalus occurs as a result of inflammation of the arachnoid villi, which absorb cerebrospinal fluid. With hemorrhage, they become inflamed or scarred from blood and particulate matter in the cerebrospinal fluid. Obstruction to absorption of cerebrospinal fluid then occurs. Obstruction less commonly occurs at the outlet of the third ventricle, the aqueduct of Sylvius, when debris and tissue reaction combine to lead to a blockage.

As stated previously, the germinal matrix is a poorly supported structure with thin-walled vessels that is adjacent to the lateral ventricles. Autoregulation of cerebral blood flow is lost in sick premature neonates. This renders the vessels of the subependymal germinal matrix vulnerable to blood flow alterations. Hemorrhage can result after a period of increased blood flow, decreased blood flow, increased central venous pressure, or with coagulation abnormalities. Most PV-IVHs occur in the first day of life, and 90 percent are identified using ultrasound by 72 hours of age.

Three clinical syndromes have been described and are thought to be related to severity of hemorrhage. A catastrophic course is the least common but most dramatic presentation. Stupor progresses to coma, shallow respirations progress to apnea, generalized seizures occur, pupils become fixed and nonreactive to light, the doll's eye maneuver is abnormal, the eyes are fixed to vestibular stimulation, and marked hypotonia is present. A falling hematocrit, hypotension, bradycardia, metabolic acidosis, and a bulging fontanel are also accompanying findings.

A less dramatic course has been described in which the neonate presents with signs of a progressively decreasing level of consciousness, hypotonia, lethargy, subtle eye movement abnormalities, and partial response to the doll's eye maneuver. The deterioration occurs over many hours, with periods of apparent stabilization followed by recurrence of abnormal signs. This progression of neurologic symptoms with

FIGURE 11-11 ▲ Sites of extracranial hemorrhage: caput, subgaleal hemorrhage, cephalhematoma.

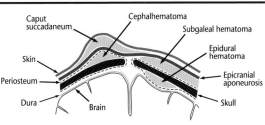

From: Sheikh, AMH. Public domain with credit.

periods of apparent stabilization may be seen over several days.

The third type of syndrome is a clinically silent course in which a screening ultrasound detects the hemorrhage.

Rarely, intraventricular hemorrhage is seen in the term neonate. In these neonates, the site of hemorrhage is most commonly the choroid plexus within the ventricle. Trauma and hypoxic events are thought to be the pathogenic mechanisms.

EXTRACRANIAL HEMORRHAGE

Two types of extracranial hemorrhage potentially complicating the neonate's course are cephalhematoma and subgaleal hemorrhage. These may lead to anemia and jaundice. Cephalhematoma is associated with the use of forceps during delivery. Subgaleal hemorrhage is associated with vacuum extraction. Cephalopelvic disproportion, prolonged labor, and tetanic contractions are also contributory factors.

Cephalhematoma is located below the periosteum and confined by the cranial sutures. The volume of blood contained within is limited because the periosteum of the cranial bone limits the potential space available for blood to expand. Cephalhematoma may contribute to jaundice, but is rarely of clinical significance from a neurologic standpoint.

TABLE 11-12 ▲ Infectious Agents Associated with Neonatal Meningitis

Bacteria	Fungi
Bacteroides fragilis	Candida
Citrobacter	**Viruses**
Escherichia coli	Cytomegalovirus
Haemophilus	Herpes simplex 1 and 2
Klebsiella	Rubella
Listeria monocytogenes	Varicella-zoster
Neisseria meningitides	Enteroviruses
Pseudomonas aeruginosa	**Protozoa**
Serratia	*Toxoplasma gondii*
Staphylococcus aureus	**Other**
Staphylococcus epidermidis	*Treponema pallidum*
Streptococcus Group B	
Streptococcus pneumoniae	

Adapted from: Bale JF, and Murphy JR. 1997. Infections of the central nervous system in the newborn. *Clinics in Perinatology* 24(4): 800. Reprinted by permission.

TABLE 11-13 ▲ Neonatal Seizures

Seizure Type	Characteristics
Subtle	Seen in term and preterm infants; apneic spells; tonic horizontal eye deviation, jerking, sustained eye opening, eyelid blinking or fluttering; sucking, drooling, oral-buccal movement; swimming, pedaling, rowing movements
Generalized tonic	Primarily seen in preterm infants; characterized by tonic extension of all limbs or by tonic flexion of arms and extension of legs
Multifocal clonic	Seen primarily in term infants; clonic movement migrating from limb to limb in a sporadic pattern (i.e., right leg, then left arm)
Focal clonic	Seen more commonly in term than in preterm infants; well-localized clonic jerking in a conscious state
Myoclonic	Seen in both term and premature infants; synchronous jerks of flexion, single or multiple, affecting upper more than lower limbs

Adapted from: Volpe JJ. 2008. *Neurology of the Newborn,* 5th ed. Philadelphia: Saunders, 211–214.

A subgaleal hemorrhage is located between the scalp (galea) and the cranial periosteum. The potential space for blood to accumulate extends from the orbital ridges to the nape of the neck.[13] A major portion of the neonate's blood volume can potentially be contained in this space, leading to severe hypovolemic shock and anemia (Figure 11-11). Clinical signs for early identification are an expanding boggy scalp, pallor, prolonged capillary refill, tachycardia, decreased responsiveness and spontaneous activity, a falling hematocrit, and signs of frank or impending shock. Seizure activity may be a late sign. The incidence of severe subgaleal hemorrhage has decreased due to the limitations on attempts at operative vaginal deliveries by the American College of Obstetricians and Gynecologists.[14]

MENINGITIS

Neonatal meningitis is associated with a variety of Gram-negative and Gram-positive bacterial organisms, as well as with viruses and fungi (Table 11-12). Neonates with bacterial meningitis often exhibit clinical signs indistinguishable from those of neonatal sepsis, including temperature instability, irritability, and poor feeding or vomiting. Neurologic signs of neonatal meningitis may include irritability, lethargy, poor tone, tremors, and seizures. The fontanel may be full, and nuchal rigidity may be present.[15] Congenital viral infections often produce growth restriction, microcephaly, skin lesions, and hepatosplenomegaly.

SEIZURES

Seizures are the most frequent sign of neonatal neurologic disorders.[8] They can be characterized by their appearance and the abnormal activity displayed (Table 11-13). The etiology of seizure activity may be central nervous system infection, metabolic derangements such as hypoglycemia and hypocalcemia, hypoxic/anoxic or ischemic-hemorrhagic events, developmental defects, or drug withdrawal. In some cases, seizures have a familial basis. When seizure activity is identified, evaluation of the cause and prompt treatment should follow rapidly. At times, it can be difficult to distinguish between seizure activity and jitteriness. Important differentiating points are that jitteriness is stimulus sensitive, consists primarily of tremorlike movement, is not associated with abnormal eye deviation or movement, and stops when the examiner passively flexes the extremity.

SUMMARY

A careful early neurologic assessment of the newborn is mandatory for optimal management. A normal exam is reassuring to the parents and the examiner. An abnormal exam serves as a guide for attempting to clarify the etiology of abnormal responses, documenting changes over time, and providing optimal care and intervention for the neonate.

REFERENCES

1. Amiel-Tison C. 1986. *A Neurologic Assessment During the First Year of Life.* Oxford: Oxford University Press, 7.
2. Prechtl H, and Beintema D. 1991. *The Neurological Examination of the Full-Term Newborn Infant,* 2nd ed. London: Cambridge University Press, 3.
3. Dubowitz L, Dubowitz V, and Mercuri E. 2007. *The Neurological Assessment of the Preterm and Full-Term Newborn Infant.* London: Heinemann, 9–11.
4. Jones KL. 2006. *Smith's Recognizable Patterns of Human Malformation,* 6th ed. Philadelphia: Saunders, 590–593.
5. Hernandez JA, and Morelli JG. 2003. Birthmarks of potential medical significance. *NeoReviews* 4(10): e263–e269.
6. Ferreira E, et al. 2007. Effects of selective serotonin reuptake inhibitors and venlafaxine during pregnancy in term and preterm neonates. *Pediatrics* 119(1): 52–59.
7. Law KL, et al. 2003. Smoking during pregnancy and newborn neurobehavior. *Pediatrics* 111(6 part 1): 1318–1323.
8. Volpe JJ. 2001. *Neurology of the Newborn,* 4th ed. Philadelphia: Saunders, 108, 178–208, 397–423, 701–703, 825–826.
9. Shalak LF, et al. 2003. Amplitude-integrated electroencephalography coupled with an early neurologic examination enhances prediction of term infants at risk for persistent encephalopathy. *Pediatrics* 111(2): 351–357.
10. Vasta I, et al. 2005. Can clinical signs identify newborns with neuromuscular disorders? *Journal of Pediatrics* 146(1): 73–79.
11. Brand MC. 2006. Part I: Recognizing neonatal spinal cord injury. *Advances in Neonatal Care* 6(1): 15–24.
12. Medlock MD, and Hanigan WC. 1997. Neurologic birth trauma: Intracranial, spinal cord, and brachial plexus injury. *Clinics in Perinatology* 24(4): 845–857.
13. Williams MC. 1995. Vacuum-assisted delivery. *Clinics in Perinatology* 22(4): 933–952.
14. American College of Obstetricians and Gynecologists. 2000. Operative vaginal delivery. ACOG practice bulletin number 17. Washington, DC: ACOG.
15. Heath PT, Nik Yusoff NK, and Baker CJ. 2003. Neonatal meningitis. *Archives of Disease in Childhood. Fetal and Neonatal Edition* 88(3): F173–F178.

BIBLIOGRAPHY

- Barness LA. 1991. *Manual of Pediatric Physical Diagnosis.* Philadelphia: Mosby.
- Brazelton TB. 1986. Neonatal Behavioral Assessment Scale. In *Clinics in Developmental Medicine,* No. 88. London: Spastics International Medical Publication; Philadelphia: Lippincott Williams & Wilkins.
- Caputo A, et al. 1978. *Primitive Reflex Profile.* Baltimore: University Park Press.
- Coen RW, and Koffler H. 2001. *Primary Care of the Newborn,* 3rd ed. Boston: Little, Brown.
- Dekaban A. 1965. *Neurology of Infancy.* Philadelphia: Lippincott Williams & Wilkins.
- Fenichel GM. 2006. *Neonatal Neurology,* 4th ed. Philadelphia: Churchill Livingstone.
- Goldbloom RB. 2002. *Pediatric Clinical Skills,* 3rd ed. Philadelphia: Saunders.
- Hill A, and Volpe J. 1989. Perinatal asphyxia: Clinical aspects. *Clinics in Perinatology* 16(2): 435–457.
- Hogan GR, and Ryan NJ. 1977. Neurological evaluation of the newborn. *Clinics in Perinatology* 4(1): 31–42.
- Napiorkowski B, et al. 1996. Effect of *in utero* substance exposure on infant neurobehavior. *Pediatrics* 98(1): 71–75.
- Noetzel M. 1989. Myelomeningocele: Current concepts of management. *Clinics in Perinatology* 16(2): 311–329.
- Painter MJ, and Bergman L. 1982. Obstetrical trauma to the neonatal central and peripheral nervous system. *Seminars in Perinatology* 6(1): 89–104.
- Roland E. 1989. Neuromuscular disorders in the newborn. *Clinics in Perinatology* 16(2): 519–547.
- Scanlon JW, Nelson T, and Grylack LJ. 1979. *A System of Newborn Physical Examination.* Baltimore: University Park Press.
- Stevenson DK, et al. 2003. *Fetal and Neonatal Brain Injury,* 3rd ed. London: Cambridge University Press.
- Taeuscher H, and Yogman M. 1987. *Follow-Up Management of the High-Risk Infant.* Boston: Little, Brown.

NOTES

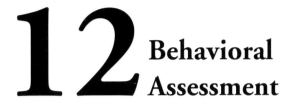

12 Behavioral Assessment

Jacqueline McGrath, PhD, RN, NNP, FNAP, FAAN

The newborn infant is truly an amazing being. Over the past several years, awareness of his capabilities and interacting behaviors has increased. Newborn behaviors can often be seen as variable and somewhat chaotic; yet they are a window into the developing brain. Assessing the neonate's neurologic status and cognitive abilities requires evaluating how he responds to and interacts with his environment. In order to respond appropriately to an infant as caregivers or parents, we must first understand his capabilities and behavioral cues and what they mean for that individual infant.

In addition to providing clues about the infant's neurologic well-being, behavioral assessment allows caregivers to design individualized, developmental care for hospitalized infants. Studies by Als and associates and by Buehler and colleagues show that appropriate, individualized developmental care of preterm infants decreases the length of hospitalization.[1,2] A meta-analysis of individualized developmental assessment and care demonstrated a statistically significant impact on the requirement for supplemental oxygen and on neurodevelopmental outcome at 9 and 12 months, but not at two years.[3] Another study indicated an enhancement of developmental outcomes

when the infant's behavioral and physiologic cues were supported in the nursery.[4,5] Although the latest (2006) Cochrane Review related to the integration of developmental care states there is not yet enough evidence to support change of practice, it also states there is no evidence to support that these interventions have negative effects.[6]

Parents and professionals have long wished and searched for accurate indicators of competence, developmental delay, or disability in infants. Untimely and/or inappropriate predictions sometimes have caused both infants and families more harm than benefit. Each approach to assessing the newborn represents the need to determine early which infants are progressing normally and which will benefit from special interventions and follow up. Parents and infants benefit from the parent's awareness and responsiveness to the infant's behavioral capabilities and temperament. Parental ability to interpret the infant's behavioral cues has been shown to strengthen parent-infant interaction during the first year of life.[4,7–9] When parents can interpret their infant's cues and respond appropriately, the infant is better able to self-regulate and control his environment as well as respond to it.[9] Providing infants with this foundation for interaction increases their learning and ability to respond to new situations.

The assessment of behavioral organization complements and elaborates on the neurologic assessment. The neurologic examination assesses the function of the central nervous system and includes assessment of muscles and reflexes within the context of the infant's state of consciousness, but the behavioral examination relies on describing the infant's observable behavior. This behavior pattern is thought to be a reflection of his underlying neurologic status.

The findings of a newborn assessment must be understood in the light of several considerations. It must be kept in mind that developmental behavior and function are not determined solely by the circumstances at birth. The human brain demonstrates a fascinating capacity to adapt and adjust to difficulties and conditions. Moreover, the future of a child's development cannot be predicted due to the structural and functional changes that will occur over time in the infant's central nervous system.

The process of infant behavioral assessment has shifted to embrace a range of competencies, rather than deficiencies. The challenge for professionals lies in offering helpful and accurate information that can facilitate parent-infant attachment. Assessment of the infant's environment and of family and social interaction must also be included to help assess the capacities and needs of infants who may be considered at risk during the perinatal period. Further, for the assessment to be most accurate, it must be repeated to determine the most current strengths and vulnerabilities of the emerging child.

APPROACH TO BEHAVIORAL ASSESSMENT

Identifying conditions of risk, describing behavior patterns, and estimating

developmental function are all important aspects of the behavioral assessment. Creditable evaluation relies primarily on the examiner's observational skills. The practitioner must observe the infant's ability to organize himself and recognize how he changes states and reacts to environmental stimuli.

It is important to follow the basic principles of physical examination when assessing the infant's behavior. Perinatal history will provide important information on factors that will affect the infant's ability to interact with the environment. Matters such as time elapsed since birth, type of labor and delivery, and drugs taken during pregnanacy and delivery by the mother must be considered. Gestational age will have a significant impact on both the behavioral findings and the infant's ability to tolerate the examination. The infant's overall health is also important; an infant with respiratory distress will exhibit different behaviors than one who is not in distress. Caregiving and activity before the exam must be considered. Research with preterm infants has demonstrated that the sequence of care and the clustering of caregiving interventions can affect the infant's responsiveness and capabilities.[10,11] These infants are easily stressed.

The environment is an important consideration that may affect the outcome of the examination. A warm, quiet, softly lit room provides the best environment in which to observe the infant's response to stimuli and his ability to control his state. Performing the exam in the presence of the infant's parents or caregivers provides a valuable opportunity for them to get to know the infant. Other supports that might be needed for some infants to perform at their best include swaddling, containment, and the use of rest periods to allow the infant to regain energy and focus for the examination. Moving to another environment away from the noise and activity of a busy nursery can also be helpful to easily stressed infants.

The infant's state of consciousness, or "state," is another important consideration.[12] The response to stimuli and behavioral cues will vary according to the state. State depends on a variety of factors, such as time of last feeding, recent events (e.g., blood tests or circumcision), and the infant's individual sleep-wake cycle. It is important to be aware of these other factors and consider them in relationship to performance during the examination. Preterm infants exhibit more variable state behaviors than term infants. The examiner needs to be flexible during the examination to obtain the most valid outcomes and conclusions.

ASSESSMENT TOOLS

Perhaps the best-known tool for behavioral assessment of the term infant is the Neonatal Behavioral Assessment Scale (NBAS) developed by Brazelton.[13] The tool was designed for use with healthy newborns from about 36 to 44 weeks gestation. A complete behavioral assessment using the NBAS takes about 30 minutes and is best administered by a trained examiner. However, even limited aspects of the examination performed by an untrained examiner can be used to provide helpful information about the infant's neurobehavioral status.[14,15] There are also several studies in which the NBAS has been done in the presence of families to enable them to see the vast capabilities of their infant.[12,16] The NBAS assesses the newborn's response to 28 behavioral items, each scored on a nine-point scale, and 18 elicited responses, each scored on a four-point continuum. These items provide information about the newborn's ability to respond and adapt to his environment. Such items as reflexes, state regulation, orientation to visual and auditory stimuli, habituation, motor performance, and interaction with caregivers are

assessed. The examination is usually done in one sitting, and items are most often presented in the same order to all infants.

The Nursing Model of the Brazelton Scale is a selected neurobehavioral assessment adapted from the NBAS for incorporation into existing nursing practice. The focus is assessment of the infant and intervention with the family.[17] The parents and nurse work together, using a nonjudgmental approach, to observe and understand specific neonatal behaviors. Specific items selected from the NBAS for the opportunity to emphasize the infant's capabilities are used by the nurse to facilitate reciprocal interaction between parents and baby. The Nursing Model of the Brazelton Scale can be used in any setting where nurses see newborn babies in the first months of life. The model is based on the assumption that the parents and newborn should be inseparable and that the family and infant require individualized attention. The nurse selects the behaviors and interactions with the baby that she feels will have the most positive impact on establishing a parental-infant bond. The nurse demonstrates and models the way parents can be most responsive to their infant. Anticipated areas of concern are addressed, and parents are taught to understand and communicate with their infant in ways that promote understanding of his behavioral needs and communications.

The nursing model focuses on motor responses and maturity, interactive skills and visual and auditory orientation, management of sleep and wake cycles, and physiologic integrity and reflexes.[17] Self-quieting activity is highlighted, and parents learn how their baby can calm himself by bringing hands to mouth, sucking, looking, and changing his position. If a baby cannot quiet himself, the nurse points out cues that signal stress or disorganization. Parents can then be aware of when their infant is stressed and modulate their reactions to him.

TABLE 12-1 ▲ Neonatal Behavioral States

State	Characteristics
Deep sleep	No eye movements No activity Regular breathing
Light sleep	Low levels of activity Rapid eye movement possible
Drowsiness	Variable activity levels Dull, heavy-lidded eyes that open and close
Quiet alert	Wide, bright eyes Attention focused on stimulus
Active alert	Increased motor activity Periods of fussiness Irregular respirations
Crying	Increased motor activity Color changes

Parents can be shown how to carefully watch for stress cues and how to intervene without either overwhelming the baby with too much stimulation or failing to offer enough intervention to soothe him.

Als and associates developed an instrument for assessing the preterm infant. Their assessment of preterm infant behavior (APIB) examines five behavioral parameters: *autonomic,* which refers to physiologic changes such as pulse, respiration, and skin color; *state,* or state of consciousness; *motor,* which assesses tone, posture, and movements; *attention/interaction,* or the ability to attend and react to the environment; and *self-regulatory,* the infant's ability to maintain state and self-console.[15,18] These parameters can be used to assess the preterm infant's ability to cope with the NICU environment. Once an infant's coping ability and organization are assessed, a plan of care that individualizes interactions for that infant can be developed.[15,18,19] As with the NBAS, training is required to become proficient at administering the complete APIB exam. However, an awareness of various behavior dynamics will increase the untrained examiner's ability

to assess the infant's well-being and provide appropriate interventions.

Another tool that has been more recently developed by Lester and Tronick for use with the preterm population is the NICU Network Neurobehavioral Scale (NNNS).[20] In the NNNS, the baseline state is a key concept because some items can be administered only if the infant is able to reach a predetermined state. This decreases the variability of examination results based on individual examiner's abilities to elicit the indicated behaviors from the infant. During the NNNS, the order of the items is more structured, and the emphasis to bring out the "best" in the infant is less apparent. This shortens the examination time and makes scoring less complex. Yet the examiner is expected to read the infant's states and behaviors and develop a rapport with him throughout the examination. The NNNS expands the scoring of the NBAS and was specifically designed for the more vulnerable preterm and/or drug-exposed infant. Examples of behavioral assessment of three different infants (well newborn, well preterm, and sick preterm) are found in Appendix B. These examples demonstrate the need for training and understanding of infant behaviors that are necessary for developing a rapport with the infant and administering a developmental assessment.

IDENTIFYING STATE OF CONSCIOUSNESS

State refers to the level of consciousness exhibited by the infant (Table 12-1). This is determined by his level of arousal and ability to respond to stimuli. The infant's behavior, function, and reaction to the environment will depend upon which baseline state he is in, ranging from deep sleep to vigorous crying. Healthy infants can use state to exert control over environmental input, but this ability is limited in the preterm or sick infant. Behavioral assessment begins with evaluating the infant's ability to control his state, move smoothly from one state to another, and maintain alertness.[14,21,22]

State is determined by observing an infant's level of arousal and accompanying behaviors or cues. Several scoring systems have been developed for identifying infant states. Brazelton's is probably the most widely used and easiest to follow, particularly in the term infant.[14] In the preterm infant, more definitive state definitions may be useful, such as those developed by Als, Holditch-Davis, and Anderson.[17,23–25] The Anderson Behavioral State Scale (ABSS) has been used often in nursing research because it is easily learned and provides interrater reliability.[24] The ABSS was devised by Gene Anderson specifically for use with preterm infants. It is based on the works of Parmalee and Stern, and Burroughs and coworkers.[26,27] The underlying theoretical framework for this state scale is different from that of other scales. Most other state scales are nominal in nature. Thus, the coding is a categorical representation of clusters of behavioral states. Hence, these state scales have been designed to capture the *qualitatively* different aspect of behavioral clusters. The ABSS was designed with consideration for the linear relationships between the states, heart rate, and energy consumption. Thus, the differences are *quantitative* or ordinal in nature.[23] The ABSS is particularly useful for preterm infants because it breaks down the typical 5 or 6 states into 12 states. This delineation more closely captures the behavioral states exhibited by preterm infants because differentiating sleep-wake states is more difficult in these subjects. For example, the ABSS has four measures of sleep, five measures of awake, and three measures of crying, allowing a more sensitive indication of infant behavioral state.

Interobserver reliability with the ABSS has been easier to establish than with other scales. ABSS scores range from 1 through 12. Activity with eyes closed (sleep) is scored from 1 to 4, representing no body movement. Scores of 1 or 2 are sleep states and are considered optimal for recovery or growth because of decreased energy expenditures. Scores of 3 or 4 are more active sleep states, with beginning awareness of the environment. Apnea due to disorganized breathing is most likely to be seen in state 3 or 4. Drowsiness with eyes open and closed at times is a score of 5. Scores of 6 or 7 are the alert states considered optimal for perception, interaction, and learning. Increasing activity with a degree of alertness are scores of 8 or 9. Scores of 10 to 12 represent increasing levels of agitation and crying. States are evaluated on the basis of their clarity and ease of identification. This may be more difficult in the preterm or ill infant, whose states may be more fleeting.[25]

SLEEP STATES

Deep sleep is characterized by closed eyes with no eye movements, regular breathing, and no spontaneous activity. There is a delayed response to external stimuli and then only a brief arousal, followed by a return to deep sleep. Isolated sucking movements or startles may be noted. Preterm infants may demonstrate a difference between very deep sleep, still sleep, and deep sleep with startles or muscle twitching.[25]

Light sleep consists of low levels of activity, with greater variability in response to external stimuli (Figure 12-1). Rapid eye movement may be observed. Preterm infants may exhibit irregular respirations. Infants in light sleep may startle or make brief fussing or crying noises. Parents may need support in delaying response to these brief episodes during the light sleep phase. Active sleep is greater in preterm infants than in term infants, who spend more time in deep sleep and alert states.[23,25]

FIGURES 12-1 through 12-9 ▲ Progression of infant through states of light sleep to crying; demonstrating time-out signals with visual stimuli.

FIGURE 12-1 ▲ Light sleep.

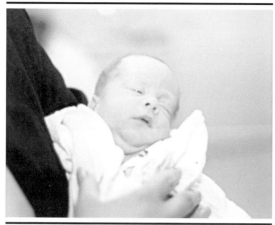

FIGURE 12-2 ▲ Drowsy.

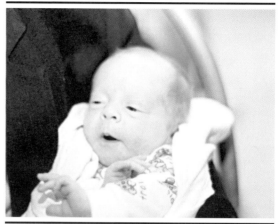

FIGURE 12-3 ▲ Quiet alert.

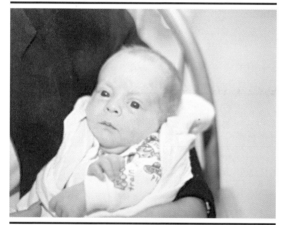

FIGURE 12-4 ▲ Signs of attentiveness.

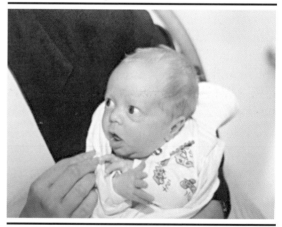

FIGURE 12-5 ▲ Hyperalert response to stimulus.

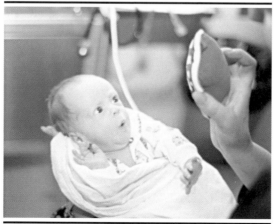

FIGURE 12-6 ▲ Self-consoling behavior; hand-to-mouth movements.

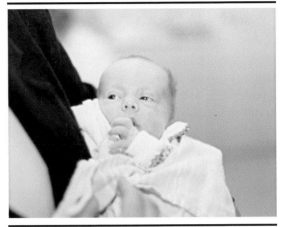

FIGURE 12-7 ▲ Sign of overstimulation in response to stimulus.

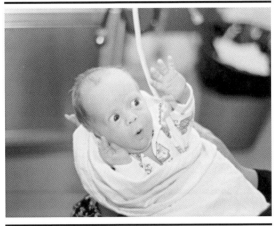

FIGURE 12-8 ▲ Sign of overstimulation in response to stimulus.

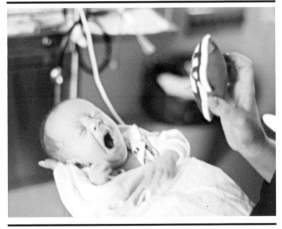

FIGURE 12-9 ▲ Crying as a response to continued stimulus.

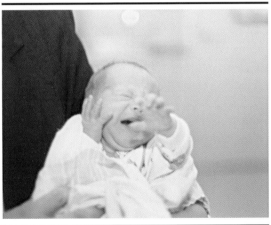

TRANSITIONAL STATE

Drowsiness is characterized by a variable activity level, with smooth movements and occasional mild startles. The eyes open and close and appear dull and heavy-lidded. The infant will react to stimuli, but the response is often delayed, or he may startle easily (Figure 12-2). From the drowsy state, the infant may either return to a sleep state or move to a more alert status. Caregivers may arouse an infant to a quiet alert state by providing an auditory or visual stimulus. Nonnutritive sucking has

also been found to be effective in calming and bringing an infant to an alert state.[23,27,28]

AWAKE STATES

Quiet alert refers to the state in which the infant interacts most with the environment. He exhibits a brightening and widening of the eyes and an alert appearance (Figure 12-3). Attention is focused on available stimuli, whether visual or auditory (Figure 12-4). A minimal amount of motor activity is noted, and respirations are regular. This state provides the greatest opportunity for infant interaction with caregivers. Term newborns commonly experience a period of quiet alertness in the first few hours after birth, providing an opportune time for parents to interact with their infant.

Preterm infants may have difficulty maintaining a quiet alert state for long. Their alert periods may be brief and fleeting. They may become "hyperalert," with an inability to decrease or end fixation on a stimulus (Figure 12-5). Preterm infants may also appear awake and alert but be unable to involve themselves in interaction.[7,18,25,29] During these periods, they are often noted to use gaze aversion to manage the overwhelming stimuli in the environment because they are so easily overloaded and stressed by the many stimuli in the NICU.[29–31]

The *active alert* state is characterized by increased motor activity, with heightened sensitivity to stimuli. The infant may have periods of fussiness, but can be consoled. Although open, the eyes are are less bright and attentive than in the quiet alert state. Respirations are irregular. The term infant may be able to use self-consoling techniques to return himself to a quiet alert state (Figure 12-6). The preterm infant will usually become distressed and unable to organize himself. Interventions such as waiting for the infant to settle, swaddling, containing, and reducing other environmental stimuli can be provided by caregivers to help the infant return to a quiet alert state.[25]

Crying is accompanied by increased motor activity and color changes. The infant is very responsive to unpleasant stimuli, both internal and external. Some infants are able to console themselves from time to time and return to a lower state, whereas others need help from caregivers. Preterm infants may exhibit a very weak cry or may be unable to cry due to intubation. They do demonstrate color changes, alterations in motor activity, and other signs

of stress, such as cry-face, apnea, vomiting, or decreased oxygen saturation.[23,25]

MAINTENANCE OF STATE

Although the states can be distinguished from one another, the infant makes frequent transitions between them. He may change from one state to another several times in the course of the examination. The term infant should display smooth transitions between states. Excessive lethargy or irritability is abnormal. The preterm or neurologically impaired infant may exhibit sudden changes between sleep and awake states, but abrupt state changes in the healthy term infant are a cause for concern.[23,25]

The ability to maintain an alert state varies among infants. Some have difficulty becoming alert initially and then are unable to maintain this state for any length of time. Others have trouble filtering out noxious stimuli and progress rapidly to active alert or crying. Swaddling or a quiet, darkened environment may help these infants remain alert and focus on a single stimulus.

The examiner should note the amount of time the infant spends in the quiet alert state or focusing on a stimulus. Infants who have difficulty remaining alert can be frustrating for caregivers, especially parents. The examiner may spend time teaching parents ways to help the infant maintain a quiet alert state.

Preterm infants have brief periods of alertness, but have difficulty maintaining this state. Brazelton describes the "cost of attention" as the amount of energy the infant must expend to maintain an alert state.[13] This cost of attention varies, depending on the health and maturity of the infant. Premature or sick infants show fatigue or stress sooner than do healthy term infants.[30,31]

Signs of stress or fatigue include color changes, irregular respirations, apnea, changes in tone, irritability or lethargy, and vomiting. The infant may change states rapidly from crying to sleep or become hyperalert. The examiner must be able to recognize these signs of stress and fatigue and discontinue the examination when appropriate. After the infant has had a period of rest, the examiner may be able to begin again. The cost to the infant or the amount of energy he expends during the examination should be noted.[13,24] The preterm or ill infant may require completion of the examination in pieces, which is not optimal; yet completion in one time period may be too much for these infants.

ORGANIZATION

Organization reflects the infant's ability to integrate physiologic and behavioral systems in response to the environment without disruption in state or physiologic functions.[7,32] Physiologic systems include such parameters as heart rate, respiratory rate, oxygen consumption, and digestion. The behavioral system includes state (attention and self-regulation) and motor activity (tone, movements, and posture).

The organized infant maintains stable vital signs, smooth state transitions, and even movements when interacting with the environment. The infant is able to self-console or be consoled easily and can habituate to or block out overwhelming stimuli. The disorganized infant will react to the environment with sudden state changes and will exhibit frantic, jittery movements, color changes, and irregular respirations. Some infants will respond with hypotonia. The ability to maintain organization depends on the infant's maturity level and overall well-being. Individual temperament may also play a role in organizational ability.

In evaluating organization of motor behavior, the practitioner assesses the infant's ability to control his motor activity and the kinds of movements he makes, both random and purposeful. Hand-to-mouth maneuvers in an attempt to self-console are purposeful movements achieved by the mature, well-organized infant (see Figure 12-6). When a cloth is placed over the face of a term neonate, he will attempt to remove it by arching, rooting, and swiping at it. As during most assessments of behavioral maturity, the preterm infant will have a limited ability to respond to stimuli with purposeful movements of muscle groups, or he may not respond at all.

Infants who are easily overwhelmed will benefit from care designed to enhance their organizational ability. Clustering care to allow for uninterrupted sleep, arousing the infant slowly, and introducing one stimulus at a time are all interventions that support the disorganized infant. However, it is important to consider those caregiving tasks that are clustered together and their effect on the infant. There is always a cost/benefit ratio to consider.[10,11] Containing the extremities, decreasing noise and lights, and handling gently are also helpful and supportive interventions.

RECOGNIZING THE SENSORY THRESHOLD

Sensory threshold refers to the level of tolerance for stimuli within which the infant can respond appropriately. When he reaches or exceeds his threshold, the infant has become overstimulated and exhibits signs of stress and fatigue (Table 12-2). Preterm and neurologically impaired infants may have low thresholds, as may some healthy term newborns. What would normally be considered routine care (e.g., talking to the infant during feeding) may be overstimulating to an infant with a low sensory threshold. These infants might do better when presented with a single stimulus.

The mature newborn has a unique ability to regulate physiologic and emotional response to a variety of stimuli. It is his way of learning to

TABLE 12-2 ▲ Signs of Overstimulation (Time-Out)

Gaze aversion

Frowning

Sneezing

Yawning

Hiccuping

Vomiting

Mottled skin

Irregular respirations

Apnea

Increased oxygen requirement

Heart rate changes

Finger splaying

Arching

Stiffening

Fussing, crying

TABLE 12-3 ▲ Signs of Approach (Attention)

Quiet alert state

Focused gaze

Dilated pupils

Regular respirations

Regular heart rate

Rhythmic sucking

Reaching or grasping

Hand-to-mouth movements

control the effects of the surrounding environment. Evaluating these reactions to the environment allows the practitioner to design a plan of care that is unique to that infant.[32–34] This also facilitates parental teaching and involvement.[9,35] Infants who are easily overwhelmed may require more frequent breaks during caregiving for the infant to have time to adapt and regulate his responses.

OBSERVING BEHAVIORAL CUES

An infant's behavior includes a variety of cues that indicate his physical, psychological, and social needs. Caregivers who respond appropriately to these cues develop a reciprocal relationship with the newborn. Responding to an infant's behavioral cues also reinforces his behavioral organization.[7,22,25]

Signs of approach (or attention) indicate that the infant is ready to interact with the caregiver or the environment. Approach behaviors include an alert, focused gaze; regular breathing; and dilated pupils. The infant may also exhibit grasping, sucking, or hand-to-mouth movements (Table 12-3; see Figure 12-6).[23,25]

Avoidance behaviors (time-out signals) indicate that the infant is becoming tired, overstimulated, or stressed and needs a break from the stimulus or interaction. Avoidance behaviors include averting the gaze, frowning, sneezing, yawning, vomiting, and hiccuping. The infant may also display finger splaying, arching, stiffening, or crying (see Figures 12-7 through 12-9 and Table 12-2). Color changes, apnea, irregular breathing, and decreased oxygen saturation also indicate the infant's need for time-out.[22,23,25] State changes may be an avoidance behavior, as demonstrated by the infant who shuts down entirely by falling asleep during repeated or prolonged painful procedures. Nurses must use these cues to provide routine care if they are to best support the infant and decrease energy consumption.[30,31]

HABITUATION

The infant's ability to alter his response to a repeated stimulus is referred to as *habituation*. When a stimulus is repeated, the infant's initial response to it will gradually disappear. Habituation provides a defense mechanism for shutting out overwhelming or disturbing stimuli. For example, health care providers often habituate to the noxious noise of the NICU.

Habituation is best assessed with the infant in a light sleep or a quiet alert state.[14,32] The stimulus can involve the visual, auditory, or tactile senses. Visual habituation can be easily assessed by shining a light briefly into the infant's eyes from 10 to 12 inches away.

Repeat the stimulus every five seconds to a maximum of ten times or until the infant ceases to respond (whichever comes first). Note the presence of startles, facial grimaces, blinking, and respiratory changes. If habituation occurs, responses will become delayed and eventually disappear. Infants who are able to habituate successfully usually do so within five to nine flashes.

The infant's ability to habituate to an auditory stimulus can be tested in the same manner, but using an object that makes a noise (e.g., a bell or rattle). Holding the object 10 to 15 inches from the baby, shake it for about one second. Reactions may include startles, facial grimaces, and respiratory changes. Note the infant's ability to decrease his reactions as the stimulus is repeated. As they do with visual habituation, most term infants decrease their reaction after five to nine repetitions.

Habituation to tactile stimulation can be determined by pressing the sole of the foot with a smooth object. Repeat the stimulus every five seconds. The infant may begin with a generalized body response, pulling both feet away. The response will gradually decrease to only the involved foot or will disappear altogether.

The ability to habituate varies among infants. Some (including those who are preterm) have difficulty tuning out noxious stimuli.[36] They are easily distracted and then become irritable and disorganized, displaying signs of stress and fatigue. Their inability to ignore other environmental sights and sounds may make interaction and feeding difficult. These infants may need to be fed in a quiet, darkened room or presented with one stimulus at a time during their quiet alert state. Teaching parents how to read their infant's cues regarding care and adaptability can facilitate a more positive relationship between the infant and the family, thus potentially increasing parent competence.

RESPONSE TO STIMULI

VISUAL STIMULI

The newborn has the ability to focus on and react to a variety of stimuli in the environment. The examiner should observe and record the infant's response to visual and auditory stimuli. For optimal evaluation, responses should be assessed with the infant in the quiet alert state.

Two tests for visual response can be performed with the newborn. The first is a response to light. When a light is directed toward the infant's eyes, an appropriate response is for him to grimace and close his eyelids. This response will lessen with habituation. The second test evaluates the ability to fixate on an object and track it. Term infants are able to fixate briefly on an object (a face or a mobile, for example). The newborn's visual field is fairly narrow, with the ability to focus on objects at a distance of about 10 to 12 inches. Objects closer or farther away will be ignored because newborns have decreased visual acuity that improves with maturation. The term newborn is able to follow or track an object horizontally about 60 degrees and vertically about 30 degrees, often with some head movement.[14,23]

The pupillary reflex develops at approximately 30 weeks gestational age. Without this reflex, premature infants have a limited ability to maintain protective lid tightening and therefore should be protected from bright lights and visual stimulation.[19] As the pupillary reflex matures, preterm infants beyond 30 weeks demonstrate both response to light and ability to fixate on simple patterns.[15] Preterm infants may take longer to fixate on an object, and they have less visual acuity than a term newborn, which accounts for this variability in response. It is important to continue monitoring light levels, protecting the infant's eyes from direct light. Behavioral response to visual stimuli should be evaluated for signs of stress and fatigue.[19] It is also important to remember that the eye exam in the preterm infant is a very noxious procedure that the infant may need supportive interventions to manage.

AUDITORY STIMULI

When in the alert state, newborns will respond to an auditory stimulus with brightening of the eyes and face and turning of the head in search of the sound. A rattle, bell, or music box will work well as an auditory stimulus. Keep in mind that a newborn may tune out a noxious auditory stimulus. With the baby's head in midline, initiate the stimulus 6 to 12 inches away from his ear, out of his visual range. He should alert and turn toward the sound; continue by alternating on each side with sounds of varying rhythm and intensity.

Preterm infants begin to orient to a soft sound source around 28 weeks gestational age, but often demonstrate sensitivity to noise and physiologic instability in the presence of loud noise. The use of soft voice and rhythmic cyclical auditory stimulation can be introduced based on the infant's behavioral response.[37] Careful attention must be paid to limiting environmental noise because it has the ability to interfere with the responses to the behavioral examination. White and associates provide design guidelines for limiting noise.[38]

EVALUATING CONSOLABILITY

Infants' abilities to quiet when in a crying state vary. The well-organized infant demonstrates observable activities to self-console during the course of examination. These include bringing the hands to the mouth, sucking on the fist or tongue, and using environmental stimuli (visual or auditory) such as a soft human voice to self-console (see Figure 12-6).[14] Infants who make limited attempts or who show decreased ability to self-console may be more irritable or sensitive to stimuli.[14,39]

Most infants will respond to consoling attempts by caregivers. Irritable infants may be easily disturbed by stimuli from the environment and may be slower to respond (or may not respond at all) to attempts to console them. The examiner should try such interventions that may lead to consoling the infant as holding, rocking, speaking quietly to the infant, swaddling or flexing his extremities near the trunk to prevent startle activity, or offering nonnutritive sucking. Decreasing such environmental stimuli as light, noise, and sudden movement may be helpful. A common mistake is trying several interventions at the same time (e.g., rocking, talking softly, *and* offering a pacifier). A combination of activities may overstimulate some infants. Therefore, limit the interventions to one at a time before using them as a group. If one intervention fails, try a different one. Note which interventions work for this particular infant so they can be used again in the future.

IDENTIFYING TEMPERAMENT

Some babies seem more difficult; others appear to be easier to care for. Infant temperament has been defined as the infant's behavioral style. It is how he behaves in relationship to the environment and caregiving he receives.[40] How the child's temperament is exhibited and perceived affects the developing relationship between the infant and mother. When there is synchrony within this dyad, there is said to be "goodness of fit." When synchrony is lacking, the infant is perceived as difficult and/or demanding by the mother (primary caregiver), and the asynchrony of the relationship predisposes the infant to long-term negative outcomes. Because she is the primary caregiver, the mother's perceptions of infant temperament are important. Maternal perceptions and beliefs about the attributes of the infant affect how she cares for her infant and the symbiotic relationship that will support the his cognitive development. Thus, infant temperament has been measured by asking mothers about their infants. How do they perceive the infant? Is he calm or demanding? How easily is he consoled or is he inconsolable? Understanding these dimensions can help the mother acquire realistic expectations for the child's behavior and perceive that he has met them.

Temperament refers to the way an individual interacts with his environment. Chess and Thomas describe nine behaviors that define variations in temperament.[40] A description of each behavior follows:

Activity level refers to motor activity such as playing, dressing, eating, crawling, and walking. Sleep-wake cycles and their durations are also used in scoring activity level. Some infants are very active, with short sleep cycles; others are more quiet.

Rhythmicity refers to the regularity of functions such as hunger, sleep-wake patterns, and elimination.

Approach or *withdrawal* describes the individual's reaction to a new stimulus such as food, a new toy, or a new person. Approach responses are positive; withdrawal responses are negative reactions to the new situation.

Adaptability is the individual's response to new situations once the initial response has passed. Adaptability examines the ability to adjust to the new situation or environment.

Threshold of responsiveness refers to the amount of stimulation required to generate a response, either positive or negative.

Quality of mood describes the overall mood of the individual or the amount of pleasant, friendly, happy behavior versus unpleasant, unfriendly, or fussy behavior.

Intensity of reaction is the level of energy in a response, whether positive or negative.

Distractibility is the ability of extraneous stimuli to interfere with the individual's current behavior.

Attention span or *persistence* refers to the length of time an individual will pursue a specific activity, especially when obstacles interfere with it.

Based on these behaviors, three categories of temperament can be defined and frequently identified in the newborn:

1. The "easy" baby demonstrates regularity, positive approaches to new situations, adaptability to change, and an overall positive mood.
2. The "difficult" baby has an irregular schedule, trouble adapting to new situations, a low threshold for stimulus, and intense, often negative moods.
3. The "slow-to-warm" infant is characterized by mild intensity, positive or negative moods, and slow adaptation to new situations and people. These infants need repeated, slow exposure to a situation before they will respond positively.

Understanding and supporting an infant to best optimize his temperament can help parents create an environment that will maximize their child's positive characteristics and minimize frustrations.[41] Parents of a slow-to-warm child can allow extra time for him to adapt to new situations. The infant with a low sensory threshold may be easier to care for if activity is limited to one or two stimuli at a time.

Summary

An infant's behavior may be difficult to elicit and interpret, but it is an integral part of the complete newborn examination. The behavioral assessment allows the examiner and the caregiver an opportunity to evaluate some aspects of the infant's neurologic status, and it helps establish guidelines for developmental care of both term and preterm infants.

Behavioral assessments can also help teach parents how to read and respond to their newborn's cues and signals. Behavioral assessment encourages a view of the infant as a whole individual—an approach that enhances care and support of infants and their families.

REFERENCES

1. Als H, Duffy FH, and McAnulty GB. 1996. Effectiveness of individualized neurodevelopmental care in the newborn intensive care unit (NICU). *Acta Paediatrica* 416(supplement): S21–S30.

2. Buehler DM, et al. 1995. Effectiveness of individualized developmental care for low-risk preterm infants: Behavioral and electrophysiologic evidence. *Pediatrics* 96(5 part 1): 923–932.

3. Jacobs SE, Sokol J, and Ohlsson A. 2002. The newborn individualized developmental care and assessment program is not supported by meta-analysis of the data. *Journal of Pediatrics* 140(6): 699–706.

4. Anderson CJ. 1981. Enhancing reciprocity between mother and neonate. *Nursing Research* 30(2): 89–93.

5. Westrup B. 2007. Newborn individualized developmental care and assessment program (NIDCAP)—Family-centered developmentally supportive care. *Early Human Development* 83(7): 443–449.

6. Symington A, and Pinelli J. 2006. Developmental care for promoting development and preventing morbidity in preterm infants. *Cochrane Database of Systematic Reviews* (2): CD001814.

7. D'Apolito K. 1991. What is an organized infant? *Neonatal Network* 10(1): 23–29.

8. Liptack GS, et al. 1983. Enhancing infant development and parent-practitioner interaction with the Brazelton Neonatal Assessment Scale. *Pediatrics* 72(1): 71–78.

9. Maguire CM, et al. 2007. Reading preterm infants' behavioral cues: An intervention study with parents of premature infants born <32 weeks. *Early Human Development* 83(7): 419–424.

10. Holsti L, et al. 2005. Prior pain induces heightened motor responses during clustered care in preterm infants in the NICU. *Early Human Development* 81(3): 293–300.

11. Holsti L, et al. 2006. Behavioral responses to pain are heightened after clustered care in preterm infants born between 30 and 32 weeks gestational age. *Clinical Journal of Pain* 22(9): 757–764.

12. Myers BJ. 1982. Early intervention using Brazelton training with middle class mothers and fathers of newborns. *Child Development* 53(2): 462–471.

13. Beal JA. 1986. The Brazelton Neonatal Behavioral Assessment Scale: A tool to enhance parental attachment. *Journal of Pediatric Nursing* 1(3): 170–177.

14. Brazelton TB. 1995. *Clinics in Developmental Medicine,* 3rd ed. London: MacKeith Press, 85–100.

15. Gorski P, Lewkowicz D, and Huntington L. 1987. Advances in neonatal and infant behavioral assessment: Toward a comprehensive evaluation of early patterns of development. *Journal of Developmental and Behavioral Pediatrics* 8(1): 39–50.

16. Lowman LB, Stone LL, and Cole JG. 2006. Using developmental assessments in the NICU to empower families. *Neonatal Network* 25(3): 177–186.

17. Karl DJ, Beal JA, and Rissmiller PN. 1995. A model for integrating the NBAS into nursing practice. In *Neonatal Behavioral Assessment Scale,* 3rd ed., Brazelton TB, and Nugent JK, eds. London: MacKeith Press, 102–107.

18. Als H, et al. 1982. Manual for the assessment of preterm infant's behavior. In *Theory and Research in Behavioral Pediatrics,* Fitzgerald HE, Lester BM, and Yogman MW, eds. New York: Plenum Press, 65–132.

19. Cole JG, et al. 1990. Changing the NICU environment: The Boston City Hospital model. *Neonatal Network* 9(2): 15–23.

20. Lester BM, and Tronick EZ. 2005. *NICU Network Neurobehavioral Scale (NNNS) Manual.* Baltimore: Brookes.

21. Zuckerman BS, and Frank DA. 1992. Infancy and toddler years. In *Developmental and Behavioral Pediatrics,* Levine MD, Carey WB, and Crocker AC, eds. Philadelphia: Saunders, 27–38.

22. Carrier CT. 2004. Developmental support. In *Core Curriculum for Neonatal Intensive Care Nursing,* 3rd ed., Verklan MT, and Walden M, eds. Philadelphia: Saunders, 236–264.

23. Holditch-Davis D, Blackburn ST, and VandenBerg K. 2007. Neurobehavioral development. In *Comprehensive Neonatal Nursing: An Interdisciplinary Approach,* 4th ed., Kenner C, and Lott JW, eds. Philadelphia: Saunders, 236–284.

24. Gill NE, et al. 1988. Effect of nonnutritive sucking on behavioral state in preterm infants before feeding. *Nursing Research* 37(6): 347–350.

25. VandenBerg KA. 2007. State systems development in high-risk newborns in the neonatal intensive care unit: Identification and management of sleep, alertness, and crying. *Journal of Perinatal & Neonatal Nursing* 21(2): 130–139.

26. Parmalee AH, and Stern E. 1972. Development of states in infants. In *Sleep and the Maturing Nervous System,* Clemente CD, Purpura DP, and Mayers FE, eds. New York: Academic Press, 199–228.

27. Burroughs AK, et al. 1978. The effect of nonnutritive sucking on transcutaneous oxygen tension in noncrying, preterm neonates. *Research in Nursing and Health* 1(2): 69–75.

28. Gill NE, et al. 1992. Nonnutritive sucking modulates behavioral state for preterm infants before feeding. Scandinavian *Journal of Caring Sciences* 6(1): 3–7.

29. McCain GC. 1992. Facilitating inactive awake states in preterm infants: A study of three interventions. *Nursing Research* 41(3): 157–160.

30. Harrison LL, Roane C, and Weaver M. 2004. The relationship between physiological and behavioral measures of stress in preterm infants. *Journal of Obstetric, Gynecologic, and Neonatal Nursing* 33(2): 236–245. (Published erratum in *Journal of Obstetric, Gynecologic, and Neonatal Nursing,* 2004, 33[3]: 389.)

31. Liaw JJ, Yuh YS, and Chang LH. 2005. A preliminary study of the associations among preterm infant behaviors. *Journal of Nursing Research* 13(1): 1–10.

32. Gorski PA, Davison MF, and Brazelton TB. 1979. Stages of behavioral organization in the high risk neonate: Theoretical and clinical considerations. *Seminars in Perinatology* 3(1): 61–72.

33. Liaw JJ, Chen SY, and Yin YT. 2004. Nurses' beliefs and values about doing cue-based care in the NICU in Taiwan. *Journal of Nursing Research* 12(4): 275-286.

34. Liaw JJ. 2003. Use of a training program to enhance NICU nurses' cognitive abilities for assessing preterm infant behaviors and offering supportive interventions. *Journal of Nursing Research* 11(2): 82–92.

35. Loo KK, et al. 2003. Using knowledge to cope with stress in the NICU: How parents integrate learning to read the physiologic and behavioral cues of the infant. *Neonatal Network* 22(1): 31–37.

36. Long LG, Lucey JF, and Phillip AG. 1980. Noise and hypoxemia in the ICN. *Pediatrics* 65(1): 61–72.

37. Hadley LB, and West D. 1999. *Developmental and Behavioral Characteristics of Preterm Infants.* Santa Rosa, California: NICU Ink.

38. White RD, et al. 2007. *Recommended Standards for Newborn ICU Design.* Report of the seventh census conference on newborn ICU design. Committee to establish recommended standards for Newborn ICU design. Accessed November 18, 2007, from http://www.nd.edu/~nicudes.

39. Budreau G, and Kleiber C. 1991. Clinical indicators of infant irritability. *Neonatal Network* 9(5): 23–30.

40. Chess S, and Thomas A. 1992. Dynamics of individual behavioral development. In *Developmental and Behavioral Pediatrics,* 2nd ed., Levine MD, Carey WB, and Croker AC, eds. Philadelphia: Saunders, 84–94.

41. Brazelton TB. 1992. *Touchpoints: Your Child's Emotional and Behavioral Development.* Reading, Massachusetts: Addison-Wesley, 76–78, 106–107.

NOTES

NOTES

13 Assessment of the Dysmorphic Infant

Michelle Bennett, MSN, RN, NNP-BC
Susan Meier, MSN, RN, NNP-BC

Most infants are born healthy, and the first clinical assessment usually reveals no physical abnormality. However, for the past 20 years, birth defects have been the leading cause of infant mortality in the U.S. Each year, approximately 3 percent of live births, or 120,000 babies, are born with major physical structural defects, and one in five infant deaths is attributed to a birth defect.[1]

Fifty to 60 percent of human congenital anomalies are of unknown etiology, and 20 to 25 percent are caused by genetic and environmental factors acting together. A smaller percentage of birth defects is the result of chromosomal aberrations, mutant genes, and environmental agents, such as viruses and drugs.[2]

The identification of dysmorphic features during the initial physical examination is a crucial first step in the continuum of care for affected infants. A thorough, systematic approach by a skilled examiner can yield important findings and direct the health care team in providing timely and appropriate care for the infant as well as resources for parents.

MATERNAL AND FAMILY HISTORIES

A complete maternal medical, gynecologic, and obstetric history should be constructed when evaluating the dysmorphic infant.

A history of adverse pregnancy outcomes including multiple miscarriages and stillbirths can be an important risk factor. Maternal age should be documented because chromosomal anomalies such as trisomy 21 occur more frequently with advancing maternal age. Pregnancies complicated by medical conditions such as diabetes mellitus or hypertension increase the possibility for fetal physical deformities. Prenatal exposure to teratogens, including medications, infections, chemicals, and illicit drugs, must be documented because certain agents exhibit specific structural abnormalities and functional diseases in the fetus. Critical periods of fetal development, dosage and duration of exposure to the teratogen, and genotype of the embryo must also be taken into consideration.[2] Results of prenatal testing, including multiple marker serum screening, maternal serum α-fetoprotein testing, chorionic villus sampling, and amniocentesis, should be recorded to identify an increased risk or a confirmed diagnosis of fetal disorders such as neural tube defects and trisomies.

A comprehensive maternal and paternal family history is also helpful. A number of congenital anomalies and medical conditions can be inherited and can therefore place an infant at risk for developing the disorder. Some

FIGURE 13-1 ▲ **Eye measurements**

Various eye measurements are depicted. **A.** Outer canthal distance. **B.** Intracanthal distance. **C.** Inter-pupillary distance (IPD), which is difficult to measure directly. The IPD can be determined with the Pryor formula: IPD = (A − B) 2 + B. **D.** Intraorbital distance. **E.** Palpebral fissure length.

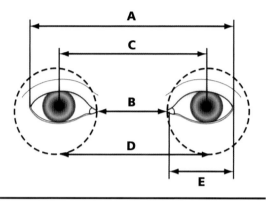

Adapted from: Cheng KP, and Biglan AW. Ophthalmology. 2007. In *Atlas of Pediatric Diagnosis,* 5th ed., Zitelli BJ, and Davis HW, eds. Philadelphia: Mosby, 727. Reprinted by permission.

of these conditions include spina bifida; hydrocephalus; muscular dystrophy; cleft lip; cleft palate; congenital heart defects; polydactyly; clubfoot; congenital hip dislocation; deafness; blindness; childhood cataracts; cystic fibrosis; dwarfism; polycystic kidney disease; and stomach, bowel, or kidney defects.

There are also genetic disorders that occur more commonly within particular ethnic groups. Descendents of Ashkenazic Jewish or French Canadian ancestors may have an increased risk of Tay Sachs disease, an often fatal disorder marked by degeneration of brain tissue and the maculae of the retinas. Infants of African American ancestry are at an increased risk of inheriting sickle cell disease, a serious condition of red blood cells that are distorted in shape and have a tendency to clump together and occlude blood vessels. Thalassemia, a group of hemolytic anemias, is increased in the Mediterranean and Asian populations.

If one or both parents are of Jewish, French Canadian, African American, Mediterranean, or Asian descent or if a medical condition occurs repeatedly in one of the partner's families, the couple may consider genetic testing prior to conceiving a child. If either partner is a carrier for a specific inheritable condition, the significance of the results can then be discussed with the couple's health care provider.

Physical Examination

The newborn infant should have a thorough physical examination within 24 hours of birth. This first examination may reveal more abnormalities than any subsequent routine examination done. First, the family, maternal, pregnancy, and perinatal histories are reviewed. The examination is performed in an area that is warm and quiet with good lighting. A systematic approach should be used. Although the exact examination sequence is not important, a consistent approach ensures that all aspects are evaluated. Assessment of gestational age should be included. Knowledge of gestational age may be important in the interpretation of physical findings, especially in infants who are noted to have intrauterine growth restriction (IUGR).

Appearance and posture

An inspection is made for deformations and obvious malformations. An abnormal facial appearance or other abnormalities may indicate the presence of a syndrome. The newborn's posture at rest usually reflects intrauterine position, sometimes called the position of comfort.

Skin

The skin is inspected for abnormalities. Areas of abnormal pigmentation, congenital nevi, hemangiomas, macular stains, or other unusual lesions should be noted.

HEAD

The shape and size of the head are inspected. The presence of abnormal hair, lacerations, abrasions or contusions, scalp defects, unusual lesions, or protuberances should be noted. An asymmetric skull that persists for longer than two to three days after birth or a palpable ridge along a suture line is abnormal and suggests craniosynostosis. Although usually occurring in normal infants, craniotabes can be a pathologic finding with syphilis and rickets.

Very large fontanels reflect a delay in bone ossification and may be associated with hypothyroidism, trisomy syndromes, intrauterine malnutrition, hypophosphatasia, rickets, and osteogenesis imperfecta.[3]

NECK

The neck is assessed for masses, decreased mobility, and abnormalities. Cystic hygroma, the most common lymphatic malformation in children, typically presents as a painless mass superior to the clavicle that transilluminates. Redundant skin in the neck may be a feature of some genetic syndromes. Examples include Turner syndrome, in which the neck appears webbed due to redundant skin along the posterolateral line, and Down syndrome, with excess skin posteriorly at the base of the neck.

FACE

The face is examined for symmetry. Facial palsies and asymmetric crying facies are most obvious when the newborn is crying and may go unnoticed in the sleeping or quiet infant. Asymmetric crying facies are the result of hypoplasia or congenital absence of the depressor anguli muscle. Only the muscles controlling movement of one side of the mouth are affected, causing asymmetry of the face with crying. However, the muscles controlling movement of the upper face are normal; so when the infant cries, the forehead wrinkles and both eyes close normally. Asymmetric

FIGURE 13-2 ▲ Ear placement.

Using the medial canthi (**A** and **B**) as landmarks, one draws a central horizontal line and extends it to a point (**C**) on the side of the face. Ears placed below this line are considered low set.

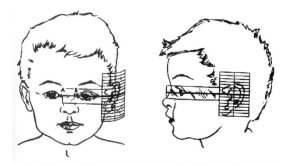

From: Saitta SC, and Zackai EH. 2005. Evaluation of the dysmorphic infant. In *Avery's Diseases of the Newborn,* 8th ed., Taeusch HW, Ballard RA, and Gleason CA, eds. Philadelphia: Saunders, 197. Reprinted by permission.

crying facies have been associated with other anomalies, particularly those of the cardiovascular system.[4] Facial palsy may also be secondary to nerve compression during delivery, which may occur as a result of forceps-assisted delivery, if delivery data support this.

EYES

If spacing appears abnormal, the distance between eyes can be measured and compared to standard values (Figure 13-1). This part of the examination is especially important if other dysmorphic features that suggest a syndrome are present. Epicanthal folds are rarely normal and usually suggest a syndrome (trisomy 21). The sclerae should be clear and white. If the sclerae appear deep blue, osteogenesis imperfecta should be considered. Glaucoma is manifested by a large cloudy cornea. Defects in the iris (coloboma) should be noted. Cataracts or retinoblastomas will present as a white pupil when the red reflex is assessed.

EARS

The ears are in normal position when the helix is intersected by a horizontal line drawn from the outer canthus of the eye perpendicular

FIGURE 13-3 ▲ Cryptorchidism.

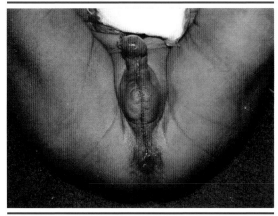

Courtesy of Presbyterian/St. Luke's Medical Center, Denver, Colorado.

to the vertical axis of the head (Figure 13-2).[5] If the helix falls below this line, the ears are low set. An ear is posteriorly rotated if its vertical axis deviates more than ten degrees from the vertical axis of the head. Malformations of the external ear are often associated with syndromes of multiple congenital anomalies that include renal malformations. The abnormalities may also indicate additional anomalies of the middle and inner ear associated with hearing loss.

NOSE AND MOUTH

A depressed nasal bridge or an extremely thin or unusually broad nose may occur in some malformation syndromes. Clefts of the soft or hard palate are visible to inspection. Palpation may be needed to detect a submucosal cleft. Macroglossia, or enlargement of the tongue, can be seen with Beckwith-Wiedemann syndrome.

CHEST

The chest is examined for size, symmetry, and structure. A malformed or small thorax may be the result of pulmonary hypoplasia or neuromuscular disorders. Pectus excavatum or pectus carinatum may occur as isolated findings or as part of congenital syndromes. Breast size and position should be noted, because widely spaced nipples occur with some genetic syndromes.

ABDOMEN

Asymmetry due to congenital anomalies or masses may first be appreciated by observation. Abnormal, absent, or misplaced kidneys are assessed by using deep palpation (see page 117 for technique). Most abdominal masses in newborns are enlarged kidneys caused by hydronephrosis or cystic renal disease.[3,6] A single umbilical artery is present in 0.3 percent of neonates, occurring more frequently in small for gestational age (SGA) infants, premature infants, and twins.[7] Approximately 40 percent of infants with a single umbilical artery have other major congenital anomalies, predominantly involving the genitourinary system, and have a significant mortality. In an otherwise normal infant, a single umbilical artery is associated with asymptomatic renal abnormalities in 7 percent of cases.[8]

GENITALIA

The genitalia are inspected immediately after birth to identify the infant's gender.

Females

The labia minora should be separated to detect whether the hymen, which normally has some opening, is imperforate. Enlargement of the uterus resulting from an imperforate hymen may be detected as a lower midline abdominal mass.

Males

Hypospadias, ventral location of the meatus, is relatively common. The meatus may be located anywhere from the proximal glans to the perineum, with more severe cases having a more proximal meatus. Infants with perineal or scrotal hypospadias and those with hypospadias of any location accompanied by nonpalpable testes should be evaluated for intersex conditions, including congenital

FIGURE 13-4 ▲ Polydactyly of the fingers.

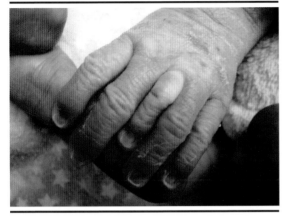

Courtesy of Presbyterian/St. Luke's Medical Center, Denver, Colorado.

FIGURE 13-5 ▲ Polydactyly of the toes.

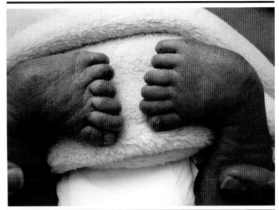

Courtesy of Presbyterian/St. Luke's Medical Center, Denver, Colorado.

adrenal hyperplasia. Epispadias, dorsal location of the meatus, is uncommon and usually associated with bladder exstrophy.

Ambiguous genitalia

Signs of ambiguous genitalia include an enlarged clitoris, fused labial folds, and palpable gonads in a phenotypic female and bifid scrotum, severe hypospadias, micropenis, and cryptorchidism (undescended testes) (Figure 13-3) in a phenotypic male. These conditions may be caused by abnormalities of sexual differentiation or congenital adrenal hyperplasia. Infants should be evaluated promptly and the appropriate gender assigned as soon as possible.

Anus

The anus and rectum should be checked carefully for patency, position, and size. Occasionally, large fistulas are mistaken for a normal anus, but if one checks carefully, it will be noted that a fistula will be either anterior or posterior to the usual location of a normal anus.[3]

Extremities

The extremities are examined for deformities and movement. The hands and feet are inspected for syndactyly (fusion of digits) and polydactyly (extra digits) (Figures 13-4 and 13-5). Syndactyly and polydactyly can be normal variants in a newborn with an otherwise normal exam, may be associated with a strong family history, or may be associated with various syndromes. The presence of a single palmar crease, or simian crease, should be noted. A single palmar crease occurs in 5–10 percent of the normal population and is common in newborns with trisomy 21. Talipes equinovarus (clubfoot) (Figure 13-6) is more common in males. The foot is turned downward and inward, and the sole is directed medially.[3] If position can be corrected with gentle force, it will resolve spontaneously. If not, orthopedic treatment and follow-up are necessary. The hips should be examined to detect developmental dysplasia of the hip.

Trunk and spine

A tuft of hair, discoloration, or hemangioma in the sacrococcygeal area may suggest an underlying vertebral anomaly. Soft tissue masses along the spine that are covered with normal skin may be lipomas or myelomeningoceles. A dimple without a visible base may indicate the presence of a pilonidal sinus or tract to the spinal cord.

FIGURE 13-6 ▲ Clubfoot.

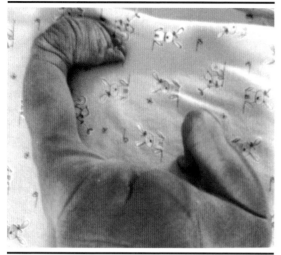

Courtesy of Presbyterian/St. Luke's Medical Center, Denver, Colorado.

FIGURE 13-7 ▲ Constriction defect from amniotic band.

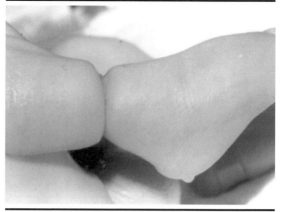

Courtesy of J. Hernandez, MD, The Children's Hospital, Denver, Colorado.

SHARING FINDINGS WITH PARENTS

When an anomaly is identified on physical examination, the infant should be shown to the parents as soon as possible. The physical finding may have been identified antenatally by ultrasound or may not have been expected. Either way, a spectrum of emotional responses from the parents is to be anticipated. Common responses of parents include guilt, intense grief, anger, denial, frustration, and a sense of isolation.[9] It is important to be sensitive to what the parents may be feeling. The defect should be shown to the parents and a factual description given, avoiding opinions or guesses. Genetic counseling should be provided to help parents answer any questions regarding the prognosis for the child and genetic risks for future pregnancies. Medical geneticists and genetic counselors have extensive knowledge of genetic disorders and congenital anomalies and are trained to provide families with psychological and emotional support. However, even a health care professional with a basic knowledge of genetics and Mendelian inheritance can be helpful when discussing the physical findings with the parents and can provide answers to general questions.

PROBLEMS IN MORPHOGENESIS

An anomaly is a structural defect, a deviation from normal. Every structural defect represents an inborn error in morphogenesis (development). Minor anomalies are unusual morphologic features that have no serious medical or cosmetic consequences to the patient. Almost any minor defect may occasionally be found as an unusual feature in a particular family. Minor external anomalies are most common in areas of complex and variable features, such as the face, ears, hands, and feet. Clinical diagnosis cannot usually be made based on a single defect. A specific diagnosis most often depends on recognition of an overall pattern of anomalies. Single minor anomalies are present in about 14 percent of newborns; 90 percent of infants with three or more minor anomalies also have one or more major defects, requiring significant surgical or cosmetic intervention.[2] Therefore, recognition of both minor and major anomalies is equally important.

Patterns of anomalies can be divided into four categories: malformation, deformation,

FIGURE 13-8 ▲ Amniotic bands resulting in finger amputation.

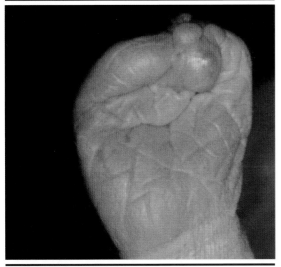

From: Clark DA. 2000. *Atlas of Neonatology.*
   Philadelphia: Saunders, 23. Reprinted by permission.

FIGURE 13-9 ▲ Hemangioma.

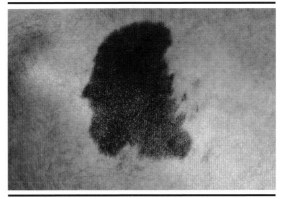

disruption, and dysplasia. A malformation is a primary structural defect in tissue formation, usually due to genetic or teratogenic reasons, that initiates a chain of subsequent defects.[5] Examples of malformations are congenital heart defects or neural tube defects. Malformations occur in all gradations, the manifestations ranging from nearly normal to more severe, and have a recurrence risk of 1–5 percent.[10]

With deformation, the fetal tissues are normally developed, but subjected to unusual mechanical forces (uterine constraint) that result in altered development. Congenital hip dislocation and clubfoot are examples of deformations that can be caused by intrauterine constraint. Most deformations have a very good prognosis with a very low recurrence risk.

Disruption represents normal developing tissue subjected to a destructive interruption. Usually, a body part rather than a specific organ is affected. Such disruptions may be vascular, infectious, or mechanical in origin. One example of this is disruption of normally

developing tissues by amniotic bands (Figure 13-7).[10] Disruptions are generally sporadic with low recurrence risks.

Dysplasia is an abnormal organization of cells into tissues and its morphological results. This can be localized, for example, a hemangioma (Figure 13-9), or generalized, such as achondroplasia (dysplasia of skeletal tissue). Dysplasias are usually not correctable, and the affected individual experiences the clinical effects of the underlying cell or tissue abnormality for life.[11] The occurrence of malformations can further be divided into several categories: syndromes, sequences, associations, and teratogenic.

GENETICS REVIEW

The nucleus of the human cell contains chromosomes, structures that include DNA and transmit genetic information during cell division and human development. Each human being has 46 chromosomes—22 pairs of autosomes and a pair of sex chromosomes (XX or XY), which determines gender. The chromosomes contain genes, the biologic units of inheritance. Genes control the physical, biochemical, and physiologic traits passed along to children from their parents. Genetic abnormalities are divided into three categories: those that influence gene dosage (chromosomal abnormalities such as trisomies), those that involve mutations in the genes themselves (over 6,000 rare single-gene disorders), and those that create a vulnerability to developmental errors that are then influenced by environmental factors (multifactorial inheritance disorders such as isolated malformations or schizophrenia).[10]

The gene mutations that cause greater than 6,000 individually rare disorders can be further classified into four categories: autosomal dominant, autosomal recessive, X-linked and mitochondrial mutations. Each individual receives two sets of chromosomes, one from each parent. Each pair of chromosomes contains a pair of genes, or alleles, that normally work together. A mutant gene is one that has altered in such a way that it can produce an abnormal trait.

Diseases caused by autosomal dominant genes are rare. A single mutant gene is dominant if it masks the effect of its paired gene and causes an obvious abnormality. The risk of the single mutant gene being passed on is 50 percent, but autosomal dominant disorders have a wide range of expression and will present in varying degrees between affected individuals due to influences of the normal paired gene, as well as the genetic and environmental background of the individual. Examples of autosomal dominant disorders are retinoblastoma and neurofibromatosis.

Autosomal recessive disorders are also rare, although the number of carriers for these diseases can be high. These disorders are inherited from normal parents who both have the same recessive mutant gene. In most cases, both parents of an affected individual are heterozygous carriers of the disease. Typically, one-fourth of their offspring will be normal heterozygotes, one-half will be normal carrier heterozygotes, and one-fourth will be homozygotes who have the disease. An example of an autosomal recessive disease is cystic fibrosis.[12]

Genes located on the sex chromosomes cause X-linked disorders. The Y chromosome does not appear to carry any disease-causing genes.

X-linked dominant traits are rare, but X-linked recessive diseases occur more commonly. A single copy of a mutant gene on the X chromosome will be expressed in the male because he has no normal partner gene. His daughters will all be carriers because they will receive his X gene, and his sons will all be normal because they receive his Y gene. Because females receive an X chromosome from each parent, they can be homozygous normal, homozygous for the X-linked disease, or heterozygous. Fifty percent of male offspring of X-linked recessive women will be affected, and 50 percent of her daughters will be carriers. Examples of X-linked disorders are Turner syndrome and Klinefelter syndrome.

Mitochondrial mutation disorders result from insufficient energy production in critical tissues. Most of these disorders present after the child is born, usually with visual loss, seizures, encephalopathy, progressive myopathy, or diabetes. The human egg is the source of mitochondria for all offspring and is therefore inherited only from the mother. Males with disorders caused by mitochondrial mutations have no risk of passing along the disorder to their offspring. Females, however, have a risk that approaches 100 percent. Female offspring of affected women will inherit some abnormal mitochondria, but may not manifest the disease.[10]

SYNDROMES

A syndrome is a collection of anomalies involving more than one developmental region or organ system or a pattern of multiple anomalies thought to be pathogenetically related.[11] Chromosomal syndromes are the usual malformation syndromes diagnosed in the neonatal period. The most common of these are trisomy 21, trisomy 18, trisomy 13, and 45,X. With the advent of the human genome project, more information is now available regarding

FIGURE 13-10 ▲ **Trisomy 21 (Down syndrome).**

Typical facies and significant decrease in tone.

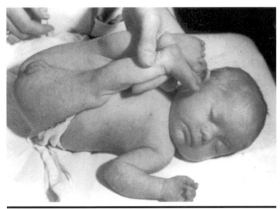

Courtesy of J. Hernandez, MD, The Children's Hospital, Denver, Colorado.

FIGURE 13-11 ▲ **Simian crease.**

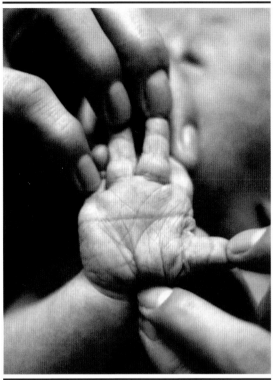

From: Clark DA. 2000. *Atlas of Neonatology.* Philadelphia: Saunders, 31. Reprinted by permission.

chromosome structure. Once thought to be associations, DiGeorge and Beckwith-Wiedemann have now been found to have chromosomal abnormalities as an underlying etiology and are more correctly categorized as syndromes.

TRISOMY 21 (DOWN SYNDROME)

The incidence of trisomy 21 is 1 in 660 newborns, making it the most common pattern of malformation in man.[10] Principal features include hypotonia, poor Moro reflex, hyperflexibility of joints, excess skin at the nape of the neck, flat facial profile (Figure 13-10), slanted palpebral fissures, and single transverse palmar (simian) creases (Figure 13-11). Associated anomalies include congenital heart defects, increased incidence of duodenal atresia, esophageal atresia, and imperforate anus. Most of the features of trisomy 21 may occur as isolated features in normal infants; therefore, it is the combination of features forming a recognizable pattern that permits early diagnosis.

TRISOMY 18 (EDWARDS SYNDROME)

The incidence of trisomy 18 is approximately 1 in 3,000 live births. There is a 3:1 preponderance of females to males. Trisomy

18 syndrome (Figure 13-12) is highly lethal with 50 percent mortality within the first week. Only 5–10 percent of affected infants will survive the first year, and they will have severe mental deficiencies.[9] Physical findings include prenatal and postnatal growth deficiency, micrognathia, overlapping digits, complex congenital heart disease, low-set ears, rocker-bottom clubfeet, and generalized hypertonicity. Associated anomalies include tracheoesophageal fistula or esophageal atresia, hemivertebrae, omphalocele, and myelomeningocele.

TRISOMY 13 (PATAU SYNDROME)

The incidence of trisomy 13 is approximately 1 in 5,000 births.[10] Trisomy 13 (Figure 13-13) is highly lethal with a median survival of seven days for infants with this syndrome. Physical findings include moderate

FIGURE 13-12 ▲ Trisomy 18.

A. Prominent occiput; short sternum; micrognathia; malformed, low-set ears. **B.** Overlapping fingers.
  C. Rocker-bottom feet.

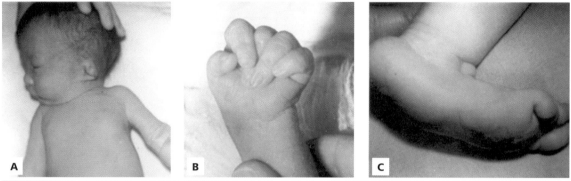

Courtesy of J. Hernandez, MD, The Children's Hospital, Denver, Colorado.

microcephaly, cleft lip, polydactyly, scalp cutis aplasia, microphthalmia, and congenital heart disease. Associated anomalies include cystic kidneys, holoprosencephaly, and rocker-bottom clubfeet. The identification of multiple midline defects is a way to recognize trisomy 13.

45,X (Turner Syndrome)

The incidence of Turner syndrome is approximately 1 in 2,500 live born females.[10] Ninety-five percent of conceptions are miscarried or stillborn. The 45,X syndrome (Figure 13-14) is usually compatible with survival if the fetus reaches term gestation. Physical findings include small stature, short webbed neck, lymphedema of the hands and feet, and ovarian dysgenesis.

DiGeorge Syndrome

DiGeorge syndrome is a chromosomal deletion of 22q11 causing absence or underdevelopment of the thymus and parathyroid glands. Estimated prevalence is 1:4,000 to 1:6,395. The male/female ratio is 1:1. Symptoms vary from patient to patient. Physical findings of DiGeorge syndrome include cardiac anomalies, usually conotruncal in nature, such as truncus arteriosus or aortic arch anomalies, small abnormally shaped ears, and mild nonspecific facial dysmorphology. Hypocalcemia is a prominent laboratory finding secondary to absence or hypoplasia of the parathyroid glands and thymus. Etiology has been associated with prenatal exposure to alcohol and isotretinoin (Accutane). There is a significant neonatal morbidity and mortality associated with the cardiac defects, immunodeficiency, and seizures related to hypocalcemia.

Beckwith-Wiedemann Syndrome

Beckwith-Wiedemann syndrome is caused by a deletion or abnormality on chromosome 11. An estimated 1 in 12,000 newborns are affected, although this sydrome may actually be more common, because infants with mild or unusual symptoms may not be diagnosed. Classified as an overgrowth syndrome, infants affected are considerably larger than normal (macrosomia) and continue to grow and gain weight at an unusual rate during childhood. It frequently presents with refractory hypoglycemia and polycythemia. Physical findings include macroglossia, omphalocele, and macrosomia. Polyhydramnios and a high incidence of prematurity are also common historical findings. Early diagnosis and aggressive treatment of hypoglycemia may prevent mental deficits.

FIGURE 13-13 ▲ Trisomy 13.

Bilateral cleft lip and palate, low-set ears, beak nose, and polydactyly.

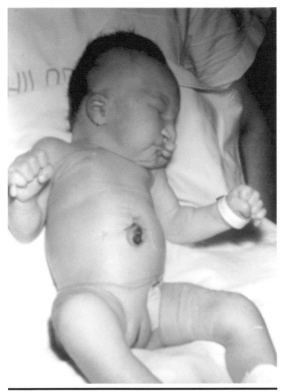

Courtesy of J. Hernandez, MD, The Children's Hospital, Denver, Colorado.

FIGURE 13-14 ▲ Turner syndrome.

Lymphedema (hands), webbed neck, low posterior hair line, low-set ears

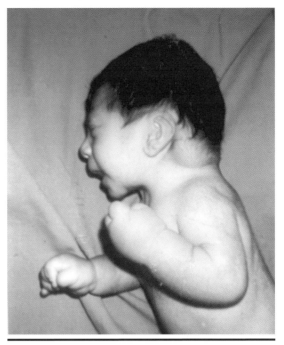

Courtesy of J. Hernandez, MD, The Children's Hospital, Denver, Colorado.

SEQUENCES

A sequence is a pattern of multiple anomalies derived from a single known or presumed structural defect or mechanical factor. The most common nonchromosomal deformation or disruption sequences diagnosed in the neonatal period are Potter oligohydramnios sequence, amniotic band sequence, arthrogryposis, and Robin sequence.

POTTER OLIGOHYDRAMNIOS SEQUENCE

The incidence of Potter sequence is 1 in 4,000 live births.[13] Almost all of these infants die in the neonatal period due to pulmonary hypoplasia. Potter sequence is a disease of severe oligohydramnios and its consequences. Renal agenesis, polycystic kidneys, urinary tract obstruction, or chronic leakage of amniotic fluid may be the cause of oligohydramnios. This results in intrauterine constraint of the fetus and pulmonary hypoplasia. Physical findings include refractory respiratory distress, frequently with concomitant pneumothoraces, clubfeet, hyperextensible fingers, large ears, low inner eye folds, and a beak nose (Figure 13-15). Anuria is typically present in the newborn. Prune belly (absent abdominal musculature, urinary tract abnormalities, and cryptorchidism) may also be an associated finding. Diagnosis is usually confirmed by renal ultrasound and autopsy findings of urinary tract abnormalities.

AMNIOTIC BAND SEQUENCE

The incidence of amniotic band sequence is 1 in 2,000–4,000 live births.[13] Early amnion rupture occurs, and small bands of amnion

FIGURE 13-15 ▲ Constraint deformities.

A. Secondary to Potter sequence: narrow, flaired thorax, folded ear. **B.** Typical Potter facies: flattened nose, ear anomalies, furrowed brow.

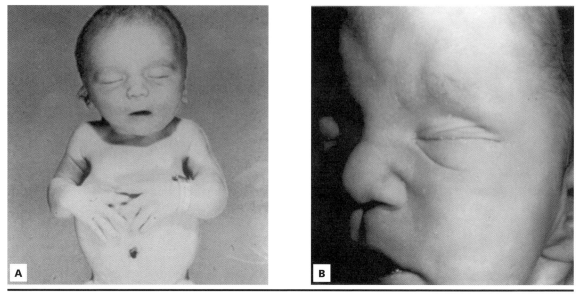

Courtesy of J. Hernandez, MD, The Children's Hospital, Denver, Colorado.

encircle developing structures, usually limbs, leading to constrictions, intrauterine amputations, and/or umbilical cord constriction (see Figure 13-7). In addition, deformational defects occur secondary to decreased fetal movement, the result of tethering of a limb by an amniotic band. The decreased fetal movement may result in scoliosis or foot deformities. No two affected fetuses will have the exact same features, and there is no single feature that consistently occurs. Examination of the placenta and membranes is diagnostic.

ARTHROGRYPOSIS (MULTIPLE JOINT FIXATIONS)

Arthrogryposis occurs in approximately 1 in 3,000 live births.[13] Physical findings include joint contractures, extensions, and dislocations. Joint contractures can be secondary to intrinsic factors affecting the fetus such as early onset of neurologic, muscle, and joint problems or to extrinsic factors such as

fetal crowding and constraint. Neurologic abnormality is the most common cause of arthrogryposis. Nonjoint-related anomalies may indicate that the arthrogryposis is part of a multiple defect syndrome. Affected infants should also be assessed for scoliosis (Figures 13-16 and 13-17) and hip dislocation.

ROBIN SEQUENCE

Robin sequence occurs in approximately 1 in 8,000 live births.[13] The initiating defect of this sequence is severe hypoplasia of the mandible causing the tongue to be posteriorly located resulting in severe upper airway obstruction and cleft palate. Physical findings include micrognathia, cleft palate, and low-set ears. Respiratory distress secondary to upper airway obstruction may be present. Many syndromes have the craniofacial features of Robin sequence. If noncraniofacial primary malformations are present, then other diagnoses should be considered.

FIGURE 13-16 ▲ Scoliosis.

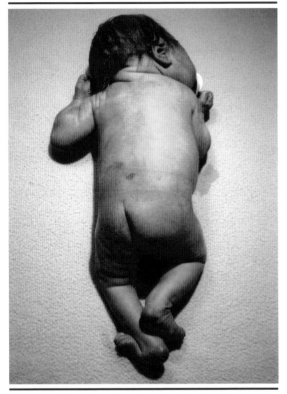

Courtesy of Presbyterian/St. Luke's Medical Center, Denver, Colorado.

FIGURE 13-17 ▲ X-ray of scoliosis.

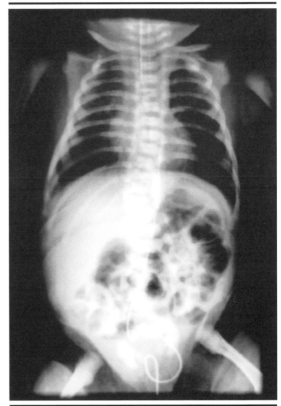

ASSOCIATIONS

Association refers to a nonrandom occurrence of multiple malformations for which no specific or common etiology has been identified.[5] The most usual associations are VATER/VACTERL, and CHARGE.

VATER/VACTERL ASSOCIATION

VATER/VACTERL is an acronym that includes **v**ertebral anomalies, **a**nal atresia, **t**racheo**e**sophageal fistula, and **r**adial and/or **r**enal dysplasia. **C**ardiac defects, single umbilical artery, **l**imb abnormalities, and IUGR are also nonrandom features of this pattern of anomalies. VATER/VACTERL occurs in 1 in 5,000 live births, and the etiology is unknown.[13] Diagnosis requires exclusion of other similar disorders, including chromosomal syndromes. Most infants diagnosed

with VATER/VACTERL have normal brain function and thus merit vigorous attempts toward rehabilitation.

CHARGE ASSOCIATION

CHARGE association includes **c**oloboma, **h**eart disease, choanal **a**tresia, **r**estricted growth and development, **g**enital anomalies, **e**ar anomalies, and/or deafness. Not all features need be present, and the extent of involvement of each system is widely variable.[11] Occurrence of CHARGE association is 1 in 10,000–15,000 live births.[13] CHARGE association often presents as a medical emergency because of the presence of choanal atresia, serious heart defects, and swallowing difficulties. Associated anomalies include cleft lip and palate as well as unilateral facial palsies. The etiology is unknown, but it has been suggested that this condition represents a chromosomal

TABLE 13-1 ▲ Teratogens Known to Cause Human Birth Defects

Agents	Most Common Congenital Anomalies
Drugs	
Alcohol	*Fetal alcohol syndrome:* intrauterine growth restriction (IUGR); mental deficiency, microcephaly; ocular anomalies; joint abnormalities; short palpebral fissures
Aminopterin	IUGR; skeletal defects; malformations of the central nervous system (CNS), notably meroanencephaly (most of the brain is absent)
Androgens and high doses of progestogens	Varying degrees of masculinization of female fetuses: ambiguous external genitalia resulting in labial fusion and clitoral hypertrophy
Busulfan	Stunted growth, skeletal abnormalities, corneal opacities, cleft palate, hypoplasia of various organs
Cocaine	IUGR; prematurity, microcephaly, cerebral infarction, urogenital abnormalities, neurobehavioral disturbances
Diethylstilbestrol	Abnormalities of the uterus and vagina; cervical erosion and ridges
Isotretinoin (13-cis-retinoic acid)	Craniofacial abnormalities, neural tube defects (NTDs) such as spina bifida cystica, cardiovascular defects, cleft palate, thymic aplasia
Lithium carbonate	Various anomalies usually involving the heart and great vessels
Methotrexate	Multiple anomalies, especially skeletal, involving the face, cranium, limbs, and vertebral column
Phenytoin (Dilantin)	*Fetal hydantoin syndrome:* IUGR, microcephaly, mental deficiency, ridged frontal suture, inner epicanthal folds, eyelid ptosis, broad depressed nasal bridge, phalangeal hypoplasia
Tetracycline	Stained teeth, hypoplasia of enamel
Thalidomide	Abnormal development of limbs (e.g., meromelia [partial absence] and amelia [complete absence], facial anomalies, systemic anomalies (e.g., cardiac and kidney defects)
Trimethadione	Developmental delay, V-shaped eyebrows, low-set ears, cleft lip and/or palate
Valproic acid	Craniofacial anomalies; NTDs, often hydrocephalus, heart and skeletal defects
Warfarin	Nasal hypoplasia, stippled epiphyses, hypoplastic phalanges; eye anomalies; mental deficiency
Chemicals	
Methylmercury	Cerebral atrophy, spasticity, seizures, mental deficiency
Polychlorinated biphenyls (PCBs)	IUGR, skin discoloration
Infections	
Cytomegalovirus	Microcephaly, chorioretinitis, sensorineural hearing loss, delayed psychomotor/mental development, hepatosplenomegaly, hydrocephaly, cerebral palsy, brain (periventricular) calcification
Herpes simplex virus	Skin vesicles and scarring, chorioretinitis, hepatomegaly, thrombocytopenia, petechiae, hemolytic anemia, hydranencephaly
Human immunodeficiency virus (HIV)	Growth failure; microcephaly; prominent boxlike forehead, flattened nasal bridge, hypertelorism, triangular philtrum and patulous (patent) lips
Human parvovirus B19	Eye defects, degenerative changes in fetal tissues
Rubella virus	IUGR, postnatal growth retardation; cardiac and great vessel abnormalities; microcephaly; sensorineural deafness; cataracts, microphthalmos, glaucoma, pigmented retinopathy; mental deficiency; newborn bleeding; hepatosplenomegaly; osteopathy; tooth defects
Toxoplasma gondii	Microcephaly; mental deficiency; microphthalmia; hydrocephaly; chorioretinitis; cerebral calcifications; hearing loss; neurologic disturbances
Treponema pallidum	Hydrocephalus, congenital deafness, mental deficiency, abnormal teeth and bones
Varicella virus	Cutaneous scars (dermatome distribution); neurologic anomalies (limb paresis [incomplete paralysis], hydrocephaly, seizures, and so on); cataracts; microphthalmia; Horner syndrome; optic atrophy; nystagmus; chorioretinitis; microcephaly; mental deficiency; skeletal anomalies (hypoplasia of limbs, fingers, toes, and so on); urogenital abnormalities
Venezuelan equine encephalitis virus	Microcephaly; microphthalmia; cerebral agenesis; CNS necrosis; hydrocephalus
Radiation	
High levels of ionizing radiation	Microcephaly; mental deficiency; skeletal anomalies; growth restriction; cataracts

Adapted from: Moore KL, and Persaud TVN. 2008. *The Developing Human: Clinically Oriented Embryology,* 8th ed. Philadelphia: Saunders, 472. Reprinted by permission.

syndrome. Most patients have some degree of mental deficiency or central nervous system defects and visual or auditory anomalies that further compromise cognitive function.

TERATOGENS

Although the human embryo is well protected in the uterus, maternal exposure to teratogens may cause developmental disruptions. A teratogen is any agent external to the fetus that causes a structural or functional disability postnatally. Teratogens can be drugs and chemicals, altered maternal metabolic states, or infectious agents (Table 13-1). Known teratogenic factors cause 5 to 10 percent of congenital anomalies. Susceptibility to a teratogen is determined by the embryologic stage of development when exposed. Each part, tissue, and organ of an embryo has a critical period during which development can be disrupted (Figure 13-18). The most critical period in development is when cell division, cell differentiation, and morphogenesis are at their peak.

FETAL ALCOHOL SYNDROME

Alcohol is thought to be the most common teratogen to which a fetus may be exposed. The incidence of this disorder in the U.S. is estimated to be 2 in 1,000 live births.[10] Common features include short palpebral fissures, epicanthal folds, a flat nasal bridge, a long, simple philtrum, a thin upper lip, small hypoplastic nails, and growth deficiency.[13] Associated anomalies are cardiac defects, ventricular septal defect being the most common, and microcephaly. Long-term effects include mental deficiency and behavioral problems.

FETAL COCAINE SYNDROME

Cocaine is one of the most commonly abused illicit drugs.[11] Infants characteristically are SGA and present with hyperirritability. No definitive physical findings have been established. There is an increased incidence

of genitourinary tract anomalies such as hydronephrosis, hypospadias, and prune belly syndrome, as well as central nervous system abnormalities such as microcephaly, porencephaly, and infarction that may occur.

ANTICONVULSANTS

Phenytoin and valproic acid are commonly prescribed for management of maternal epilepsy; however, both are teratogens. Fetal hydantoin syndrome is characterized by a typical facies (a broad, low nasal bridge, hypertelorism, epicanthal folds, ptosis, and prominent, malformed ears).[13] Exposed infants also have a high incidence of hypoplasia or aplasia of the fifth fingernail and toenail.

Fetal valproate syndrome features consist of a prominent or fused metopic suture, epicanthal folds, midface hypoplasia, anteverted nostrils, oral cleft, cardiac defects, hypospadias, and psychomotor delay.

INFANTS OF DIABETIC MOTHERS

Maternal altered metabolic states can lead to a higher risk of abnormalities in the newborn. Poorly controlled maternal diabetes mellitus with persistent hyperglycemia and ketosis, particularly during embryogenesis, is associated with a two- to threefold higher incidence of birth defects.[2] Infants of diabetic mothers (IDMs) present with anomalies in approximately 1 in 2,000 births. Common anomalies include holoprosencephaly (failure of the forebrain to divide into hemispheres), meroencephaly (partial absence of the brain), sacral agenesis, vertebral anomalies, congenital heart defects, limb defects, and cleft palate. Improved diabetic control during gestation dramatically decreases the incidence of IDM-related malformations, but does not reduce it back to baseline.[13]

INFECTIOUS DISEASES

Congenital anomalies also may be associated with certain infections during pregnancy.

FIGURE 13-18 ▲ Embryonic and fetal development.

Schematic illustration of critical periods in human prenatal development. During the first two weeks of development, the embryo is usually not susceptible to teratogens; a teratogen damages either all or most of the cells, resulting in death of the embryo, or damages only a few cells, allowing the conceptus to recover and the embryo to develop without birth defects. [____] *denotes highly sensitive periods* when major defects may be produced (e.g., amelia, absence of limbs, neural tube defects such as spina bifida cystica). [____] indicates stages that are less sensitive to teratogens when minor defects may be induced (e.g., hypoplastic thumbs).

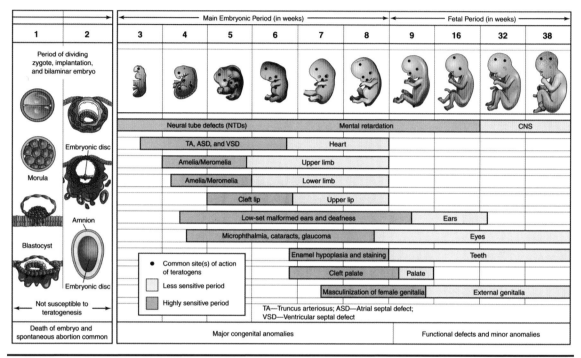

From: Moore KL, and Persaud TVN. 2008. *The Developing Human: Clinically Oriented Embryology,* 8th ed. Philadelphia: Saunders, 473. Reprinted by permission.

The common and best-understood infections are represented by the acronym TORCH, which stands for **t**oxoplasmosis, **o**ther agents (including syphilis), **r**ubella, **c**ytomegalovirus, and **h**erpes simplex. Common anomalies are IUGR, microcephaly, chorioretinitis, intracranial calcification, microphthalmia, and cataracts.[11]

RESOURCES

The World Wide Web is a powerful tool to utilize when searching for information regarding birth defects, including specific conditions, diagnosis, prevention and screening, research, and national organizations. An abundance of reliable and up-to-date information from expert sources can be accessed in a short time. Each of the sources listed below provides links to alternate websites if additional information is desired. To begin a general search, access the following reputable websites:

- March of Dimes Birth Defects Foundation
  http://www.marchofdimes.com/
  professionals/14332_1206.asp
- National Institute of Child Health and
  Human Development
  http://www.nichd.nih.gov/health/topics/
  birth_defects.cfm
- Centers for Disease Control and
  Prevention
  http://www.cdc.gov/ncbddd/bd/faq1.htm

- National Newborn Screening and Genetics Resource Center
  http://genes-r-us.uthscsa.edu/
- Organization of Teratology Information Services
  http://otispregnancy.org/hm
- Online Mendelian Inheritance in Man
  http://www.ncbi.nlm.nih.gov/sites/entrez?db=OMIM
- Medline Plus
  http://www.nlm.nih.gov/medlineplus/birthdefects.html
- GeneTests
  http://genetests.org/
- The Genetic Alliance
  http://www.geneticalliance.org/

SUMMARY

The approach to the evaluation of the dysmorphic infant is multifaceted and begins with a thorough history and physical exam. With experience, the examiner's identification of physical findings on the continuum of normal to abnormal is enhanced. A general knowledge of genetics and common disorders is helpful when counseling parents. Multiple resources including genetic counselors and Internet websites are available to health care professionals and parents who are involved in providing care to the dysmorphic infant.

REFERENCES

1. March of Dimes. 2007. Birth Defects Monitoring Program. Retrieved July 21, 2007, from Perinatal Data Snapshots www.marchofdimes.com/peristats.
2. Moore KL, and Persaud TVN. 2008. *The Developing Human: Clinically Oriented Embryology,* 8th ed. Philadelphia: Saunders, 457–486.
3. Gomella TL. Newborn physical examination. 2004. In *Neonatology: Management, Procedures, On-Call Problems, Diseases, and Drugs,* 5th ed., Gomella TL, et al., eds. New York: Lange, 29–38.
4. Rioja-Mazza D, et al. 2005. Asymmetric crying facies: A possible marker for congenital malformations. *Journal of Maternal-Fetal & Neonatal Medicine* 18(4): 275–277.
5. Hudgins L, and Cassidy SB. 2006. Congenital anomalies. In *Neonatal-Perinatal Medicine: Diseases of the Fetus and Infant,* 8th ed., Martin RJ, Fanaroff AA, and Walsh MC, eds. Philadelphia: Mosby, 561–582.
6. Pulito AR. 2004. Surgical diseases of the newborn. In *Neonatology: Management, Procedures, On-Call Problems, Diseases, and Drugs,* 5th ed., Gomella TL, et al., eds. New York: Lange, 572–584.
7. Thummala MR, Raju TN, and Langenberg P. 1998. Isolated single umbilical artery anomaly and the risk for congenital malformations: A meta-analysis. *Journal of Pediatric Surgery* 33(4): 580–585.
8. Lissauer T. 2006. Physical examination of the newborn. In *Neonatal-Perinatal Medicine: Diseases of the Fetus and Infant,* 8th ed., Fanaroff AA, Martin RJ, and Walsh MC, eds. Philadelphia: Mosby, 513–528.
9. Klaus MHY, Kennell JH, and De Pompei PM. 2006. Care of the mother, father, and infant. In *Neonatal-Perinatal Medicine: Diseases of the Fetus and Infant,* 8th ed., Fanaroff AA, Martin RJ, and Walsh MC, eds. Philadelphia: Mosby, 645–659.
10. Jones KL. 2006. *Smith's Recognizable Patterns of Human Malformation,* 6th ed. Philadelphia: Saunders, 2, 7, 14, 18, 76, 646, 796, 810.
11. Saitta SC, and Zackai EH. 2005. Evaluation of the dysmorphic infant. In *Avery's Diseases of the Newborn,* 8th ed., Taeusch HW, Ballard RA, and Gleason CA, eds. Philadelphia: Saunders, 194–203.
12. McCance KL, and Huether SE. 2006. *Pathophysiology: The Biologic Basis for Disease in Adults and Children,* 5th ed. Philadelphia: Mosby, 138.
13. Hall BD. 2004. Common multiple congenital anomaly syndromes. In *Neonatology: Management, Procedures, On-Call Problems, Diseases, and Drugs,* 5th ed., Gomella TL, et al., eds. New York: Lange, 373–380.

NOTES

NOTES

14 Pain Assessment in the Newborn

Marlene Walden, PhD, RN, CCNS, NNP-BC
Carol Turnage Carrier, MSN, RN, CNS

Over the last several decades, there has been an increased awareness of the importance of assessing and managing pain in hospitalized newborns. One only has to spend time in the NICU to observe how frequently newborns encounter postoperative, procedural, and disease-related pain throughout their hospital stay. Although neonates cannot verbally communicate pain, they do display physiologic and behavioral cues that caregivers can use as objective and valid indicators of the infant's pain experience.[1] Caregivers must know the potential causes of pain and use a high index of suspicion when gauging the infant's response cues for the presence, absence, or intensity of pain.[2,3] The assessment of the infant's response cues is an essential first step to optimally addressing the infant's pain.

APPROACH TO PAIN ASSESSMENT

Pain assessment in the newborn and especially the preterm neonate presents a challenge to even the most skilled clinician. Dependence on a pain score to identify pain consistently and accurately will lead to undertreated neonates due to the number of variables that affect physiologic and behavioral responses to painful stimuli. Pain assessment tools are useful insofar as a normal baseline is known and the score is interpreted based on a change from baseline parameters. If a patient is admitted in pain or baseline parameters are abnormal, the pain score may be misinterpreted, and undertreatment or overtreatment may occur. More information is required for interpreting pain in neonatal patients.

Infants in neonatal intensive care may or may not respond to pain with clear signals for a variety of reasons such as low energy reserves, sedation, paralysis, and vague or unclear behavioral cues due to illness and/or prematurity. Therefore, a number of factors must be considered in assessing neonatal pain. A complete approach to assessment is required for the neonatal nurse to adequately determine the presence of pain, interpret the findings, and take action as an advocate for her patients (Figure 14-1). The process involves data collection, a systematic approach to evaluation, and a method of documentation.

DATA COLLECTION

Assessment of pain in infants depends on the collection of various types of data, including demographic and historic data, current physiologic and behavioral data, and risk factors for pain (Table 14-1). For successful interpretation and intervention, nursing judgment and

FIGURE 14-1 ▲ Pain assessment algorithm, generalized.

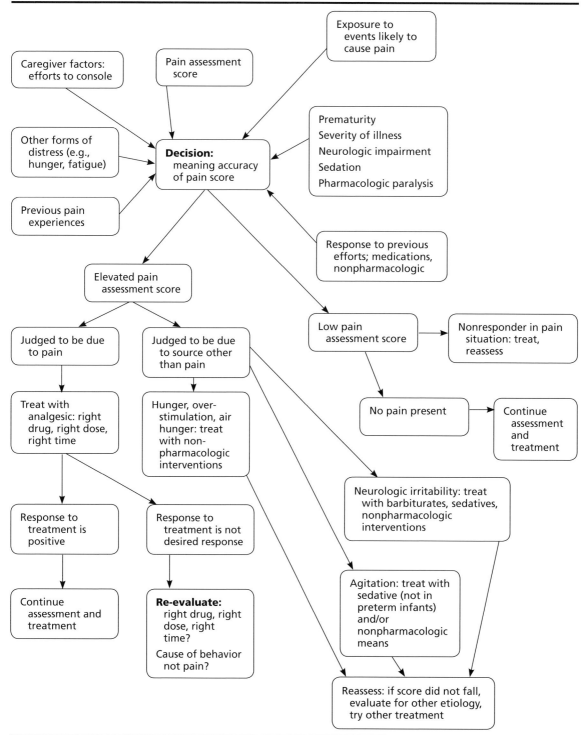

Adapted from: Hummel P, and van Dijk M. 2006. Pain assessment: Current status and challenges. *Seminars in Fetal & Neonatal Medicine* 11(4): 242. Reprinted by permission.

TABLE 14-1 ▲ Data collection for pain assessment.

Nursing Judgment		
• Experience		
• Familiarity with infant's physical/behavioral baseline		
• Knowledge, skills, and attitude regarding pain		
↓	↓	↓
Infant	**History/Current Status**	**Risk for Pain**
Age	Baseline vital signs	Disease/illness
• Postmenstrual	Baseline behavior	Procedures (e.g., chest tube, peripherally inserted central catheter placement)
• Gestational	Current vital signs and behaviors	
Behavioral state	Physical assessment	Tests
• Sleep	Previous pain scores	Surgery
• Awake	Current pain scores	Wounds
• Drowsy	Vital sign and pain score trends	Indwelling tubes/lines
Acuity	Risk for pain	Immobility
• Disease/illness	• Procedures	
• Wound/incision	• Tests	
Irritability and consolability	• Recent surgery	
Neurologic status	Prior pain experience	
	Medications	

communication, both written and verbal, are vital.[4] Without the whole process, pain may go unobserved and untreated.

SYSTEMATIC APPROACH TO EVALUATION

Data collection is only part of the process; it is what a nurse does with the data that will determine whether pain is viewed as being present. Judgment comes from education about neonatal pain, experience, and a belief that pain assessment is essential for quality care in the NICU. Once the critical component of nursing judgment is present, the nurse can provide a convincing argument for pain intervention to medical staff. An overall approach to pain assessment that is systematic and provides guidance for nursing practice is shown in Table 14-2.[5,6]

In a quasi-experimental study, 24 pediatric nurses were asked to assess pain after viewing videotapes of infants (birth to 12 months) and reading written clinical information. Their pain assessments were compared with assessments by 60 pediatric nurses who viewed the same videotapes but without the written background data. The nurses who only viewed the videotapes rated the pain level as significantly lower than those who also read background clinical information. These nurses were similar in age and experience, demonstrating that clinical information is important for the identification of pain, particularly in nonverbal

TABLE 14-2 ▲ Infant Pain Assessment Process

1. Acknowledging pain cues/signs
2. Hypothesizing the reason for distress
3. Analyzing assessment data using nursing judgment
4. Evaluating effectiveness of comfort measures
5. Assessing consolability following comfort measures
6. Speculating on the pain intensity
7. Providing pain medication when indicated
8. Reassessing at appropriate intervals for analgesic effectiveness or medication tolerance

Adapted from: Fuller BF. 1998. The process of infant pain assessment. *Applied Nursing Research* 11(2): 62–68.

FIGURE 14-2 ▲ **Pain scales with vital signs graph for trending pain signs.**

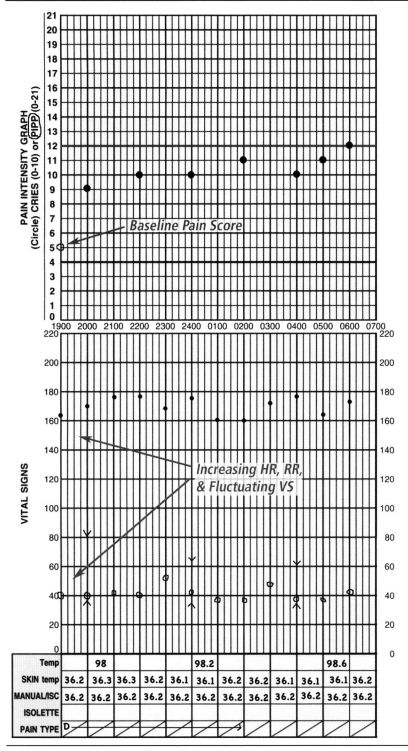

Key: D, disease; HR, heart rate; RR, respiratory rate; VS, vital signs

patients. Nurses from the video only group also judged infants from 0 to 3 months as having lower pain levels than those 10 to 12 months.[7] Therefore, judgment of pain requires the nurse to have complete information, especially for infants who demonstrate weak pain signals.

DOCUMENTATION

Documentation of pain data should be done in a way that helps the caregiver analyze an infant's pain and the response to intervention immediately and over time. A single pain score provides immediate information about pain, but does not support analysis of fluctuating scores, adequacy of pain control, gradually increasing pain, or emerging tolerance to a particular medication, dose, or dose interval. Individual scores are useful when an acute event causes elevated pain scores. However, gradually increasing scores may be missed until the score is high enough to rate intervention. By that time, pain management may be more difficult. A documentation design that can be used in print or electronic format is a graph for plotting pain scores over 12 to 24 hours. Formats in this layout offer a practical solution to the busy clinician. Subtle changes are easier to see if the documentation method allows for an overview of vital signs along with pain scores, as is the case when using a graphic display (Figure 14-2). Nurses familiar with the infant's baseline assessment of vital signs and behaviors will be able to note the subtle variations over time, which may lead to better identification and management of pain.

ASSESSMENT OF PAIN

Pain assessment relies on the careful observational skills of the examiner. Pain can be assessed using behavioral measures or physiologic measures, but the best assessment is done when a multidimensional approach is employed.

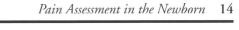

FIGURE 14-3 ▲ Characteristic of "cry face."

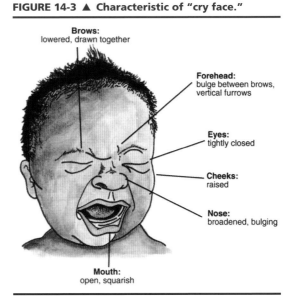

Brows: lowered, drawn together

Forehead: bulge between brows, vertical furrows

Eyes: tightly closed

Cheeks: raised

Nose: broadened, bulging

Mouth: open, squarish

From: Wong D. 1995. *Whaley & Wong's Nursing Care of Infants and Children,* 5th ed. Philadelphia: Mosby, 1070. Reprinted by permission.

BEHAVIORAL INDICATORS

The clinician can observe the infant's facial activity, crying, and body movements to assess for the possibility that the infant is experiencing pain. A "cry face" (Figure 14-3) consisting of subtle changes in the infant's facial expressions such as brow bulge, eye squeeze, and nasolabial furrow is the most specific indicator of acute pain in newborns.[8–12] Gestational age and behavioral state will have a significant impact on the infant's facial expressions, with younger and sleeping infants having a diminished or delayed response.

The clinician can also observe and listen to the infant's cry. Different types of cry—such as high pitched, harsh, intense—may communicate the urgency or severity of distress.[13,14] Absence of cry or objective signs of pain does not necessarily mean that the infant is not in pain, but may only signal that the infant's response capability has been depleted.[12,15–18]

Individual body movements can also provide helpful information about the infant's pain experience. Infants, particularly healthy term

FIGURE 14-4 ▲ Premature Infant Pain Profile (PIPP).

Infant study number: _____

Date/time: _____

Event: _____

Process	Indicator	0	1	2	3	Score
Chart	Gestational age	36 weeks and more	32 weeks to 35 weeks, 6 days	28 weeks to 31 weeks, 6 days	28 weeks and less	
Observe infant 15 seconds before event Observe baseline Heart rate ___ Oxygen saturation ___	Behavioral state	Active/awake Eyes open Facial movements	Quiet/awake Eyes open No facial movements	Active/sleep Eyes closed Facial movements	Quiet/sleep Eyes closed No facial movements	
Observe infant 30 seconds after event	Heart rate maximum ___	0–4 beats/ minute increase	5–14 beats/ minute increase	15–24 beats/ minute increase	25 beats/minute or more increase	
Observe infant 30 seconds after event	Oxygen saturation minimum ___	0–2.4% decrease	2.5–4.9% decrease	5.0–7.4% decrease	7.5% or more decrease	
Observe infant 30 seconds after event	Brow bulge	None 0–9% of time	Minimum 10–39% of time	Moderate 40–69% of time	Maximum 70% of time or more	
Observe infant 30 seconds after event	Eye squeeze	None 0–9% of time	Minimum 10–39% of time	Moderate 40–69% of time	Maximum 70% of time or more	
Observe infant 30 seconds after event	Nasolabial furrow	None 0–9% of time	Minimum 10–39% of time	Moderate 40–69% of time	Maximum 70% of time or more	
					Total Score	

Adapted from: Stevens B, et al. 1996. Premature Infant Pain Profile: Development and initial validation. *Clinical Journal of Pain* 12(1): 22. Reprinted by permission.

newborns, may use reflexive limb withdrawal in response to noxious stimuli to signal pain.[19] Because of inadequate muscle strength, posture, tone, and movement compared to term newborns, preterm neonates have less vigorous and robust pain responses.[15,16,20] Other observed behaviors exhibited by preterm neonates include increased flexion and extension of arms and toe and finger splay.[21–23]

Physiologic Indicators

Infants may also communicate pain through physiologic changes. The clinician can often observe vital sign changes on the infant's cardiorespiratory monitor to assess an infant's pain. Newborns will acutely respond to pain of handling or procedures with increases in heart rate and blood pressure while oxygen saturation decreases.[11,24] Although vital signs may be the sole method of assessing pain in pharmacologically paralyzed, sedated, or severely neurologically impaired infants, these assessments may not be valid if pain is prolonged because changes in vital signs cannot be maintained.[11]

Assessment Tools

Pain assessment is best accomplished using a published pain assessment tool with known reliability and validity that has been demonstrated to be clinically useful and feasible in the clinical setting. The clinician should also

FIGURE 14-5 ■ CRIES: Neonatal postoperative pain assessment score.

	Scoring Criteria for Each Assessment			
	0	1	2	Infant's Score
Crying	No	High pitched	Inconsolable	
Requires O₂ for saturation >95%	No	<30%	>30%	
Increased vital signs*	HR and BP within 10% of preoperative value	HR or BP 11–20% higher than preoperative value	HR or BP 21% or more above preoperative value	
Expression	None	Grimace	Grimace/grunt	
Sleepless	No	Wakes at frequent intervals	Constantly awake	
			Total score†	

* BP should be done last.

† Add scores for all assessments to calculate total score.

Key: BP = blood pressure; HR = heart rate.

© S. Krechel, MD, and J. Bildner, RNC, CNS. Neonatal pain assessment tool developed at the University of Missouri–Columbia. Reprinted by permission.

consider choosing an instrument based on a similar infant population, setting, and type of pain.[25] In order to best assess trends over time, the clinician should use the same tool over consecutive assessments when evaluating pain in a given newborn.

At least 35 different pain assessment instruments exist.[25] Perhaps the three best validated ones are the Premature Infant Pain Profile (PIPP) developed by Stevens and associates, the CRIES developed by Bildner and Krechel, and the Neonatal Infant Pain Scale (NIPS) developed by Lawrence and colleagues.[26–28]

The PIPP (Figure 14-4) was originally developed to measure procedural pain, but recently has also been used in newborns to assess postoperative pain.[29,30] Although the PIPP may be presumed to be valid only with preterm neonates, it has been tested in neonates ranging in age from extremely preterm up to 40 weeks postconceptional age. The PIPP incorporates two contextual factors that may account for the infant's less robust pain responses that can result from immaturity or behavioral state.

By scoring infants who are younger or asleep higher on the PIPP, the adjusted scores do not penalize those known to be less capable of mounting a robust response to noxious stimuli. The PIPP contains two physiologic indicators (i.e., heart rate and oxygen saturation) and three facial indicators (i.e., brow bulge, eye squeeze, and nasolabial furrow). Physiologic and behavioral indicators are fairly straightforward to score when scoring procedural pain, but are often more challenging if used to score ongoing pain. If no clear 15-second baseline period is available for scoring, the clinician must sometimes judge baseline parameters using either preoperative vital signs or estimated vital signs before the known painful event. Although total scores vary between 18 and 21, depending on the infant's gestational age, scores between 7 and 12 usually signify mild to moderate pain requiring nonpharmacologic comfort measures. Scores greater than 12 indicate moderate to severe pain requiring pharmacologic pain intervention in addition to comfort measures.

The CRIES (Figure 14-5) is another instrument that has been used extensively to assess pain in the newborn. CRIES is an acronym for the five parameters it measures: **C**rying, **R**equires oxygen to maintain saturation greater than 95 percent, **I**ncreased vital signs, **E**xpression, and **S**leepless. Although it was originally developed to assess postoperative pain in infants between 32 and 36 weeks

FIGURE14-6 ▲ Neonatal Infant Pain Scale (NIPS).

	Before Time*		During Time*					After Time*		
	1	2	1	2	3	4	5	1	2	3
Facial expression 0: Relaxed 1: Grimace										
Cry 0: No cry 1: Whimper 2: Vigorous										
Breathing patterns 0: Relaxed 1: Change in breathing										
Arms 0: Relaxed/restrained 1: Flexed/extended										
Legs 0: Relaxed/restrained 1: Flexed/extended										
State of arousal 0: Sleeping/awake 1: Fussy										
Total										

* Time is measured in one (1) minute intervals.

gestational age, studies have recently documented its clinical utility in gauging procedural pain in preterm and term neonates.[31–33] Infants previously requiring oxygen are more difficult to score using the CRIES instrument. It provides no specific guideline for infants previously requiring oxygen, so nursing judgment is required to systematically adjust scores in this category to account for increases in oxygen levels above baseline values. In addition, if the CRIES is used for procedural pain assessment, baseline vital signs immediately before the procedure can be used for scoring the category of "increased vital signs." Total scores for the CRIES range from 0 to 10, with scores less than 4 indicative of mild pain requiring nonpharmacologic pain relief measures and 5 or greater consistent with moderate to severe pain requiring pharmacologic intervention in conjunction with comfort measures.

The NIPS (Figure 14-6), like the PIPP, was originally developed to assess procedural pain in preterm and term newborns, but recent literature also validates its utility with postoperative pain.[34,35] The NIPS examines five behavioral parameters (i.e., facial expression, crying, arms, legs, and state of arousal) and one physiologic parameter (i.e., breathing pattern). Total score ranges from 0 to 7. Scoring of the NIPS does not contain physiologic parameters requiring cardiorespiratory monitoring; therefore, this tool is particularly useful in assessing pain in healthy term infants. Although guidelines for pain interventions based on total score are not provided by the developers of the NIPS, all pain instruments in neonates are based on the premise of increasing pain intensity.

Therefore, in tools without scoring guidelines for pain management, when pain scores reach the midrange of the total possible points for that tool (i.e., approximately 4 or greater with the NIPS), the clinician may infer that the infant is experiencing moderate to severe pain and pharmacologic intervention for that pain is warranted.

SPECIAL POPULATIONS

The evidence base on pain assessment is still limited for extremely low for gestational age (ELGA), neurologically impaired, pharmacologically paralyzed or sedated, and other special populations of infants.

EXTREMELY LOW FOR GESTATIONAL AGE INFANTS

Gestation at birth and postmenstrual age both affect pain response, with more robust responses to pain stimuli noted with advancing gestation and postmenstrual age.[36] The ELGA infant's lack of response does not necessarily indicate a lack of pain perception, but may be due to factors such as exhaustion, minimal energy reserves, protective apathy (resulting from the infant's repeated attempts to communicate that he/she is in pain with no response from caregivers), or disease progression.[15,37]

Preterm and term infant responses to pain differ from those of two- and four-month-old infants, who show no difference between each other in pain responses. Preterm infants demonstrate longer latency for cry and have higher pitched cries; term newborns show more tautness of tongue than either preterm or older infants. The two- and four-month-old infants have more vertical mouth position than preterm or term newborns, who display more horizontal mouth action.[38]

Facial actions in both preterm and term infants have been demonstrated to show more sensitivity and specificity to pain than physiologic parameters and some behaviors such as

crying may be influenced by a variety of conditions such as hunger, agitation, stressful environment, and repositioning.[36,39] In addition, the degree of response and ability to maintain a grimace depend on gestational age, postmenstrual age, and energy to mount a sustained response.

ELGA infants who are less than 27 weeks postconceptional age have pain responses similar to more mature infants, although a decreased intensity of responses is noted. The preterm infant's pain response is affected by severity of illness, previous pain experiences, number of painful procedures, and medications. Cry is not a sensitive indicator for pain in ELGA infants because many are intubated or lack the energy for crying.[40]

NEUROLOGICALLY IMPAIRED INFANTS

A survey of direct care staff suggests there is a generalized perception that, as the level of neurologic impairment increases from mild to moderate to severe, progressively less pain is experienced by the infant compared to infants without impairment.[41]

Stevens and colleagues conducted a study using Delphi methodology to gain group consensus among 14 pediatric pain experts on pain indicators thought to be characteristic of infants at risk for neurologic impairment (low, moderate, severe risk). The highest level of agreement among experts on pain indicators in infants at risk for neurologic impairment was on brow bulge, facial grimace, eye squeeze, and inconsolability. The expert panel also agreed that, for the severe risk group, heart rate changes and decreased oxygen saturation were important indicators of pain.[42]

Another study found infants at a postmenstrual age around 32 weeks with Grade IV intraventricular hemorrhage or cystic periventricular leukomalacia by ultrasound showed no signs of an altered pain response compared with matched controls, although infants with

FIGURE 14-7 ▲ EDIN Pain Scale—Assessment of prolonged pain in premature infants.

Indicator	Score/Description	Results
Facial activity	0: Relaxed facial activity	
	1: Transient grimaces with frowning, lip purse, and chin quiver	
	2: Frequent grimaces, lasting grimaces	
	3: Permanent grimaces resembling crying or blank face	
Body movements	0: Relaxed body movements	
	1: Transient agitation, often quiet	
	2: Frequent agitation but can be calmed down	
	3: Permanent agitation with contraction of fingers and toes and hypertonia of limbs or infrequent, slow movements and prostration	
Quality of sleep	0: Falls asleep easily	
	1: Falls asleep with difficulty	
	2: Frequent, spontaneous arousals, independent of nursing, restless sleep	
	3: Sleeplessness	
Quality of contact with nurses	0: Smiles, attentive to voice	
	1: Transient apprehension during interactions with nurses	
	2: Difficulty communicating with nurses, cries in response to minor stimulation	
	3: Refusal to communicate with nurses, no interpersonal rapport, moans without stimulation	
Consolability	0: Quiet, total relaxation	
	1: Calms down quickly in response to stroking or voice or with sucking	
	2: Calms down with difficulty	
	3: Disconsolate, sucks desperately	
	TOTAL SCORE =	

Adapted from: Debillon T, et al. 2001. Development and initial validation of the EDIN scale, a new tool for assessing prolonged pain in preterm infants. *Archives of Disease in Childhood. Fetal Neonatal Edition* 85(1): F37. Reprinted by permission.

parenchymal brain injury demonstrated significantly more tongue protrusion upon heel lance. The researchers also noted that pain responses of these infants may change as they grow and develop. Abnormal pain responses later in infancy may become apparent as neurodevelopmental abnormalities that blunt or alter biobehavioral reactivity emerge.[43]

PHARMACOLOGICALLY PARALYZED OR SEDATED INFANTS

Infants receiving moderate to heavy sedation or paralytic agents cannot mount a behavioral response to pain. Risk factors for pain should be carefully considered, and physiologic measures of pain should be used in the absence of behavioral indicators.[44,45] Unfortunately, there

are no available pain instruments for use with this special NICU population.

INFANTS WITH PERSISTENT OR CHRONIC PAIN

Prolonged or persistent pain is not well described due to limited research, especially in the preterm population. Most of the research on neonatal pain consists of an acute pain stimulus (heel lance) or postoperative pain.[46] In one study, 22 ventilated preterm infants, randomized to receive morphine or placebo, were assessed for ongoing or persistent pain by clinical staff including nurses and doctors. Infants on morphine therapy were correctly identified by staff 71 percent of the time. Pain-related facial expressions (grimacing), high activity levels, poor response to handling or routine care, and insufficient ventilatory synchrony were associated more with infants on placebo than those receiving morphine.[47]

Initial validation with the EDIN (Echelle Douleur Inconfort Nouveau-Ne [neonatal pain and discomfort scale]) scale for assessing prolonged pain in preterm infants is promising, but requires additional research.[48] Five behavioral indicators with increasing scores indicating prolonged pain comprise this scale: facial activity, body movements, quality of sleep, quality of nurse-infant interaction, and consolability (Figure 14-7).

More subdued responses may be seen in infants with chronic pain or a complete shutdown when pain exceeds the infant's ability to respond, as with any overwhelming stimulation.[36,46] This may be due to the ongoing nature of persistent or chronic pain, where the usual pain signals don't result in relief resulting in a negative feedback loop.

Infants Exposed to Psychotropic Medications

Infants exposed prenatally or postnatally through breast milk to selective serotonin reuptake inhibitors (SSRIs) and benzodiazepines demonstrate significantly decreased facial action and less cardiac reactivity during heel lance than those not exposed to psychotropic medications. Mean heart rate was significantly lower during recovery from heel lance for the SSRI-exposed infants.[49,50]

Infants Undergoing Opioid Weaning

Screening for pain should continue during opioid weaning. One might suspect recurring pain in infants with increased neonatal abstinence scores who frequently need extra doses of opioids above the weaning dose for symptom management. Although alternate dosing of opioids and benzodiazepines have not been studied in neonates during weaning, this

combination might diminish the pain response in infants still experiencing pain. Pain screening with a validated tool in combination with neonatal abstinence scoring can alert the clinician to the presence of pain because some indicators are different on each instrument. For example, facial grimacing, a sensitive indicator of pain, is not on abstinence scoring tools.

Infants at End of Life

Currently, there is no appropriate tool sensitive to neonatal pain at the end of life. Choice of an assessment tool depends on the individual patient (e.g., a preterm infant might be best evaluated using the PIPP to account for gestational age). Often, infants who are terminally ill do not have the energy to express pain behaviorally. Significant impairment of the terminal infant's communication ability could compromise comfort. Physiologic indicators may be the only available parameters, and these might be affected by the dying infant's condition. Therefore, it is reasonable to use physiologic indicators, risk factors for pain, and an infant's general condition to help determine pain at this time.[44]

After ventilator withdrawal, there is great variation in the provision of analgesics during and after the procedure, with many infants receiving no analgesia. Infants with major chromosome abnormalities, congenital anomalies, and necrotizing enterocolitis (NEC) were more likely to receive analgesia than those with other diagnoses or for whom further treatment was considered futile.[51,52] The provision of analgesics is frequently based on obvious risk factors for suffering as life support is withdrawn or for known painful conditions. Frequently, infant behaviors are not documented as the reason for administering pain medications.[53] As stated, the inability to demonstrate behavioral pain responses leaves the clinician without clear indices for assessment. Therefore, it may be necessary to consider that infants have increasing pain intensity as death becomes imminent. Clearly, a population that receives little or no analgesia at a time when most older children and adults receive compassionate analgesia indicates a different standard of care and warrants a close examination of clinical practice.

INFANTS WITH DISEASES OR CONDITIONS WARRANTING PAIN ASSESSMENT

One way to think about particular conditions is whether it would be painful to an older child or adult. If that answer is "yes," then pain needs to be frequently assessed. Tests, procedures, or wound care may increase the level of pain and require careful observation to determine the need for a bolus of pain medication. Some conditions such as epidermolysis bullosa (EB) require varying amounts of pain management from ongoing baseline pain control to control of acute pain when dressings are changed. A study of 140 randomly selected children and 374 adults with various types and subtypes of EB found that only 12 to 13 percent reported no pain. Individuals with more extensive EB and EB subtypes reported pain levels greater than 5 on a 10-point pain scale.[54]

Another study of 35 children, ages 5 to 18, with osteogenesis imperfecta found they experienced moderate to severe pain related to fractures and less intense pain when no fractures were present. With nonverbal patients, it would be easy to assume that they have no pain when they have no fractures.[55] This would lead to undertreatment of pain in this population. These patients may experience acute pain during repositioning or other care not usually considered painful.

In a retrospective chart review of 25 infants with NEC, it was noted that infants averaged 13–19 painful events per day for five days. Although the unit standard was to document two PIPP scores a day, the compliance was less than 8 percent. For two days after NEC was diagnosed, only 30 percent of infants had pain scores documented in the medical record. From day 3 through day 5, PIPP scores were documented on 60 percent of the infants. On day 1 of diagnosis, 48 percent of infants were given no analgesia, and on day 2 that fell to 24 percent. After day 2, the frequency of analgesic treatment slowly declined.[56] In this study, the use of opioid analgesics for NEC was low possibly in association with inadequate screening assessments for pain.

Many conditions in the NICU result in prolonged pain that may affect the nature of biobehavioral responsiveness, and the onus of responsibility is on the clinician to appropriately determine if the infant is in pain. When pain is questionable, a compassionate clinician can always err on the side that pain is present, initiate a trial of analgesic therapy, and evaluate infant response.

PARENTS' VIEWS ON PAIN

Surveys of parents on pain assessment and management for their infant in the NICU provide some guidance concerning their needs associated with neonatal pain. One survey of 257 parents from nine NICUs in the United Kingdom and U.S. showed dissatisfaction of 64 percent of parents because they received no information about infant pain. Thirty percent of parents were disappointed with the information they had received. Only 18 percent of parents reported being taught by NICU staff how to identify their infant's pain signals. Seventy percent of parents wrote comments on ways they identified their infant's pain signs, with crying (37 percent), movements (31 percent), or facial expression (21 percent) the most commonly reported. Very few parents used skin color or cardiorespiratory monitor data for pain assessment.[57]

Interviews and focus groups with parents show that their infant's pain is a source of stress and that health team members have an important role in alleviating that stress.[58] The ability to participate in parenting their infant seems to provide a coping mechanism that relieved some of the distress associated with the pain their infant endured in the NICU. Parents felt there was a difference between their perceptions of their infant's pain and those of NICU staff. This disparity increased their anxiety, as did the concern that staff might not intervene when presented with signs of pain by their infant after the parents left the NICU. These issues heightened parental stress; whereas support by NICU staff, parenting opportunities, and information or resources relieved it.

SUMMARY

Pain assessment is an essential prerequisite to optimal pain management. Pain is best assessed when a multidimensional approach is employed using a valid and reliable instrument. Balancing pain assessment data with the infant's risk factors for pain and contextual modifiers that may impact how the infant communicates pain will ensure that pain is recognized early and interventions are implemented in a timely manner.

REFERENCES

1. Anand KJ, and Craig K. 1996. New perspectives on the definition of pain. *Pain* 67(1): 3–6.
2. Agency for Health Care Policy and Research. 1992. *Acute Pain Management in Infants, Children, and Adolescents: Operative or Medical Procedures and Trauma. (Quick Reference Guide for Clinicians.)* Rockville, Maryland: U.S. Department of Health and Human Services.
3. Walden M, and Gibbins S. 2008. *Pain Assessment and Management: Guideline for Practice,* 2nd ed. Glenview, Illinois: National Association of Neonatal Nurses.
4. Foster RL. 2001. Nursing judgment: The key to pain assessment in critically ill children. *Journal of the Society of Pediatric Nurses* 6(2): 90–93, 96.
5. Fuller BF. 1998. The process of infant pain assessment. *Applied Nursing Research* 11(2): 62–68.
6. Hummel P, and Puchalski M. 2001. Assessment and management of pain in infancy. *Newborn & Infant Nursing Reviews* 1(2): 114–121.
7. Fuller BF, Neu M, and Smith M. 1999. The influence of background clinical data on infant pain assessments. *Clinical Nursing Research* 8(2): 179–187.
8. Gibbins S, and Stevens B. 2003. The influence of gestational age on the efficacy and short-term safety of sucrose for procedural pain relief. *Advances in Neonatal Care* 3(5): 241–249.
9. Grunau RV, and Craig KD. 1987. Pain expression in neonates: Facial action and cry. *Pain* 28(3): 395–410.
10. Grunau RV, Johnston CC, and Craig KD. 1990. Neonatal facial and cry responses to invasive and non-invasive procedures. *Pain* 42(3): 295–305.
11. Hummel P, and van Dijk M. 2006. Pain assessment: Current status and challenges. *Seminars in Fetal & Neonatal Medicine* 11(4): 237–245.
12. Stevens BJ, Johnston CC, and Horton L. 1993. Multidimensional pain assessment in premature infants: A pilot study. *Journal of Obstetric, Gynecologic, and Neonatal Nursing* 22(6): 531–541.
13. Fuller BF. 1991. Acoustic discrimination of three types of infant cries. *Nursing Research* 40(3): 156–160.
14. Porter FL, Porges SW, and Marshall RE. 1988. Newborn cries and vagal tone: Parallel changes in response to circumcision. *Child Development* 59(2): 495–505.
15. Johnston CC, et al. 1999. Factors explaining lack of response to heel stick in preterm newborns. *Journal of Obstetric, Gynecologic, and Neonatal Nursing* 28(6): 587–594.
16. Johnston CC, et al. 1995. Differential response to pain by very premature infants. *Pain* 61(3): 471–479.
17. Stevens BJ, Johnston CC, and Horton L. 1994. Factors that influence the behavioral pain responses of premature infants. *Pain* 59(1): 101–109.
18. Walden M. 2007. Pain in the newborn. In *Comprehensive Neonatal Nursing: An Interdisciplinary Approach,* 4th ed., Kenner C, and Lott J, eds. Philadelphia: Saunders, 360–371.
19. Franck LS. 1986. A new method to quantitatively describe pain behavior in infants. *Nursing Research* 35(1): 28–31.
20. Craig KD, et al. 1993. Pain in the preterm neonate: Behavioral and physiological indices. *Pain* 52(3): 287–299. (Published erratum in *Pain,* 1993, 54[1]: 111.)
21. Grunau RE, et al. 2000. Are twitches, startles, and body movements pain indicators in extremely low birth weight infants? *Clinical Journal of Pain* 16(1): 37–45.
22. Holsti L, et al. 2004. Specific Newborn Individualized Developmental Care and Assessment Program movements are associated with acute pain in preterm infants in the neonatal intensive care unit. *Pediatrics* 114(1): 65–72.
23. Morison SJ, et al. 2003. Are there developmentally distinct motor indicators of pain in preterm infants? *Early Human Development* 72(2): 131–146.
24. Sweet SD, and McGrath PJ. 1998. Relative importance of mothers' versus medical staffs' behavior in the prediction of infant immunization pain behavior. *Journal of Pediatric Psychology* 23(4): 249–256.
25. Duhn LJ, and Medves JM. 2004. A systematic integrative review of infant pain assessment tools. *Advances in Neonatal Care* 4(3): 126–140.
26. Stevens B, et al. 1996. Premature Infant Pain Profile: Development and initial validation. *Clinical Journal of Pain* 12(1): 13–22.
27. Bildner J, and Krechel SW. 1996. Increasing staff nurse awareness of postoperative pain management in the NICU. *Neonatal Network* 15(1): 11–16.

28. Lawrence J, et al. 1993. The development of a tool to assess neonatal pain. *Neonatal Network* 12(6): 59–66.

29. McNair C, et al. 2004. Postoperative pain assessment in the neonatal intensive care unit. *Archives of Disease in Childhood. Fetal and Neonatal Edition* 89(6): F537–F541.

30. El Sayed MF, et al. 2007. Safety profile of morphine following surgery in neonates. *Journal of Perinatology* 27(7): 444–447.

31. Ahn Y. 2006. The relationship between behavioral states and pain responses to various NICU procedures in premature infants. *Journal of Tropical Pediatrics* 52(3): 201–205.

32. Belda S, et al. 2004. Screening for retinopathy of prematurity: Is it painful? *Biology of the Neonate* 86(3): 195–200. (Comment in *Biology of the Neonate,* 2006, 89[3]: 197.)

33. Herrington CJ, Olomu IN, and Geller SM. 2004. Salivary cortisol as indicators of pain in preterm infants: A pilot study. *Clinical Nursing Research* 13(1): 53–68.

34. Rouss K, et al. 2007. Long-term subcutaneous morphine administration after surgery in newborns. *Journal of Perinatal Medicine* 35(1): 79–81.

35. Suraseranivongse S, et al. 2006. A comparison of postoperative pain scales in neonates. *British Journal of Anaesthesia* 97(4): 540–544.

36. Ranger M, Johnston CC, and Anand KJ. 2007. Current controversies regarding pain assessment in neonates. *Seminars in Perinatology* 31(5): 283–288.

37. Tronick EZ, Scanlon KB, and Scanlon JW. 1990. Protective apathy, a hypothesis about the behavioral organization and its relation to clinical and physiologic status of the preterm infant during the newborn period. *Clinics in Perinatology* 17(1): 125–154.

38. Johnston CC, et al. 1993. Developmental changes in pain expression in premature, full-term, two- and four-month-old infants. *Pain* 52(2): 201–208.

39. Anand KJ. 2007. Pain assessment in preterm neonates. *Pediatrics* 119(3): 605–607.

40. Gibbins S, et al. 2008. Comparison of pain responses in infants of different gestational ages. *Neonatology* 93(1): 10–18.

41. Breau LM, et al. 2006. Judgments of pain in the neonatal intensive care setting: A survey of direct care staffs' perceptions of pain in infants at risk for neurological impairment. *Clinical Journal of Pain* 22(2): 122–129.

42. Stevens B, et al. 2006. Identification of pain indicators for infants at risk for neurological impairment: A Delphi consensus study. *BMC Pediatrics* 6: 1–9.

43. Oberlander TF, et al. 2002. Does parenchymal brain injury affect biobehavioral pain responses in very low birth weight infants at 32 weeks' postconceptional age? *Pediatrics* 110(3): 570–576.

44. Walden M, Sudia-Robinson T, and Carrier CT. 2001. Comfort care for infants in the neonatal intensive care unit at end of life. *Newborn and Infant Nursing Reviews* 1(2): 97–105.

45. Walden M. 2004. Pain assessment and management. *Core Curriculum for Neonatal Intensive Care Nursing,* 3rd ed., Verklan MT, and Walden M, eds. Philadelphia: Saunders, 375–391.

46. Herr K, et al. 2006. Pain assessment in the nonverbal patient: Position statement with clinical practice recommendations. *Pain Management Nursing* 7(2): 44–52.

47. Boyle EM, et al. 2006. Assessment of persistent pain or distress and adequacy of analgesia in preterm ventilated infants. *Pain* 124(1-2): 87–91.

48. Debillon T, et al. 2001. Development and initial validation of the EDIN scale, a new tool for assessing prolonged pain in preterm infants. *Archives of Disease in Childhood. Fetal and Neonatal Edition* 85(1): F36–F41.

49. Oberlander TF, et al. 2002. Prolonged prenatal psychotropic medication exposure alters neonatal acute pain response. *Pediatric Research* 51(4): 443–453.

50. Oberlander TF, et al. 2005. Pain reactivity in 2-month-old infants after prenatal and postnatal serotonin reuptake inhibitor medication exposure. *Pediatrics* 115(2): 411–425.

51. Partridge JC, and Wall SN. 1997. Analgesia for dying infants whose life support is withdrawn or withheld. *Pediatrics* 99(1): 76–79.

52. Moro T, et al. 2006. Neonatal end-of-life care: A review of the research literature. *Journal of Perinatal and Neonatal Nursing* 20(3): 262–273.

53. Abe N, Catlin A, and Mihara D. 2001. End of life in the NICU. A study of ventilator withdrawal. MCN. *American Journal of Maternal Child Nursing* 26(3): 141–146.

54. Fine JD, et al. 2004. Assessment of mobility, activities and pain in different subtypes of epidermolysis bullosa. *Clinical and Experimental Dermatology* 29(2): 122–127.

55. Zack P, et al. 2005. Fracture and non-fracture pain in children with osteogenesis imperfecta. *Acta Paediatrica* 94(9): 1238–1242.

56. Gibbins S, et al. 2006. Pain assessment and pharmacologic management for infants with NEC: A retrospective chart audit. *Neonatal Network* 25(5): 339–345.

57. Franck LS, et al. 2005. Parents' views about infant pain in neonatal intensive care. *Clinical Journal of Pain* 21(2): 133–139.

58. Gale G, et al. 2004. Parents' perceptions of their infant's pain experience in the NICU. *International Journal of Nursing Studies* 41(1): 51–58.

Notes

Antepartum Tests and Intrapartum Monitoring

Kimberly Horns LaBronte, PhD, RN, NNP-BC

COMMON ANTEPARTUM TESTS

ASSESSMENT OF FETAL ACTIVITY

Assessment of fetal activity, or movement counts by the mother, is a noninvasive technique for monitoring fetal well-being. This is thought to be an effective method of reducing fetal stillbirth.[1] Usually, monitoring begins at 28 weeks gestation.[2,3] For this evaluation, the mother rests for one hour daily at the same time each day in a quiet room. During that rest period, she records the fetal movements on an activity chart. Most practitioners consider a baseline of four fetal movements per hour acceptable.[2] If fewer than four fetal movements are detected, further testing is indicated.

Amniocentesis is advised for mothers over 35 years of age to screen for chromosomal abnormalities and for those with known hereditary disorders or carrier states (i.e., cystic fibrosis) to identify a potential genetic/chromosomal disorder in the fetus. Pregnancies affected by Rh disease are monitored by examining the amniotic fluid for optical density. A low serum α-fetoprotein level or positive triple screen in the mother may indicate that trisomy 21 (Down syndrome) is present in the fetus and may suggest the need for amniocentesis for chromosomal analysis. Other indications for amniocentesis for chromosomal analysis are known consanguinity in the parents and a previous child with a chromosomal or hereditary disease. Amniocentesis traditionally is performed at 18 to 20 weeks gestation, but some practitioners may offer it at 13 to 14 weeks gestation.[1,2] There is an increased risk of rupture of membranes if the test is performed before 13 weeks gestation.[2] For chromosomal analysis, the cells acquired from the amniotic fluid can take from 10 to 14 days for karyotyping. At later gestational ages, amniocentesis can be used to evaluate fetal lung maturity.

Chorionic villus sampling is indicated for suspected chromosomal or biochemical defects in the fetus. It has the advantage of earlier diagnostic analysis than when amniocentesis is used. Sampling can be by the transabdominal or transcervical approach.[1,2] Chorionic tissue has the same genotype as the fetus, and testing can be performed at 10 to 12 weeks. Results are available within 24 hours because living tissue is analyzed.

Ultrasound examination is useful in helping to determine gestational age, for detecting altered or abnormal growth, and for identifying the presence of malformations. In the first trimester, it can be used to locate the gestational sac and the embryo or embryos and to

TABLE A-1 ▲ Biophysical Profile Scoring: Variables and Scoring Criteria

Biophysical Variable	Normal (score = 2)	Abnormal (score = 0)
Fetal breathing movements (FBM)	At least 1 episode of FBM of at least 20 seconds duration in 30 minutes of observation	Absent FBM or no episodes of more than 20 seconds in 30 minutes
Gross body movements	At least 2 discrete body/limb movements in 30 minutes (episodes of active continuous movement are considered to be a single movement)	Less than two episodes of body/limb movements in 30 minutes
Fetal tone	At least 1 episode of active extension with return to flexion of fetal limb(s) or trunk; opening and closing of hand considered normal tone	Either slow extension with return to partial flexion or movement of limb in full extension or absent fetal movement or partially open fetal hand
Qualitative pockets of amniotic fluid (AF) volume	At least 1 pocket of AF that measures at least 2 cm in vertical axis	Either no pockets or a pocket of less than 2 cm in vertical axis
Reactive fetal heart rate (FHR) episodes	At least 2 episodes of FHR accelerations of at least 15 beats per minute and of more than 15 seconds duration associated with fetal movement in 20 minutes	Fewer than 2 accelerations of FHR or accelerations of less than 15 beats per minute in 20 minutes

Adapted from: Manning FA. 1999. The fetal biophysical profile. *Obstetrics and Gynecology Clinics of North America* 26(4): 560. Reprinted by permission.

determine crown to rump length. Pregnancy can be detected by ultrasound as early as five weeks from the last menstrual period. In the second and third trimesters, ultrasound can be used to evaluate for fetal loss, fetal age, a four-chamber heart, abnormalities of the bladder, kidneys, brain, spine, and extremities. Placental maturity can be determined by grading the placenta from Grade 0 to Grade III. Changes in the chorionic plate, placental surface, and basal layers of the placenta can be evaluated to provide supporting information to help date the pregnancy or when deciding on the timing for cesarean section. Biparietal diameters of ≥9.3 cm with a Grade III placenta have been consistent with a mature fetus in the absence of maternal diabetes.[4] The status of amniotic fluid volume can be evaluated, and the umbilical cord can be inspected.[1] Hydrops fetalis can also be detected and monitored.

Increasingly, ultrasound is used in the first trimester for early detection of trisomy 21. Fetal **nuchal fold** (the space between the back of the neck and the overlying skin) **translucency** is a test done to measure nuchal

fold thickness in the fetus. A measurement over 3 mm is related to the abnormal collection of fluid in this area and is associated with trisomy 21. The combination of advanced maternal age, increased nuchal fold thickness, and elevated maternal serum levels of free β-human chorionic gonadotropin and pregnancy-associated plasma protein are highly predictive of trisomy 21. Risk is calculated using maternal age, the head to bottom measurement of the baby, and the thickness of the nuchal fold. The overall Down syndrome detection rate is 71 percent, and the false positive rate is 2.4 percent.[1]

Another ultrasound finding of Down syndrome is short long bones (femur and humerus). The nuchal fold thickness is also increased in cases of Turner syndrome (karyotype XO) due to webbing of the neck, when a cystic hygroma is present in this area, and with congenital heart disorders of the great arteries.[5]

Fetal fibronectin is the "glue" that helps attach the membranes surrounding the infant to the lower part of the uterus. Shortly before labor (or sometimes during labor), this lower part of the uterus begins to change shape, causing the membranes to separate from the uterine wall. When this happens, fibronectin is released and mingles with a woman's cervical and vaginal secretions. The fetal fibronectin test measures the absence or presence of fibronectin levels in these secretions. When a positive fetal fibronectin value is found and added to the clinical sign of cervical shortening, the combined findings are a powerful positive predictor of preterm labor and impending birth.[6]

Doppler velocimetry evaluates blood flow in the umbilical arteries during diastole. A decrease in diastolic flow indicates an increase in downstream placental resistance. Absent or reversed flow is an ominous sign and may indicate uteroplacental insufficiency.[7] This test is used to detect a compromised fetus in diabetic, chronic hypertensive, and preeclamptic pregnancies. Doppler velocimetry is also used to detect twin-to-twin transfusion *in utero.*

The **nonstress test** (NST) is an indirect test of placental function that assesses fetal heart rate acceleration and variability. External fetal monitoring is done, and uterine activity is monitored. Observations of the baseline fetal heart rate, accelerations, and decelerations are made. Fetal movements and changes in fetal heart rate with movement are assessed. Generally, patients are monitored for 20 to 60 minutes.[2,8] Fetal movements can be spontaneous, or they can be induced by manipulation of or vibroacoustic stimulation to the mother's abdomen.[2] Accelerations in the fetal heart rate of at least 15 beats per minute correlate positively with fetal well-being. The results are classified as reactive, which indicates that two accelerations in fetal heart rate of at least 15 beats per minute occurred with fetal movement in a 20-minute period, or nonreactive, which indicates that no or fewer than two periods of fetal heart rate acceleration occurred. If

test results are nonreactive, testing time may be increased, or the test may be repeated later the same day.[2] In some cases, a contraction stress test or a biophysical profile will be the next step.

A **contraction stress test** is a method of determining fetal well-being by evaluating the response of fetal heart rate to uterine contractions. It is a nonspecific test of placental reserve. Uterine contractions normally increase fetal heart rate variability and may result in increased fetal movement. Uterine contractions are induced by oxytocin (Pitocin) or by nipple stimulation. Three contractions in a ten-minute period are evaluated. A negative test indicates the absence of late deceleration of the fetal heart rate with contractions. A positive test shows late deceleration in fetal heart rate with contractions. In cases of positive stress tests and suspicious or technically poor tests, a biophysical profile may be ordered.[2,8,9]

The **biophysical profile** is a more extensive evaluation of the fetus using ultrasound in addition to NST. Scoring and recommended management approaches are explained in Tables A-1 and A-2. In addition to NST, ultrasound evaluations of fetal breathing, gross and fine movement, tone, and the amniotic fluid index are obtained.[10,11]

Alpha-fetoprotein is evaluated at 15–18 weeks of gestation to screen for neural tube defects, which are associated with elevated levels of this protein. Maternal serum or amniotic fluid can be used to determine levels. High levels are also associated with multiple gestation, congenital nephritis, exstrophy of the bladder, omphalocele, gastroschisis, intrauterine growth restriction, and fetal death. A lower than normal level is associated with trisomies 21, 18, and 13. **Unconjugated estriol and human chorionic gonadotropin levels** may be evaluated with the α-fetoprotein level.[11] A lower than normal unconjugated estriol level with an elevated human chorionic

TABLE A-2 ▲ Interpretation of Fetal Biophysical Profile Score Results and Recommended Clinical Management

Score	Interpretation	Risk of Fetal Death/ 1,000/Weeks Undelivered	Management
10 of 10	Nonasphyxiated	0.565	Conservative
8 of 10; normal AFV*	Nonasphyxiated	0.565	Conservative
8 of 8 (nonstress test not done)	Nonasphyxiated	0.565	Conservative
8 of 10; decreased AFV	Chronic compensated asphyxia	20–30	If mature (≥37 weeks): deliver If immature: serial testing twice a week
6 of 10; normal AFV	Possible acute fetal asphyxia	50	If mature (≥37 weeks): deliver If immature: repeat test in 24 hours and deliver if score remains ≤6 of 10
6 of 10; decreased AFV	Chronic asphyxia, with possible acute asphyxia	>50	If ≥32 weeks: deliver If <32 weeks: test daily
4 of 10; normal AFV	Acute asphyxia likely	115	If ≥32 weeks: deliver If ≤32 weeks: test daily
4 of 10; decreased AFV	Chronic asphyxia, with acute likely	>115	If ≥26 weeks: deliver
2 of 10; normal AFV	Acute asphyxia almost certain	220	If ≥26 weeks: deliver
0 of 10	Gross severe asphyxia	550	If ≥26 weeks: deliver

* AFV = amniotic fluid volume

Adapted from: Manning FA. 1999. Fetal biophysical profile. *Obstetrics and Gynecology Clinics of North America* 26(4): 564. Reprinted by permission.

gonadotropin level in the second trimester correlates with trisomies 21 and 18 in the fetus.[11] These tests, along with an ultrasound positive for increased nuchal fold translucency, are sometimes referred to as **triple markers** for trisomies 21 and 18. Use of the triple-marker tests along with the indicator of maternal age has led to a prediction rate accuracy of 60–90 percent for trisomy 21.[1,11]

Maternal serum estriol levels increase as pregnancy advances. Estriol rises rapidly until 24 weeks gestation, more slowly between 24 and 32 weeks, and then resumes a rapid rise until term. A sharp or progressive decrease indicates fetal compromise. In the past, serial assays were used to determine if the fetus was compromised; currently, this method is seldom used. Falsely low levels are seen with maternal corticosteroid use and with impaired maternal renal and hepatic function.

Human placental lactogen is a hormone released by cytotrophoblasts into the maternal circulation. Production increases until about 37 weeks of gestation and then may stabilize or decrease slightly. Low levels can indicate uteroplacental insufficiency and are seen with maternal hypertension. Serial levels are recommended. Because high placental lactogen levels are seen in multiple gestation, erythroblastosis fetalis, and poorly controlled diabetes, however, levels are not helpful indicators in women with these conditions. The normal range for human placental lactogen levels near term is 5.4 to 7 mcg/mL.[8,9]

Hemoglobin A$_{1c}$ (HgbA$_{1c}$) peptide levels are used for monitoring diabetic pregnancies and reflect net hyperglycemia over previous weeks. Higher first-trimester levels are associated with a greater incidence of congenital anomalies and cardiac defects and reflect poor metabolic control.[1] Tight control of blood sugar before pregnancy and in the first trimester is recommended to avoid hyperglycemic exposure of the fetus. HgbA$_{1c}$ levels should be less than 8 percent and blood glucose levels, below 150 mg/dL.[1]

The **lecithin-sphingomyelin ratio (L/S ratio)** is used to determine fetal lung maturity and is done on amniotic fluid. Levels of 2 or higher indicate fetal lung maturity. Falsely high levels are seen if blood, meconium, or vaginal secretions contaminate the amniotic fluid. Mature L/S ratios are not always accurate in the diabetic pregnancy and in those affected by erythroblastosis fetalis. Use of a lung profile with a phosphatidylglycerol (PG) level (see below) is more accurate in determining fetal lung maturity in these pregnancies.[1,8,9]

The **shake test,** done on amniotic fluid, is a rapid and inexpensive bedside screening test for lung maturity. Lung maturity is indicated by a complete ring of bubbles in a dilution of amniotic fluid and ethanol. Persistence of an intact ring of bubbles at the air-liquid interface after 15 minutes is considered positive, indicating pulmonary maturity. Contamination of the fluid with blood or meconium results in false positives.[1]

The **lung profile** evaluates amniotic fluid for the L/S ratio and for PG and phosphatidylinositol levels. PG appears in the amniotic fluid as phosphatidylinositol begins to fall. The presence of PG indicates mature lungs and is not affected by a diabetic or erythroblastotic pregnancy. Contamination of the amniotic fluid does not alter test accuracy. Some institutions may use the lung profile for the L/S ratio and PG measurement only.[1,12]

A commercial test, the **AmnioStat-FLM-PG** (Irvine Scientific Products, Santa Ana, California) is available and detects PG in a sample of amniotic fluid. The test takes approximately 15 minutes and is not affected by contamination with blood or meconium. A positive test indicates pulmonary maturity.

The **TDx FLx FLM II assay** (Abbott Laboratories, Abbott Park, Illinois) is an automated fetal lung maturity test that also can be performed in less than an hour. This test determines the relative concentrations of surfactant and albumin in a sample of amniotic fluid. The manufacturer's recommended interpretation of the surfactant/albumin values is as follows:[13,14]

▶ A value <30 mg/g is considered definitely immature.

▶ A value between 30 and 50 mg/g is considered transitionally immature and risky.

▶ A value in the range of 50–70 mg/g is considered transitionally mature and should be treated with caution.

▶ A value >70 mg/g indicates lung maturity.

INTRAPARTAL MONITORING

Fetal heart rate monitoring is commonly used during labor to identify fetal distress. The beat-to-beat fetal heart rate is recorded, with simultaneous recording of uterine activity. The normal baseline fetal heart rate is 120 to 160 beats per minute (bpm) and should be accompanied by good baseline fetal heart rate variability. The following fetal heart rate abnormalities may occur.

Decreased or lost beat-to-beat variability can result from fetal hypoxia. It is also seen when narcotics, sedatives, or analgesic drugs have been administered to the mother. A decrease in variability can be seen with fetal sleep. Other factors that can lead to decreased or lost variability are administration of magnesium sulfate to the mother, fetal immaturity, and fetal tachycardia.[12,15]

Fetal tachycardia, indicated by a fetal heart rate greater than 160 bpm, can be associated with maternal fever, chorioamnionitis, and certain medications such as atropine, terbutaline, and others that may cause a decrease in uterine blood flow. A small percentage of fetuses whose mothers are hyperthyroid demonstrate tachycardia. Rates of 200–300 bpm are seen with fetal supraventricular tachycardia. Tachycardia is frequently seen in the recovery phase following fetal bradycardia related to a hypoxic episode, but can also been seen with the gradual onset of fetal hypoxemia.

Fetal bradycardia is indicated by a heart rate less than 120 bpm. It is often referred to as physiologic, not related to hypoxemia, if accompanied by good baseline variability. Some practitioners think that a baseline fetal heart rate of 90–120 bpm with good variability represents a normal heart rate.[1,2] Sustained low heart rates with normal variability can also be seen with fetal heart block, fetal central nervous system anomalies, and administration to the mother of β-adrenergic receptor blocking drugs such as propranolol. Loss of variability with bradycardia can be associated with fetal hypoxia.

Early fetal heart rate decelerations are a benign response to uterine pressure on the fetal head. Baseline fetal heart rate and variability are normal.

Variable decelerations of fetal heart rate are caused by umbilical cord compression as uterine contraction activity peaks. Transient fetal hypoxemia and acidosis occur with compression of the arteries.

Late decelerations reflect fetal hypoxemia. Initially, the late deceleration pattern may be mediated by the vagus nerve, but with continued, prolonged hypoxia, the heart rate is low because of myocardial depression. Other factors leading to this pattern are maternal hypotension; hypercontractility of the uterus due to oxytocin; regional anesthesia; and major

TABLE A-3 ▲ Normal Arterial Umbilical Blood Gas Values for Term and Premature Infants

Value	Term n = 3,520	Premature n = 1,015
pH	7.25 ± 0.07	7.28 ± 0.089
PCO$_2$ (mmHg)	50.30 ± 11.1	50.20 ± 12.3
HCO$_3^-$ (mmol/liter)	22.00 ± 3.6	22.40 ± 3.5
BE* (mmol/liter)	–2.70 ± 2.8	–2.50 ± 3.0

* BE = Base excess

Adapted from: Riley RJ, and Johnson JWC. 1993. Collecting and analyzing cord blood gases. *Clinical Obstetrics and Gynecology* 36(1): 13. Reprinted by permission.

maternal emergencies such as hemorrhage, seizures, or respiratory arrest.[15]

Sinusoidal patterns of fetal heart rate appear as baseline oscillations of fetal heart rate similar to a sine wave, with fixed periodicity and loss of variability. They are associated with severe fetal anemia and are seen with Rh-sensitized fetuses and with large fetofetal transfusion; fetomaternal transfusion; and fetal hemorrhage, as into a cavernous hemangioma.[1,15]

Umbilical and fetal scalp pH has been a confusing and difficult predictor of poor Apgar scores, fetal distress, and neonatal outcome. It is now known that the former cutoff for pH <7.2 is not an appropriate predictor.[1] Even an umbilical cord blood pH of 7.0 can have equivocal correlations with neurologic outcomes and Apgar scores. Normal mean umbilical pH at the end of labor is 7.27–7.28.[1]

Cord blood gases are often obtained following delivery of depressed neonates and those with abnormal monitoring results during the intrapartum period. Information from the cord blood gases often aids understanding of the events surrounding the birth of a neonate with low Apgar scores. Cord blood gases are routinely obtained in many institutions.[1,15] Normal values are listed in Table A-3.

REFERENCES

1. Creasy RK, Resnick R, and Iams J, eds. 2009. *Maternal-Fetal Medicine: Principles and Practice,* 6th ed., Philadelphia: Saunders.

2. Gomella TL. 2004. *Neonatology: Management, Procedures, On-Call Problems, Diseases, and Drugs,* 5th ed., Gomella TL, et al., eds. New York: McGraw-Hill, 1–8.

3. Shaffer BL, and Parer JT. 2007. Antepartum fetal monitoring. In *Management of High-Risk Pregnancy: An Evidence-Based Approach,* 5th ed., Queenan JT, Spong CY, and Lockwood CJ, eds. Boston: Blackwell, 95–103.

4. Miller DA. 2002. Antepartum fetal surveillance. In *Management of Common Problems in Obstetrics and Gynecology,* 4th ed., Mishell DR, Goodwin TM, and Brenner PF, eds. Malden, Massachusetts: Blackwell Science, 187–191.

5. Kuller JA, Strauss RA, and Cefalo RC. 2001. Preconceptional and prenatal care. In *Obstetrics and Gynecology: Principles for Practice,* Ling FW, and Duff P, eds. New York: McGraw-Hill, 48–49.

6. Tekesin I, Wallweiner D, and Schmidt S. 2005. The value of quantitative ultrasound tissue characterization of the cervix and rapid fetal fibronectin in predicting preterm delivery. *Journal of Perinatal Medicine* 33(5): 383–391.

7. Farmakides G, et al. 1994. Doppler velocimetry. Where does it belong in evaluation of fetal status? *Clinics in Perinatology* 21(4): 849–861.

8. Abuhamad A, and Nyberg D. 2007. Sonographic dating and standard fetal biometry. In *Management of High-Risk Pregnancy: An Evidence-Based Approach,* 5th ed., Queenan JT, Spong CY, and Lockwood CJ, eds. Boston: Blackwell, 286–298.

9. Fanaroff AA, Kiwi R, and Shah D. 2001. Antenatal and intrapartum care of the high-risk neonate. In *Care of the High-Risk Neonate,* 5th ed., Klaus MH, and Fanaroff AA, eds. Philadelphia: Saunders, 1–44.

10. Knuppel RA, and Druckker JE. 1993. *High-Risk Pregnancy: A Team Approach,* 2nd ed. Philadelphia: Saunders, 531–532.

11. Manning FA. 1999. Fetal biophysical profile. *Obstetrics and Gynecology Clinics of North America* 26(4): 557–577.

12. Kjos SL. 2002. Fetal lung maturation, respiratory distress, and antenatal steroid therapy. In *Management of Common Problems in Obstetrics and Gynecology,* 4th ed., Mishell DR, Goodwin TM, and Brenner PF, eds. Malden, Massachusetts: Blackwell Science, 202–205.

13. Herbert WNP, et al. 1993. Role of the TDx FLM assay in fetal lung maturity. *American Journal of Obstetrics and Gynecology* 168(3 part 1): 808–812.

14. Russell JC, et al. 1989. Multicenter evaluation of TDx test for assessing fetal lung maturity. *Clinical Chemistry* 35(6): 1005–1010.

15. Huddleston JF. 1999. Intrapartum fetal assessment. A review. *Clinics in Perinatology* 26(3): 549–568.

NOTES

NOTES

Assessing Behavioral
Organization in Infants

Jacqueline McGrath, PhD, RN, NNP, FNAP, FAAN

This appendix describes sample assessments of behavioral organization in three categories of newborns: the healthy term newborn, the healthy preterm newborn, and the immature, extrasensitive, or depressed preterm newborn. It details the types of responses examiners often see in these three categories and explains what these responses mean. These examples were first described by VandenBerg in the previous edition and have been slightly modified for this publication because they were already excellent examples of the variability of assessment in these different types of infants.

The behavioral assessment is intended to identify an infant's current level of balance and smooth, integrated functioning. In other words, it is designed to identify in what situations and with what supports the infant appears to function smoothly, be relaxed, and be comfortable—that is, to exhibit organized behavior. It is also the purpose of the assessment to describe the threshold of disorganization indicated in the infant's behaviors of defense and avoidance. The degree and kind of stress and the intensity of frustration or defense that the infant experiences can be indicators of the degree of energy the infant has available. The behavioral assessment must also determine if there is any leeway in the infant's responses.

For example, if the infant can tolerate being moved from the examiner's shoulder (where he is flexed, tucked, and resting calmly) to her lap without an onslaught of disorganized behaviors (such as extended arms and hands, grimaces, and fussiness), then he is organized, even if he is working hard to achieve that organization. If disorganization is unavoidable, even when sensitive handling is provided, the infant needs a great deal more preparatory support before, during, and even after caregiving, with minimal activity during handling.

It is the job of the organizational assessment to describe the degree of organization in the infant's behavioral repertoire (smooth functioning) and where, when, and how these behaviors turn to disorganized ones (stressful reactions). Are there changes in the infant's color, breathing, or movement patterns as he is moved? Or can he be moved from one place to another with minimal adjustments and limited cost to his systems? What strategies does the caregiver need to employ to help the infant function smoothly? The organizational assessment provides data for answering all these questions.

As Described in Chapter 12, several tools have been developed to describe and quantify neurobehavioral organization and function of both term and preterm newborns. In many intensive care nurseries and follow-up clinics, neurobehavioral assessment is an essential part of the comprehensive care of the high-risk newborn. Evaluating behavior is a useful concept because it facilitates understanding of the infant's ability to cope with his or her environment and develop and conserve energy reserves for recovery. Evaluation also allows for the development of interactional capacities, including alerting and orienting to caregivers' faces and objects in the environment.

ASSESSING THE TERM NEWBORN

The first exam uses the Newborn Behavioral Assessment Scale (NBAS).[1] The NBAS is appropriate to use with term infants and can be administered until the end of the second month of life. Supplementary items are also available for use with healthy preterm newborns. This examination is not appropriate for infants requiring neonatal intensive care or recovering from it.

The examination is structured with a preferred order of presentation of items. The infant's state plays a major role in the evaluation; therefore, observing the state of consciousness becomes the starting point. This sample evaluation describes some of the major responses of a healthy term newborn, but space does not permit description of the entire examination. Administration of the NBAS items requires specific training if the examiner is to obtain reliable results. This description highlights some of the behaviors that would be encountered in the examination of a healthy term newborn.

Initially, the examiner evaluates level of state by observing respirations, eye movements, startles, and body movements. A specific scoring system is utilized to describe the initial state and the predominant states throughout the examination. In addition, the range and variety of state changes are noted. Once

state is observed, habituation is evaluated. Habituation is the degree to which the nervous system reduces or inhibits responsiveness to a repeated stimulus until shutdown. A flashlight is passed across the sleeping infant's closed eyes ten times, and the degree of response and response decrement is noted. The assessment is repeated with a rattle and then a bell to note the infant's ability to shut out sound after repeated presentations. A typical response would be a startle or dramatic movement to the first stimulus, followed by some decreasing reaction to each of the remaining ten presentations. A range of responses is possible, but overall, one would like to see the infant react strongly at first and then show a reduction of reaction over time. Next, the supine sleeping infant is uncovered slowly and the response to this change is noted. One may see no change, postural changes, color or breathing changes, or state changes. Next, a series of reflexes is evaluated with the infant still in a supine position. First the reflexes of the hands and feet, including plantar grasp, Babinski, heel prick, ankle clonus, passive tone in legs and arms, rooting response, sucking reflex, and glabella reflex. Each item is presented in a specific pattern with a watchful eye for change and variable responses.

Because the infant is supine, he can be undressed gently as palmar grasp and pull-to-sit reflexes are tested. The infant is then picked up with his head facing away from the examiner, and standing and stepping reflexes are tested. The infant is then placed prone on the bed to evaluate the crawling reflex. Next, the infant is picked up to evaluate incurvation, tonic deviation of head and eyes, and nystagmus. He is held to evaluate cuddliness. Vestibular reactions are assessed by placing a cloth over the infant's eyes and evaluating the defensive movement pattern. Tonic neck reflex and Moro reflex are then tested.

By this time in the examination, the examiner can begin to define what is necessary to help this infant stay in a calm, alert state. When the infant does alert, the social interactive package can be administered. To set the stage for administration of these items, evaluate state, check room temperature and lighting, and have a comfortable chair available. Gently move the infant to the examiner's lap. Ideally, this change will not disrupt the alertness that has been achieved by the infant. The examiner then presents a red ball, a rattle, and the examiner's face alone, voice alone, and the two together. The responses that are evaluated are the degree of visual fixation, gazing, and any avoidance reactions, turning away, or nonresponsiveness. In addition, the examiner may see the degree of recognition of voice and sound in the infant's turning with head and/or eyes to "see" the sound off to the side of each ear.

Throughout the administration of these items, the examiner is vigilant in watching for state changes (i.e., change in the quality of alertness, becoming fussy, or crying). All state changes (if they last at least 15 seconds each) are recorded. The lability of crying and alertness is scored along with irritability. The degree of excitation and ease in consoling the infant are important (self-quieting and consolability). As crying or fussiness develops, the examiner does not immediately stop the cry, but gives the infant a chance to self-quiet, then offers a series of supports to see what level of support quiets the infant. The examiner watches for any attempts or strategies used by the infant to organize himself and quiet himself (such as hands to mouth, bracing a foot, or sucking). The buildup to a full, intense, cry state becomes important so that the examiner can see the degree of self-quieting, as well as what it takes to calm the infant. If, at any time, any physiologic instability is observed, the examiner terminates the exam.

Throughout the examination, the examiner is scoring the infant's best performance. The examination moves from presentation of simple to more vigorous stimuli. A typical term newborn may show a variety of responses, from smooth responses that appear to come steadily and without cost or effort to vigorous activity levels with intense upset, demonstrating a need to be comforted. Some infants are more difficult to comfort than others. They may need specific levels of stimulation to elicit their ability to use the comforting resources available to them. "Normal" encompasses a wide range, and all of these responses can fall within normal limits.

CASE EXAMPLE

Jenna is a normal three-day-old newborn. Her mother, Helena, had recovered from her delivery and was eager to get to know her baby, but had been told that babies do not see well for the first few weeks. Helena had many questions when the nurse came in to discuss Jenna with her. The nurse noted that Jenna's mother had already learned several things about Jenna: how she liked to suck on her fist, what made her cry, and even how to calm her successfully. When the nurse pointed out Jenna's alertness and explained that Jenna could see her mother even at this early stage, Helena seemed skeptical. The nurse suggested that because Jenna was awake now, Helena should hold her in front of her and move her face out of Jenna's vision, call her name, and talk to her. As soon as Jenna heard her mother's voice, her eyes shifted in the direction of her mother's face. Encouraged to keep talking, Helena was extremely pleased as Jenna continued to look and search until she found her mother's face and voice. As Jenna gazed at her mother, the nurse pointed out that if she kept Jenna's face within ten inches of her own face, Jenna could focus and look (Figures B-1 and B-2). Helena and Jenna sat gazing at each other, enthralled, for several minutes. After these minutes, her nurse, who had

FIGURE B-1 ▲ Jenna gazes at her mother's face.

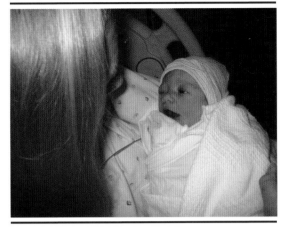

FIGURE B-2 ▲ Jenna gazes at her father's face in full alert state.

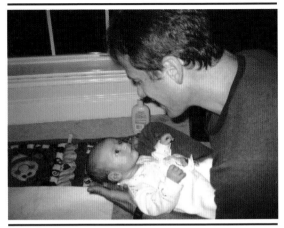

remained quiet while letting them get to know each other, explained that Jenna could indeed see and even hear and look for her mother's voice and face. She suggested that this be a game they could play. Helena was absolutely amazed and proud at the same time, marveling at her baby's capacity to interact at such a young age.

ASSESSING PRETERM INFANT BEHAVIOR

The Assessment of Preterm Infant behavior (APIB) was created to provide a comprehensive functional assessment of the behavior and development of the less mature newborn.[2] Its purpose is to determine how infants cope with the intense environment of the NICU and the degree of organization of the central nervous system. The assessment seeks to describe the unique way in which each individual infant interacts, copes with, and integrates experience from the world around him. The degree of organization rather than maturation of the central nervous system is the focus because in this model the infant is seen as being in continuous interaction with the environment.

This assessment is intended to identify an infant's current level of balanced and smooth integrated function. In other words, identifying in which situations and with what supports the infant appears to function smoothly and is relaxed and comfortable enables the caretaker to promote organized behavior. It is also the purpose of the assessment to enable the examiner to describe the threshold of disorganization indicated in the infant's behaviors of defense and avoidance. The degree and kind of stress and intensity of frustration or defense that the infant experiences can be indicators of the degree of energy the infant has available. The assessment will also show if there is any leeway in the infant's responses. For example, if the infant can tolerate being turned over to supine from prone (where he is flexed, tucked, and resting calmly) without demonstrating disorganized behaviors (such as extended arms and hands, grimaces, and fussiness), then he is organized, whatever difficulty he has achieving this state. If the infant cannot display organized behavior when being handled sensitively, he requires greater preparatory support before, during, and after caregiving and minimal activity.

Training in the APIB is available by contacting Heidelise Als, PhD, Neurobehavioral Infant and Child Studies, Children's Hospital, 320 Longwood Avenue, Boston, Massachusetts 02115.

FIGURE B-3 ▲ Containment helps the preterm infant to stay organized.

Alejandra, as her mother holds her close and contains her, curls her fingers around her mother's finger, holds on, and can suck on her hand and "hold" her mother's face.

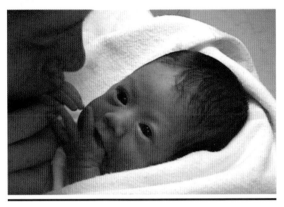

FIGURE B-4 ▲ Alert state.

Alejandra focuses and scans the outer edges of her mother's face with a clear calm alert state.

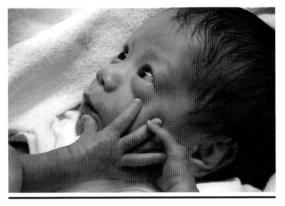

Assessing The Healthy Preterm Newborn

Assessing the organizational function of a healthy preterm newborn follows much the same approach as examining the term infant, but the expected responses are different. The following example represents a healthy preterm newborn who was an appropriate weight for gestational age when delivered at 33 weeks and who is now 36 weeks postmenstrual age. The infant is considered a "feeder and grower," is maintained in a small open crib in the nursery, and is breastfed every two to four hours.

As the examiner begins the evaluation of this infant, she is positioned supine with support to maintain flexion and midline. Her hips and legs are flexed, with rolled blankets for support. One hand is placed on top of the infant's face and the other arm extended along the side of her body. The infant is breathing regularly and has stable oxygen saturation levels. Her color is pink and she is in deep sleep. Her nicely flexed body position, regular breathing, and good color indicate organized sleep. Assessment of habituation responses with several equal flashes from a flashlight yields an intense startle at first shine,

followed by brief squirming and returning to sleep. The second and third flashes trigger a slightly delayed but less intense response. The fourth flash yields a cycle of activity starting with the startle, and then all arms and legs react, followed by a brief stoppage and then a recycling of less intense movements. The next flash yields a facial movement only, and then stillness. The infant's breathing is regular, but color is pale around the eyes and nose. The next two flashes produce no reaction. Thus, the infant had some difficulty inhibiting the motor arousal with one cycle of response, but was able to eventually settle into sleep and shut out the remaining light stimuli. Using a rattle as an auditory sound stimulus, the examiner repeats a similar sequence of ten trials. The first response shows a movement, with subsequent responses subsiding, and eventually the infant successfully inhibits the motor response. The second auditory stimulus of a bell produces no response, and the infant cannot be aroused. This means that the sequence can end because the infant has shut down successfully. These are appropriate habituation responses for a healthy preterm newborn.

The next part of the assessment evaluates movement, posture, and tone. Begin by placing the infant on her back. As she is touched,

FIGURE B-5 ▲ Organized preterm infant.

Alejandra can sustain looking at her mother while being talked to. Her mother holds her hands and contains her entire body. Alejandra focuses only on her mother's face.

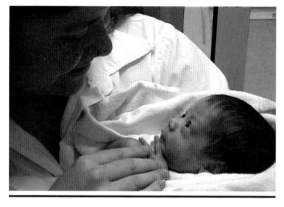

FIGURE B-6 ▲ Disorganized preterm infant.

Alejandra squirms on the bed and has difficulty tucking and calming on her own. She shows her stress by extending her arms and fingers in jerky movements over and over.

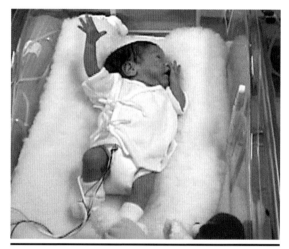

her color changes across her face, her hands become blue, and her trunk appears mottled. She makes jerky arm and leg movements in all directions. The infant awakens and squirms. The examiner places her hand on the soles of the infant's feet and contains them, allowing the leg movements to slow, which softens the arm movements. As the examiner bends over the infant and talks quietly, her eyes open and she fixates on the examiner's face.

Now that the infant is calmer and is able to use motor inhibition to quiet her state and movement pattern, the examiner touches the sole of her foot and begins a series of reflexive tests. As the infant's feet are touched, she once again becomes active with uncontrolled activity of arms, legs, and trunk, resulting in prolonged tremors. The infant also begins breathing irregularly, and her color changes, so that she appears very pale. She does not fuss or cry, but it is clear that the examiner's tactile stimulation has aroused the motor system beyond the infant's capacity to regain any control on her own. As the infant is placed on her stomach, she squirms and attempts to regain control. By pressing her feet against the bottom wall of the incubator and putting her

hands to her face, the infant is able to inhibit the squirming and motor movements. Her color and breathing once again come under control.

The examiner wraps the infant and lifts her to assess social skills. The examiner places the infant's face about 12 inches away from hers. The infant opens her eyes wide and actively avoids the examiner, turning away. The examiner speaks softly, keeping her face unavailable and out of the infant's visual field. The baby seems to relax, and her hands open and close rhythmically, her face softens, her mouth begins to purse, and eventually the infant turns her head in the direction of the voice. As the infant continues to focus, looking and staying alert, her arms, hands, and head lift toward the examiner in a generalized approach movement. At the height of this approach, she yawns and sneezes and then settles into a resting state. Then the examiner presents the rattle to the infant and sees a different response. She startles, and frowns, and pales. The examiner presents the sound again, but more softly, and the infant turns to the left, in the direction of

FIGURE B-7 ▲ Disorganized preterm infant.

Alejandra tries to suck on her fingers. She cannot do so and becomes upset and splays her fingers.

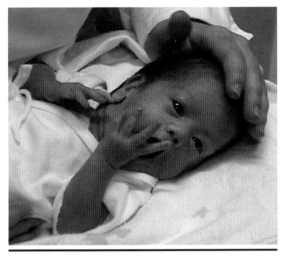

the sound. The infant appears more relaxed and with great effort shifts her eyes to search in the direction of the rattle. Even though her movements remain smooth, she becomes paler and frowns again, indicating the cost of this maneuver to her nervous system.

These responses indicate that although this infant can process and respond to the information, it is very taxing for her. Being held wrapped and being placed on the examiner's lap help the infant to respond. She can show her ability to be selective, choosing the animate social voice to turn to and avoiding the more difficult inanimate auditory stimulus of the rattle. The infant's responses give the overall impression of a well-organized healthy preterm newborn. She is capable of communicating within a range of behaviors in which she can function smoothly without stress to her systems. Her sleep is stable, and her ability to visually and auditorily process stimuli indicates that she can handle stimuli without becoming upset or irritable. With the onset of a stimulus that is too loud, the infant's autonomic system is taxed, and she becomes pale, but the assistance of being wrapped and

supported on the examiner's lap, along with a slower presentation of the stimulus, affords the infant an opportunity to smoothly regulate her motor and autonomic systems. This infant is able to avoid overwhelming input with some degree of specificity by rejecting taxing and costly stimulation.

If this infant is given a supportive environment, several developmental achievements can be predicted for the next two to three months. First, her intense sensitivity to activity will lessen, and her autonomic nervous system will mature to a degree so that sleeping and wakefulness will become more regular. She is already able to become alert and begin some social interaction, but she has a low threshold for stimulation. She demonstrates the capacity for consistent modulation of his ability to self-regulate when the stimulation is appropriate. As the infant's organization increases, the examiner should see arousal of her motor system after tactile stimulation lessens. The infant has demonstrated that she can modulate her arousal when the examiner provides containment (putting her hands on the infant's feet, wrapping her, and letting her press her feet against a surface). The infant has also shown that her movements become smoother when motor arousal is diminished. Additional signs of motor organization include the ability to bring fingers to mouth and to fold hands under chin and keep them together. The infant is also demonstrating the ability to make a transition from one state to another without becoming upset. Figures B-5 through B-9 show a preterm infant in an organized state, and disorganized state, with some instances of infant cues.

ASSESSING THE IMMATURE, FRAGILE PRETERM INFANT

Some infants may show a range of immature or highly sensitive reactions to handling and environmental stimuli. At one extreme of

FIGURE B-8 ▲ Disorganized preterm infant unable to cope with outside stimulation.

Alejandra fusses diffusely (disorganized state) when her head is stroked and waves her arms and extends her fingers.

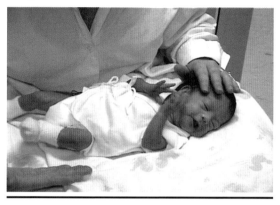

FIGURE B-9 ▲ Preterm infant signals "time out."

Alejandra turns away from her mother's face and extends her fingers in a "time-out" gesture, indicating that she is overwhelmed.

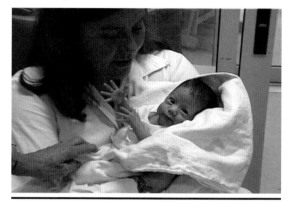

the continuum of preterm functioning is the hyperreactive infant who reacts to all stimuli, lacking any ability to shut them out and protect himself. This infant appears to be "at the mercy of the stimuli."[1–3] As a result of this overreaction and a great sensitivity to incoming stimuli, his autonomic system pays a severe cost in stress.[1,2] This infant overreacts to sound or to being touched with a series of startles and limb extensions, followed by uncontrollable flailing, arching, and squirming. Soon he is in an unbreakable cycle that goes on until he either stops breathing or drops his oxygen saturation level or heart rate. This is costly to the infant because it uses energy and delays his ability to consolidate the regulation of his motor and state systems.[1–3] This infant's high reactivity interferes with his growth and may lead to failure to thrive.

Unlike the hyperreactive preterm infant, the lethargic, depressed infant does not respond to stimuli.[1–3] This preterm newborn appears to want to preserve his fragile autonomic regulation. Because he will not respond and does not put any energy into attempted interactions, he does not develop or activate new pathways or take in new information. Therefore, he

develops a rigid or minimal range of response. This infant lies unresponsive and uncommunicative. He appears depressed to his caregivers and is unable to respond to their efforts to communicate with him.

Some premature infants exhibit a combination of these two types of response patterns, demonstrating an overreactive range of sensitivity at times and later becoming unavailable if overwhelmed by the constant environmental stimuli of light and noise. In some disorganized infants, the pattern of protest takes the form of resistant squirms, turning away, pushing away, and avoidance of being held. These behaviors can be channeled into a more modulated level of interaction if the caregiver slowly introduces caregiving activities, allowing the infant time to ease into them.[4] For example, taking very tiny breaks while preparing the infant for feeding or a bath can provide just the pace the infant needs to remain involved.

SUMMARY

An appropriate behavioral assessment describes the infant's abilities to utilize intervention support and delineates what kinds of facilitation will be necessary to ensure smooth functioning. If the infant can mount a defense against overloading inputs, then a stable and more organized response range will emerge, and the next developmental agenda will be realized. The new capacities become competencies, and the next level of development occurs.[5-6]

The ability to understand and reveal the infant's full range of responses and defenses becomes essential when parents of a newborn infant begin to read his behaviors as meaningful communications. The nurse's role is to help parents become attuned to the infant's responses and reactions. If parents can interpret the behaviors and understand the infant's message, they can generate appropriate interactions. When parents and caregivers can support the infant based on his behavioral cues, the infant becomes aware of his own competence and can improve his overall autonomy while his caregivers continue to develop their understanding of his unique individuality as he progresses.

REFERENCES

1. Brazelton TB, and Nugent JK. 1995. *Neonatal Behavioral Assessment Scale,* 3rd ed. London: Mac Keith Press.
2. Als H, et al. 1982. Assessment of preterm infant behavior (APIB). In *Theory and Research in Behavioral Pediatrics,* vol. 1, Fitzgerald HE, and Yogman M, eds. New York: Plenum Press, 63–133.
3. Als H. 1985. *Manual for the Naturalistic Observation of Newborn Behavior: Preterm and Full Term Infants.* Boston: The Children's Hospital.
4. Als H. 1984. Newborn behavioral assessment. In *Progress in Pediatric Psychology,* Burns WJ, and Lavigne JV, eds. New York: Grune and Stratton.
5. Holditch-Davis D, Blackburn ST, and VandenBerg K. 2007. Neurobehavioral development. In *Comprehensive Neonatal Nursing: An Interdisciplinary Approach,* 4th ed., Kenner C, and Lott JW, eds. Philadelphia: Saunders, 236–284.
6. Brazelton TB, Parker WB, and Zuckerman B. 1976. Importance of behavioral assessment of the neonate. *Current Problems in Pediatrics* 7(2): 1–82.

NOTES

Notes

Glossary of Terms

Abduction: Drawing a limb or limbs away from the midline of the body or the digits away from the axial line of the limb. The lower the neonate's gestational age, the greater the amount of hip abduction seen.

Acetabulum: The cup-shaped cavity in which the femoral head articulates.

Achondroplasia: Congenitally shortened lower extremities, seen when the ratio of upper body length to lower body length exceeds 1.7:1.

Acrocyanosis: Bluish discoloration of the palms of the hands and the soles of the feet. This condition is normal in otherwise normal neonates immediately after birth, but should not persist longer than 48 hours. Also sometimes called *peripheral cyanosis.*

Active alert state: A wakeful state of infant consciousness characterized by increased motor activity and sensitivity to stimuli. The eyes are less attentive than in the quiet alert state, and periods of fussiness may be seen. In this state, preterm infants may become distressed and unable to focus.

Active sleep: A sleeping state of infant consciousness characterized by low activity but with some response to external stimuli (startle, brief crying noises). Rapid eye movements may be seen.

Adduction: Drawing a limb or limbs toward the midline of the body or the digits toward the axial line of the limb. In the neonate, hip adduction increases with gestational age.

Adventitious breath sounds: Abnormal breath sounds or sounds not normally found within the lungs.

Agenesis: Absence or failure of development of any organ or part.

Allis's sign: A procedure for observing femoral length. With the infant's feet flat on the bed and the big toes and femurs aligned, flex the infant's knees. Face the feet and observe the height of the knees. A positive Allis's sign is present if one knee is higher than the other.

Anal wink: Reflexive contraction of the anal sphincter in response to gentle stroking of the anal area. This reflex aids inspection of sphincter placement and tone in the newborn. Also called *anocutaneous reflex.*

Anencephaly: A defect in the newborn's skull (beginning at the vertex and extending, in some cases, to the foramen magnum) resulting from defective closure of the anterior neural tube. Hemorrhagic and fibrotic cerebral tissue protrudes, uncovered, through the defect. Generally, anencephaly involves the forebrain and some amount of the upper brainstem. The infant displays an underdeveloped cranial vault, shallow orbits, and protruding eyes. Abnormalities of other systems are also seen.

Anomaly: A deviation from normal, especially a defect of congenital or hereditary origin.

A **minor anomaly** is one that is of little cosmetic significance and requires minimal or no intervention. Many deformations fall into this category. A **major anomaly** is cosmetically significant and requires medical intervention. Most malformations and disruptions are categorized as major anomalies. The greater the number of minor anomalies seen in an infant, the higher the risk of a major anomaly also being present.

Anterior axillary line: A reference line (used to describe the location of physical findings) that passes vertically through the anterior axillary fold.

Anterior vascular capsule of the lens: Within the first 24 to 48 hours of life, transient embryologic vascular systems that nourish the eye during active intrauterine growth can be seen on the anterior vascular capsule of the preterm infant's lens using an ophthalmoscope. Because these systems appear at week 27 and disappear by the end of week 34 of gestation, the degree of their presence in the neonate's lens can be used to determine gestational age.

Aphonia: Loss of the voice.

Apical impulse: The forward thrust of the left ventricle during systole, usually seen in the newborn in the fourth intercostal space at or left of the midclavicular line. An apical impulse downward and to the left suggests left ventricular dilatation. A very sharp apical impulse indicates high cardiac output or left ventricular hypertrophy.

Aplasia cutis congenita (ACC): A congenital abnormality of unknown cause, aplasia cutis congenita most often appears on the scalp (over the parietal bones or near the sagittal suture) and is characterized by the absence of some or all layers of the skin. It may be an isolated defect or may be associated with chromosomal disorders such as trisomy 13.

Apnea: A lapse of 20 seconds or more between respiratory cycles, with bradycardia or color changes. Apnea is commonly seen in premature neonates, and is outgrown as the infant approaches term. It is abnormal in near-term or term infants.

Appropriate for gestational age (AGA): An infant whose weight, length, and/or occipital-frontal circumference falls between the tenth and the ninetieth percentiles for gestational age when plotted on a standard growth chart.

Areola: The darkened area surrounding the nipple. In a full-term infant, it is raised and stippled, with 0.75–1 cm of palpable breast tissue. The distance between the outside of the two areolae should be less than 25 percent of the chest circumference.

Arnold-Chiari malformation: A congenital anomaly marked by inferior displacement of the medulla and fourth ventricle into the upper cervical canal and elongation and thinning of the upper medulla and lower pons, along with interior displacement of the lower cerebellum through the foramen magnum into the lower cervical canal. It is generally associated with hydrocephalus and myelomeningocele.

Arrhythmia: An irregularity in the heart rhythm. Arrhythmias are common—and usually benign—in the newborn. **Sinus arrhythmia** is characterized by irregularity of the R-R interval with an otherwise normal cardiac cycle. **Premature atrial beat**, seen in perhaps a third of healthy term and premature infants, is an early beat arising from a supraventricular focus, with normal ventricular conduction. **Premature ventricular beat** is an early beat arising from an irritable ventricular focus, with abnormal ventricular conduction producing a wide QRS complex.

Arthrogryposis: Congenital limitation of movement of limbs due to nonprogressive contracture of the joint.

Ascites: Accumulation of serous fluid in the peritoneal cavity.

Asphyxia, perinatal: Acidosis, hypoxia, and hypercapnia caused by lack of oxygen and carbon dioxide exchange and decreased perfusion in the fetus or the newborn. It may result in hypoxic-ischemic encephalopathy.

Association: A combination of defects that occur together more frequently than would be normal by chance, but that is less fixed than the pattern seen in a syndrome. Associations are generally named by acronyms formed from the initial letter of each defect in them.

Atelectasis: Incomplete expansion of all or part of a lung.

Atresia, anal: Congenital absence of the anal canal and/or orifice, indicated by lack of stool passage, progressive abdominal distention, and finally vomiting. Also called *imperforate anus.*

Atresia, bilateral choanal: Obstruction of the posterior nasal passages. Infants affected are cyanotic at rest and pink when crying because they are breathing through an open mouth.

Atresia, esophageal: Congenital lack of continuity of the esophagus, characterized by excessive salivation.

Auscultation: A physical assessment technique involving listening for body sounds—chiefly those of the heart and lungs, but also those of the pleura and abdomen. *Direct* auscultation is performed without the aid of a stethoscope; *indirect (mediate)* auscultation involves use of the stethoscope.

Avulsion: A tearing away.

Barrel chest: An abnormality of the bony structure of the chest in which the anterior-posterior diameter of the chest is greater than normal. It is seen with TTN, meconium aspiration, and hyperinflation.

Behavioral assessment: Evaluation of the infant's ability to interact with the environment; includes assessment of organization, changes in state of consciousness, response to stimuli, and evaluation of motor maturity, and muscle tone, strength, and coordination.

Behavioral cues: Signs infants give to indicate their physical, psychological, and social needs. **Signs of attention** (also called *signs of approach*) indicate a readiness to interact. These cues include an alert, focused gaze, and regular breathing; they may also include grasping, sucking, or hand-to-mouth movements. **Time-out signals** (also called *avoidance behaviors*) indicate the need for a respite from interaction. These cues include an averted gaze, frowning, sneezing, yawning, vomiting, and hiccups, sometimes accompanied by finger splaying, arching, and stiffening. Color changes, apnea, irregular breathing, and decreased oxygen saturation levels may also be seen.

Bell's palsy: Paralysis of the facial nerve with a resultant characteristic distortion of the face—unilateral.

Biparietal diameter (low profile type):

Biparietal diameter (low flattening type):

Bones, cranial: There are four cranial bones: the *frontal, occipital, parietal,* and *temporal.* See Figure 5-3 for locations.

Bowel sounds: Metallic, tinkling sounds heard every 15–20 seconds when the four abdominal quadrants are auscultated beginning within 15 minutes after birth. Hyperactive sounds immediately after feeding, with the intensity of the sounds diminishing as the next feeding approaches, are normal. Auscultation of *friction rubs* (resembling the sound of rubbing a finger over a cupped hand held near the ear) may indicate peritoneal irritation. When heard in the newborn over the lung fields, bowel sounds are likely referred sounds from the abdomen. If they persist, however, they could indicate diaphragmatic hernia.

Brachial plexus palsy: A functional paralysis of part or all of the arm, resulting from birth trauma and more common in large babies. It is caused by stretching injuries to the components of the brachial plexus during delivery. The upper arm is more commonly affected than the lower or the entire arm. The Moro reflex is absent on the affected side, but the grasp reflex remains. If the nerve roots are not injured, neurologic function returns within several days of birth as hemorrhage and edema resolve.

Brachycephaly: Broad skull shape caused by craniosynostosis (premature fusion) of the coronal suture, limiting forward growth of the skull.

Bradycardia, sinus: A heart rate less than 80 beats per minute in a newborn. Transient bradycardia, with origin in the sinus node, is commonly seen in both full-term and premature newborns, generally in response to vagal stimulation.

Bradypnea: Excessively slow respirations. In the neonate, persistent respirations of less than 40 per minute are associated with central nervous system depression from such factors as maternal drug ingestion, asphyxia, or birth injury.

Branchial sinus: An abnormal opening seen anywhere along the sternocleidomastoid muscle. It may communicate with deeper structures, with potential for infection.

Bronchial breath sounds: Seldom heard in the neonate, bronchial sounds are the loudest of the normal breath sounds. They are found over the trachea and are marked by a short inspiration and a longer expiration.

Bronchopulmonary dysplasia (BPD): Chronic neonatal lung disease characterized by bronchiolar metaplasia and interstitial fibrosis.

Bronchovesicular breath sounds: Normally found over the manubrium and the intrascapular regions, bronchovesicular sounds are intermediate in intensity between bronchial and vesicular breath sounds. In these sounds, inspiration and expiration are equal in quality, intensity, pitch, and duration.

Bruit: (1) A murmur-like sound auscultated over the fontanels or the lateral skull. It may signify intracranial arteriovenous malformation in an infant with congestive heart failure. (2) A sound, resembling a systolic murmur, heard with dilated, tortuous, or constricted vessels during auscultation of the skull. It is produced by the vibration of vessel walls within the skull, caused by flow disturbances that interfere with the normal laminar flow through the vessels. Bruits may be heard with Sturge-Weber syndrome. (3) If heard over the newborn's abdomen and not eliminated by changing the infant's position, bruits may indicate umbilical vein or hepatic vascular system abnormalities, renal artery stenosis, or hepatic hemangiomas.

Brushfield spots: White specks scattered linearly around the circumference of the iris. These spots are associated with Down syndrome, but may also be seen as a normal variant.

Bulla: An elevation of the skin filled with serous fluid (a vesicle) greater than 1 cm in diameter.

Café au lait spot (patch): A tan or light brown macule or patch with well-defined borders. One patch is found in up to 19 percent of normal children, and these patches are of no pathologic significance when they are less than 3 cm in length and less than six in number. A greater number of patches or patches larger than 3 cm may indicate a cutaneous neurofibromatosis, an autosomal dominant genetic disorder.

Candida diaper dermatitis: A moist, erythematous rash caused by or associated with *Candida albicans* and consisting of small white or yellow pustules over the buttocks and perianal region (and occasionally the thighs).

Canthus: The angle at either end of the opening between the eyelids. The eye has two canthi, the inner (adjacent to the nose) and the outer.

Capillary filling time: A measurement used to assess cardiac perfusion in the newborn. Press the infant's skin with a finger until it blanches; then count the seconds required for the color to return. This should take no more than three to four seconds in a normal infant. Check filling time in both a central and a peripheral area.

Caput: The head.

Caput succedaneum: Edema occurring in and under the presenting part of the fetal scalp during delivery, generally due to pressure restricting venous and lymph flow. The edema has poorly defined edges, pits on pressure, and usually crosses suture lines. It resolves within a few days. Caput succedaneum is the most common form of birth trauma to the head.

Cephalhematoma: Collection of blood (hemorrhage) between the periosteum and the skull, generally resulting from birth trauma. The edges are clearly demarcated and bounded by suture lines. Cephalhematomas are most commonly seen over the parietal and occipital bones. Over time, a cephalhematoma may liquefy and become fluctuant on palpation; resolution can take weeks to months.

Chordee: Ventral bowing of the penis, which produces a downward curvature on erection. It is often seen with hypospadias.

Chromosomal aneuploidy: Too many or too few chromosomes, resulting in a genetic malformation. Normal infants have 46 chromosomes (22 pairs of autosomes and 2 sex chromosomes). Forms of aneuploidy include monosomy and trisomy.

Clavicle: One of the pair of bones linking the sternum with a scapula. Commonly called the *collarbone.*

Cleft lip: A congenital defect in the upper lip.

Cleidocranial dysostosis: Syndrome characterized by congenital complete or partial absence of the clavicles. Defective cranial ossification, large fontanels, and delayed suture closure are often seen with complete absence of clavicles. This anomaly is characterized by excessive scapulothoracic motion.

Clonic: Relating to or characterized by clonus.

Clonus: Involuntary repetitive muscle contraction and relaxation.

Clubfoot *(talipes equinovarus)*: One of the common congenital deformities of the foot, seen more often in male infants than in female, and varying in severity. The forefoot is adducted and points medially, there is pronounced varus of the heel, and the foot and toes point downward. In unilateral presentation, the affected foot is smaller, with thickened joints.

Coloboma: A malformation characterized by absence of or a defect in the tissue of the eye. It is sometimes seen as a keyhole-shaped pupil and associated with other anomalies.

Congenital absence of the radius: A bilateral anomaly in half the infants who exhibit it, radial absence presents with a deviated hand and wrist, a shortened forearm with a bowed ulna, an absent or hypoplastic thumb, and limited elbow movement. The condition may require surgery.

Congenital absence of the tibia or fibula: This unusual anomaly more frequently affects the fibula than the tibia and is more often unilateral than bilateral. There may be partial or complete absence of the bone. Foot deformity and leg length discrepancies are generally seen in the absence of either long bone.

Congenital constricting bands (Streeter dysplasia): Bands of tissue (thought to be amniotic in origin) encircling one or more extremities of the newborn. These bands can produce shallow indentations of the soft tissue or constrictions severe enough to cause partial or complete amputation of the extremity. Treatment depends on the severity; a surgical consultation may be required.

Congenital heart disease (CHD): A spectrum of cardiac anomalies present at birth. There is increased risk of CHD in infants of mothers with CHD, in infants with an older sibling who has CHD, and in low birth weight infants. An increased incidence of CHD is also associated with extracardiac anomalies, including those of the gastrointestinal, renal, and urogenital systems; tracheoesophageal fistulas; and diaphragmatic hernias.

Consolability: An infant's ability to quiet himself when in the crying state or to respond to attempts by a caregiver to quiet him. An infant with well-developed organization generally exhibits self-consoling behaviors, including bringing the hands to the mouth, sucking on the fist or tongue, or using environmental stimuli as a distraction.

Consolidation: An area of increased lung tissue density.

Cost of attention: A term used by T.B. Brazelton to describe the amount of energy an infant must expend to maintain an alert state of consciousness. The cost of attention depends on both the health and maturity of the infant.

Crackles: Adventitious breath sounds involving a series of brief crackling or bubbling sounds. (Crackles were previously termed *rales*.) **Fine crackles,** usually heard at the end of inspiration, resemble the sound made by rubbing a lock of hair. They may be associated with RDS or BPD. **Medium crackles** sound like a carbonated fizz. They are believed to reflect the passage of air past sticky surfaces, as found with pneumonia or TTN. **Coarse crackles** (also called *rhonchi*) are loud, bubbly sounds associated with mucus or fluid accumulation in the large airways.

Craniosynostosis: Premature fusion of one or more sutures, stopping bone growth perpendicular to the suture but permitting it parallel to the suture.

Craniotabes: Areas of soft (demineralized) bone in the skull, usually in the occipital and parietal bones along the lambdoidal suture. Craniotabes is sometimes seen with hydrocephalus.

Cremasteric reflex: Contraction of the cremaster muscle resulting in a drawing up of the ipsilateral testis when the inner thigh is stroked or stretched longitudinally.

Cri du chat syndrome: A chromosomal disorder in which the short arm of the fifth chromosome is missing. It presents with a catlike cry in the newborn and other associated anomalies.

Crust: Dried serous exudate, blood, or pus.

Crying: A wakeful state of infant consciousness characterized by crying (in term infants), increased motor activity, color changes, and exaggerated response to unpleasant stimuli. Some term infants console themselves by returning to a lower state of consciousness. Preterm infants may have a very weak (or even absent) cry, but exhibit the other signs of stress indicative of this state.

Cryptorchidism: Failure of one or both testes to descend into the scrotum. It can be unilateral (most often occurring on the right side) or bilateral. In full-term infants who present with undescended testes at birth, about half show descent by six weeks of age;

in 75 percent of preterm infants, the testes descend by three months of age. Testes do not usually descend spontaneously after nine months of age. Inguinal hernia is commonly seen with cryptorchidism.

Cutis marmorata: Bluish mottling or marbling of the skin in response to chilling, stress, or overstimulation, usually disappearing when the infant is warmed.

Cyanosis, central: Bluish discoloration of the skin and mucous membranes due to significant arterial oxygen desaturation. It presents when at least 5 g of unbound (to oxygen) hemoglobin are present per 100 mL of blood. An important indicator of congenital heart disease, cyanosis due to cardiac causes does not improve on administration of 100 percent oxygen and also increases with crying. In cyanotic infants without increased respiratory effort, the cause of the cyanosis is most likely congenital heart disease. Central cyanosis may also occur in the presence of persistent pulmonary hypertension, lung disease, sepsis, or neurologic disease. Central cyanosis must be differentiated from acrocyanosis (peripheral cyanosis) and circumoral cyanosis, both of which are normally seen in the first few days after birth.

Cyanosis, circumoral: Bluish discoloration of the lips and area surrounding the mouth.

Darwinian tubercle: A normal variant appearing as a small nodule on the upper helix of the ear.

Deep sleep state: A sleeping state of infant consciousness characterized by closed eyes, regular breathing, and lack of spontaneous activity. Response to external stimuli is delayed.

Defect, single-gene: A genetically caused malformation. The form of inheritance may be dominant (carried by one gene from one parent), recessive (requiring one gene from each parent), or X-linked (carried on the X chromosome and expressed in male offspring, with female offspring being carriers).

Deformation: A congenital abnormality caused by pressure exerted by mechanical forces on the fetus generally late in gestation after the major organ systems are formed. The source of the pressure is generally uterine constraint (maternal or fetal). Most deformations occur to the musculoskeletal system.

Depigmentation lesion: A white, macular lesion with an irregular, leaflike border. These lesions may be early indicators of tuberous sclerosis, a progressive degenerative neurologic disease.

Dermis: Inner, vascular layer of the skin containing fibrous and elastic tissues, sweat and sebaceous glands and ducts, hair follicles and shafts, blood vessels, and nerves. Also called *corium.*

Developmental dysplasia of the hip: An abnormality in which the hip joint develops abnormally, causing instability of the hip ranging from minimal to dislocation. The causes of congenital hip dysplasia may include lack of acetabular depth, laxity of the ligaments, and/or intrauterine breech position. Congenital hip dysplasia is more often seen in Caucasian than in African American or Asian infants; it is more common in females than in males, and the left hip is affected more often than the right. In multiple births, it is more common in the first born. A positive Allis's sign may indicate congenital hip dysplasia. It is associated with other orthopedic anomalies and deformities.

Diaphragmatic hernia: Protrusion of abdominal contents through an opening in the diaphragm.

Diastasis recti: A palpable midline gap between the rectus muscles of the abdominal wall. Bulging may be seen when the infant cries.

Diastasis recti is often seen in otherwise normal infants and is benign unless a hernia is present.

Diastole: Dilation of the heart (particularly of the ventricles), coincident with the interval between the second (S2) and the first (S1) heart sounds.

Disruption: A congenital abnormality caused by the breakdown of normal tissue *in utero.* Most disruptions result from amniotic bands wrapping around fetal extremities or entering the fetus' mouth.

Doll's eye maneuver: Used to evaluate movement of the eyes as the head is turned. The infant's head is gently rotated from side to side; the eyes should deviate away from the direction of rotation, i.e., turning the head to the right, the eyes should deviate to the left.

Dorsiflexion: Flexion toward the back, as in flexion of the foot so that the forefoot is higher than the ankle.

Drowsiness: The transitional state of infant consciousness between sleep and wakefulness. The infant exhibits a variable activity level, with dull, heavy-lidded eyes that open and close periodically. Movements are smooth, and there is response to stimuli, but not immediately.

Dysmorphogenesis: Abnormal development of form or structure, as seen in congenital malformations. Dysmorphic features are also called *anomalies.*

Ecchymosis (plural: ecchymoses): A non-blanching area of subepidermal hemorrhage, initially bluish black in color, then changing to greenish brown or yellow. Ecchymoses may be seen on the labia of female infants and the scrotal area of male infants after breech deliveries.

Edema: Abnormally large amounts of fluid in the intercellular tissue spaces of the body, usually the subcutaneous tissues. Most newborns have some edema around the face and

eyes due to excess fluid volume after delivery. After difficult deliveries, edema of the scalp or in dependent areas is often seen. In *pitting edema,* indentations produced by pressure remain for prolonged periods.

Ejection click: A snappy, high-frequency heart sound normal during the first 24 hours of life; after that, it is considered abnormal. If present, it is best heard just after the first heart sound and resembles in timing, but not in quality, a widely split S1 heart sound.

Embryonic period: The third to the eighth week of pregnancy, the period during which differentiation and major organ system development take place. Insults to the embryo during this period can result in major anomalies in the newborn.

Encephalocele: A restricted disorder of anterior neural tube closure producing a defect in the skull called *cranium bifidum.* In some cases, a skin-covered protrusion (sac) containing meninges and cerebral spinal fluid (and sometimes cerebral tissue) is present. In other cases, the defect appears as a small tissue-covered opening (often surrounded by tufts of abnormal hair) on the skull, with no protrusion of skull contents. The most common location for encephaloceles is the midline of the occipital bone, but they are also seen in the parietal, temporal, or frontal nasopharyngeal areas. Size varies from tiny to massive; severity depends on location, size, and the contents of the protrusion. Skull x-rays can identify the cranium bifidum, and transillumination and ultrasound help identify the contents of the protrusion.

Encephalopathy, hypoxic-ischemic: A syndrome resulting from perinatal asphyxia. It can be categorized as **mild** (associated with irritability, jitteriness, and hyperalertness), **moderate** (characterized by lethargy, hypotonia, decreased spontaneous movement, and seizures), or **severe** (characterized by coma, flaccidity, disturbed brainstem function, and seizures). The pattern of limb weakness displayed by an affected infant reflects the area of the brain injured by the asphyxia. In term neonates, injury to the parasagittal areas (resulting in weakness of the shoulder girdle and proximal upper extremities) or the middle cerebral artery (presenting as hemiparesis) predominates. In the premature newborn, injury is often to the periventricular area, resulting in weakness in the lower extremities.

Epicanthal fold: A vertical fold of skin on either side of the nose that covers the lacrimal caruncle. These folds are normal in Asian infants but suggestive of Down syndrome in neonates of other races.

Epidermis: Outermost layer of the skin, itself composed of five layers. The top layer is the *stratum corneum* (dead cells that are constantly being sloughed off and replaced); lower layers contain keratin-forming cells and melanocytes.

Epispadias: Location of the urethral meatus on the *dorsal* surface of the penis. It is a less common abnormality than hypospadias. In **balanic epispadias,** the meatus is found at the base of the balanus (glans); in **penile epispadias,** it is on the penile shaft; and in **penopubic epispadias,** it is found, not on the penis at all, but directly below the symphysis pubis.

Epstein's pearls: Epidermal inclusion cysts seen in the newborn at the junction of the hard and soft palates of the mouth and on the gums. They usually disappear by a few weeks of age.

Erb's palsy: Damage (generally due to birth trauma) to the upper spinal roots C5 and C6, resulting in paralysis of an arm (but usually without involvement of the hand). See also **Brachial plexus palsy.**

Erythema toxicum neonatorum: A benign rash consisting of small white or yellow papules or vesicles with an erythematous base. Seen in up to 70 percent of term infants between 24 and 48 hours of age, the rash occurs most often on the face, trunk, or extremities.

Everted: Turned out and away from the midline of the body.

Exophthalmos: Abnormal protrusion of the eyeball. It may be associated with hyperthyroidism.

Expected date of confinement (EDC): Delivery due date. Generally 280 days (40 weeks) from the onset of the mother's last menstrual period.

Exstrophy of the bladder: A visible fissure between the anterior abdominal wall and the urinary bladder. In male infants, it is commonly accompanied by epispadias.

Extension: The straightening of a limb at a joint.

Familial traits: Unusual features (subtle or significant) identified by a family as characteristic of its phenotype.

Fasciculation: The spontaneous localized contraction of a group of fibers in a motor unit, visible through the skin. In Werdnig-Hoffmann disease, these continuous and rapid twitching movements can be seen in the tongue.

Fetal period: The ninth week of pregnancy through birth. The fetus becomes more and more resistant to teratogens as this period progresses.

Fibrils: Tiny fibers or filaments connecting the dermis and the epidermis.

Fistula, rectourethral: An abnormal connection between the rectum and the urethra, indicated by the presence of meconium in the urethral orifice.

Fistula, rectovaginal: An abnormal connection between the rectum and the vagina, indicated by the presence of meconium in the vaginal orifice.

Flexion: The act of bending or the condition of being bent. The bending of a limb at a joint. In the neonate, the degree of arm, knee, and hip flexion is indicative of gestational age.

Flexion contracture: Resistance of a muscle to passive flexion. The newborn's hips generally have a flexion contracture; when the right hip is flexed to stabilize the pelvis and flatten the lumbar spine, a flexion contracture of the left hip may be seen. The infant's elbow also shows a flexion contracture for the first few weeks of life, making it difficult to examine.

Fontanel: A membrane-covered space (soft spot) in the infant's skull reflecting incomplete ossification of the skull. Fontanels occur where two sutures meet. The **anterior fontanel** occurs at the intersection of the metopic, coronal, and sagittal sutures. The **posterior fontanel** occurs where the sagittal and lambdoidal sutures meet. The **sphenoid fontanel** is at the juncture of the coronal and squamosal sutures. The **mastoid fontanel** occurs at the intersection of the squamosal and lambdoidal sutures. A defect of the parietal bone along the sagittal suture may appear to be—but is not—a true fontanel (third fontanel). It may be a normal variant or may be associated with Down syndrome or congenital hypothyroidism.

Forcep marks: Red, bruised, or abraded areas on the cheeks, scalp, and face of infants born after application of forceps. Observation of forcep marks calls for examination for facial palsy, fractured clavicles, skull fractures, or other complications of birth trauma.

Frog leg position: A resting posture, normal in premature neonates of 36 or fewer weeks gestation, in which the legs are abducted and the lateral thigh rests against the bed surface. This position is abnormal if seen in newborns older than 36 weeks gestational age.

Funnel chest (pectus excavatum): An abnormality of the bony structure of the chest in which the sternum is indented. It is seen in infants with Marfan syndrome and rickets.

Gastroschisis: Protrusion of abdominal contents and other organs through an abdominal wall defect lateral to the midline; the protrusion is not covered by a membrane. A gastroschisis is associated with fewer congenital malformations than is an omphalocele.

Gestational age: The length of time between fertilization of the egg and birth of the infant.

Glabella: The area above the nose and between the eyebrows (bridge of the nose).

Growth parameters: Measurements used to determine whether an infant is small, appropriate, or large for gestational age. The three parameters are weight, length, and occipital-frontal head circumference.

Habituation: A newborn's ability to alter his response to a repeated stimulus, decreasing and finally eliminating the response on repetition of the stimulus. Habituation is a defense mechanism.

Harlequin sign: A sharply demarcated red color in the dependent half of the body, with the superior half of the body appearing pale, when the infant is placed on his side. Rotating the infant to the other side reverses the coloring. Harlequin color change occurs in both healthy and sick infants but is more common in low birth weight infants. It has no pathologic significance.

Heart rate: The normal heart rate for a full-term neonate is 80–160 beats per minute.

Heart sounds: **S1,** the first heart sound, is best heard at the mitral or tricuspid area. It is usually loud at birth, but decreases in intensity by two days of life. **S2,** the second heart sound, is best heard at the aortic or pulmonic area. It is usually single at birth but is split in two-thirds of infants by 16 hours of age and in 80 percent by 48 hours of age. Wide splitting of S2 is abnormal. **S3,** commonly heard in premature infants with a PDA, is best heard at the apex of the heart during early diastole. **S4,** a pathologic sound, is heard at the apex of the heart in infants with conditions characterized by decreased compliance.

Heave: A point of maximum impulse that is slow rising and diffuse, generally associated with ventricular dilation or volume overload. Also called a *lift.*

Helix: The upper and outer margin of the pinna of the ear.

Hemangioma, cavernous: A raised, lobulated, soft and compressible bluish-red tumor, with poorly defined margins. The cavernous hemangioma consists of large, mature vascular elements lined with endothelial cells and involves the dermis and subcutaneous tissues of the skin. It increases in size during the first 6–12 months of life, and then involutes spontaneously. Two syndromes—Kasabach-Merritt and Klippel-Trenaunay-Weber—may be associated with cavernous hemangiomas.

Hemangioma, strawberry: A raised, lobulated, soft and compressible bright red tumor, with sharply demarcated margins, on the head, neck, trunk, or extremities. (Tumors occurring in the throat can obstruct the airway.) Caused by dilated capillaries, with associated endothelial proliferation in the dermal and subdermal layers of the skin, the strawberry hemangioma occurs in up to 10 percent of newborns. It gradually increases in size for about six months and then spontaneously regresses over a period of up to several years.

Hemiparesis: Muscle weakness or partial paralysis affecting one half of the body.

Hepatomegaly: Enlargement of the liver.

Hermaphroditism: Anomalous differentiation of the gonads, with presence of both ovarian and testicular tissue and ambiguous morphologic sex criteria. Hermaphroditism is suspected when only one testis is confirmed in a male-appearing infant. See also **Pseudohermaphroditism.**

Hernia, epigastric: Protrusion of fat through a defect on the midline above the umbilicus and below the sternum, presenting as a firm palpable mass. Palpation may elicit a pain response. Surgical intervention is necessary.

Hernia, femoral: A small bulge adjacent and medial to the femoral artery. It is more common in females than in males.

Hernia, inguinal: Muscle wall defect in the inguinal area through which bowel loops or gonads enter the scrotal sac (in males) or the soft tissues (in females). The hernia usually presents as bulging in the groin area and is more common in male than in female infants.

Hernia, umbilical: Skin- and subcutaneous-tissue-covered protrusion of part of the intestine at the umbilicus. It is seen with some frequency in low birth weight and African-American male infants and in infants of other races with hypothyroidism. The hernia usually reduces by two years of age, but intervention is required with strangulation of abdominal contents or large size.

Holosystolic: Occurring throughout systole. Also called *pansystolic.*

Hydranencephaly: Partial or complete absence of the cerebral hemispheres, with the space being filled with cerebrospinal fluid.

Hydrocele: A circumscribed collection of clear fluid in the scrotum, which may resolve spontaneously by six months of age. A hydrocele may communicate with the inguinal canal, however, and may be associated with a hernia. **Hydrocele of the cord** presents as a palpable sausage-shaped, smooth bulge above the testes.

Hydrocephalus: Accumulation of cerebrospinal fluid (often under increased pressure) within the skull, due to obstruction of the cerebrospinal fluid pathways causing dilation of the cerebral ventricles. It may be congenital or may develop after birth and is characterized by head enlargement, forehead prominence, brain atrophy, mental deterioration, and convulsions. The skull is often globular in shape.

Hydrometrocolpos: Collection of secretions in the vagina and uterus due to an imperforate hymen. It may be palpated as a small midline lower abdominal mass or a cystic movable mass as the quantity of secretions increases.

Hygroma, cystic: The most commonly seen neck mass in newborns, a cystic hygroma is soft, fluctuant, and can range from only a few centimeters in size to massive. It is usually seen laterally or over the clavicle and transilluminates well.

Hymenal tag: A small appendage or flap on the hymen, normal in female infants. It disappears in several weeks.

Hyperplasia, sebaceous gland: Numerous white or yellow papules (less than 0.5 mm in size) on the nose and upper lips. These enlarged sebaceous glands spontaneously decrease in size with age and require no treatment.

Hypertelorism: Widely spaced eyes—those with greater than a palpebral fissure length between them.

Hypertonia: Increased resistance of the skeletal muscles to passive stretching. In the presence of hypertonia, passive manipulation of the limbs often increases the tone.

Hypertrophy: Enlargement or overgrowth of an organ or part.

Hypertrophy of the clitoris: The most common genitourinary abnormality in female infants, suggesting pseudohermaphroditism.

Hypoplastic nails: Nails that are incompletely developed. Edema of the hands can give the appearance of hypoplastic nails.

Hypospadias: Location of the urethral meatus on the **ventral** surface of the penis. In **balanic (glanular) hypospadias,** the meatus is located at the base of the balanus (glans). In **penile hypospadias,** the meatus is found between the glans and the scrotum. It is often accompanied by chordee, flattening of the glans, and an absent ventral foreskin. In **penoscrotal (perineal) hypospadias,** the meatus is found at the penoscrotal junction. Gender ambiguity is associated with penoscrotal hypospadias, as is bifid scrotum, small penis with a large meatus, and undescended testes.

Hypotelorism: Closely spaced eyes—those with less than a palpebral fissure length between them.

Hypotonia: Depressed postural muscle tone.

Inner canthal distance: The measurement between the inner canthi of the two eyes. If the eyes are normally spaced, this distance should be equal to the length of the palpebral fissure.

Inspection: A physical assessment technique involving careful visual attention to, measurement of, and notation of the status of external body parts and systems, for the purpose of forming a judgment.

Intrauterine growth restricted (IUGR) neonate: A newborn who did not grow *in utero* at the expected rate for weight, length, or occipital-frontal head circumference. Although the term is often used synonymously with small for gestational age (SGA), the two terms do not necessarily mean the same thing. A neonate may be growth restricted but may not fall below the tenth percentile for gestational age.

Inverted: Turned inward toward the midline of the body.

Jaundice: Yellow coloring of the skin and whites of the eyes, generally appearing first on the head and face and then progressing toward the feet. Jaundice is due to excess bilirubin in the blood (hyperbilirubinemia).

Jitteriness: A series of movements seen at times in normal preterm neonates and in normal term neonates with vigorous crying. (Persistent jitteriness may indicate a disorder.) Jitteriness is characterized by rapid movements of equal amplitude in alternating directions, generally occurs in response to a stimulus, can be stopped by flexing and holding the involved extremity, and is not associated with abnormal eye movements or other signs of seizure. Jitteriness must be distinguished from seizure activity. See also **Seizure.**

Karyotype: Representation by diagram of the chromosomal characteristics of an individual or species.

Karyotyping: Chromosomal evaluation.

Keratin: An insoluble, fibrous protein that is the main component of certain protective and/or supportive elements of the body, including the nails, hair, and epidermis.

Klippel-Feil syndrome: Defects of the cervical vertebrae, resulting in a shorter-than-normal neck with limited motion and asymmetry in rotation and lateral flexion.

Klumpke's palsy: Damage (generally due to birth trauma) resulting in paralysis of the forearm. See also **Brachial plexus palsy.**

Kyphosis: A spinal abnormality in which the curvature of the thoracic spine is excessively convex. Commonly called *hunchback.*

Lacrimal caruncle: The red area at the inner canthus of the eye.

Lanugo: A fine, soft, downy hair covering the fetus *in utero* and sometimes the neonate. It first appears at about 20 weeks gestation, covering most of the body including the face. Most of it disappears by 40 weeks gestation.

Large for gestational age (LGA): An infant whose weight falls above the ninetieth percentile for gestational age when plotted on a standard growth chart.

Lesion: Any discontinuity of tissue or change in the structure or function of an organ or part due to disease or trauma.

Leukoplakia: A white spot or patch on the tongue or mucous membranes in the mouth, which cannot be wiped off and that does not clinically represent any other condition.

Light sleep state: See Active sleep.

Lipoma: A benign tumor composed of fat cells.

Lordosis: A spinal abnormality in which the curvature of the lumbar and cervical spine is excessively concave. Commonly called *swayback.*

Low birth weight: An infant who weighs less than 2,500 g at birth.

Macrocephaly: Excessive head size (an occipital-frontal circumference above the ninetieth percentile for gestational age, with otherwise normal weight and length percentiles). Macrocephaly can be familial or it may be due to hydrocephalus or associated with dwarfism or osteogenesis imperfecta.

Macrodactyly: An enlarged finger or toe. It is seen in otherwise normal infants, or it may indicate neurofibromatosis.

Macroglossia: An abnormally large tongue.

Macrostomia: An abnormally large oral opening.

Macule: A discolored, flat, nonpalpable spot or patch less than 1 cm in diameter.

Malacia: Abnormal softening of tissues.

Malformation: A congenital defect arising from abnormal tissue. The cause of the tissue abnormality may be intrinsic (genetic) or extrinsic (environmental).

Manubrium: Uppermost portion of the sternum.

Mediastinum: A space within the chest cavity containing the heart, esophagus, trachea, mainstem bronchi, thymus, and major blood vessels.

Melanosis, transient neonatal pustular: Small pigmented macules (often surrounded by very fine white scales) caused by the rupture of superficial vesiculopustular lesions 12–48 hours after birth. The condition—seen in up to 5 percent of African-American and about 0.2 percent of Caucasian infants—is benign and generally resolves by three months of age.

Meningocele: A lesion associated with spina bifida in which more than one vertebra is involved. The meninges protrude through the bony defect and are covered by a thin atrophic skin. The spinal roots and nerves are normal.

Metatarsus adductus: A common congenital foot anomaly caused by intrauterine positioning. It may be positional (flexible) or structural (fixed). In the structural type (with bony abnormalities), there is limited abduction of the forefoot, and the heel is in a valgus position. In the positional type, the forefoot abducts easily, and the heel is in a varus or neutral position.

Microcephaly: Abnormal smallness of the head (an occipital-frontal circumference below the tenth percentile for gestational age), generally due to poor brain growth.

Micrognathia: An abnormally small lower jaw, seen in Robin sequence and other syndromes.

Micropenis: Abnormally small penis. Micropenis suggests congenital hypopituitarism when seen with certain other anomalies or conditions. Also called *penile hypoplasia.*

Microstomia: An abnormally small oral opening. It may be seen with some trisomies.

Midclavicular line: A reference line (used to describe the location of physical findings) passing vertically through the clavicle.

Midsternal line: A reference line (used to describe the location of physical findings) bisecting the suprasternal notch.

Milia: Multiple yellow or pearly white papules about 1 mm in size. These epidermal cysts, found on the brow, cheeks, and nose of up to 40 percent of newborns, are caused by accumulation of sebaceous gland secretions and spontaneously resolve during the first few weeks of life.

Miliaria: Changes in the skin caused by obstruction of the sweat ducts. Miliaria is generally associated with excessive warmth and/or humidity and is classified into four types, based on severity. **Miliaria crystallina** occurs when sweat escapes into the epidermal stratum corneum, causing formation of clear, thin vesicles 1–2 mm in diameter. **Miliaria rubra,** commonly called *prickly heat,* presents as small erythematous papules and occurs when continued obstruction of the sweat ducts causes release of sweat into adjacent tissues of the epidermis. **Miliaria pustulosa** occurs with continued occlusion of the sweat ducts, as leukocytes infiltrate the vesicles. Unresolved miliaria pustulosa can lead to **miliaria profunda,** secondary infection of the deeper dermal portions of the sweat glands.

Mongolian spot: A large gray or blue-green macule or patch caused by melanocyte infiltration of the dermis. This pigmented lesion, generally found on the buttocks, flanks, or shoulders, is seen in up to 90 percent of African-American, Asian, and Hispanic and up to 10 percent of Caucasian infants.

Morphogenesis: Differentiation of cells and tissues in the early embryo that establishes the form and structure of the various organs and parts of the body.

Mottling: Blotchy skin showing areas of different color. It may indicate cardiogenic shock in the neonate.

Mucocele: A mucous retention cyst (distended cavity containing mucus) presenting as a translucent or bluish swelling under the tongue.

Murmur: A prolonged heart sound caused by turbulent blood flow. Documenting the timing, location, intensity, radiation, quality, and pitch are all important to the evaluation of the origin of a murmur, as is the age of the newborn. There are two types of murmurs: *innocent* and *pathologic;* see **Murmurs, innocent** and **Murmurs, pathologic.**

Murmur, continuous: A pathologic murmur, heard through both systole and diastole, present in about a third of premature infants with a PDA and also in full-term or premature infants with arteriovenous fistulas.

Murmur, continuous systolic (crescendo systolic): An innocent murmur heard in up to 15 percent of newborns, beginning within the first 8 hours of life. It is best heard in the upper left sternal border.

Murmur, early soft midsystolic ejection: An innocent murmur often heard in premature infants, beginning within the first week or two of life and disappearing by the eighth week. Medium- to high-pitched, it is best heard in the upper left sternal border, with wide radiation.

Murmur, loud systolic ejection: A pathologic murmur that presents within hours of birth, generally due to aortic or pulmonary stenosis or coarctation of the aorta.

Murmur, systolic ejection: An innocent murmur heard in more than half of all newborns, beginning within the first day of life and lasting up to a week. It can be described as "vibratory" and is best heard along the mid- and upper left sternal border.

Murmurs, innocent: Innocent murmurs have no pathologic cause within the heart or great vessels. They are generally systolic, symptomless, and common in normal newborns during the first 48 hours of life when they are associated with decreasing pulmonary vascular resistance and with closure of the PDA. They include **systolic ejection murmurs, continuous systolic (crescendo systolic) murmurs,** and **early soft midsystolic ejection murmurs.**

Murmurs, pathologic: Pathologic murmurs are due to cardiovascular disease. When they present is dependent on their cause and on normal changes associated with transitional circulation. Many do not appear until pulmonary vascular resistance falls. Absence of a murmur does not rule out CHD; as many as a fifth of the infants who die from CHD by one month of age do not have murmurs. Pathologic murmurs include **loud systolic ejection murmurs** and **continuous murmurs.**

Muscle tone, phasic: The brief, forceful contraction of a muscle in response to a short-duration, high-amplitude stretch. In the newborn, phasic tone is evaluated by testing the resistance of the extremities to movement (scarf sign and arm and leg recoil) and by assessing the activity of the deep tendon reflexes (biceps and patellar reflexes).

Muscle tone, postural: The long-duration, low-amplitude stretch of a muscle in response to gravity. In the newborn, the traction response (pull-to-sit maneuver) is used to evaluate postural tone. Depressed postural tone is called *hypotonia.*

Myelomeningocele: A lesion associated with spina bifida in which bilateral broadening of the vertebrae or absence of the vertebral arches is seen. The lesion is most often seen in the lumbar spine and is characterized by protrusion of meninges and spinal roots and nerves, along with fusion of remnants of the spinal cord and an exposed neural tube. The higher the defect on the spine, the greater the degree of paralysis. Hydrocephalus is frequently seen with a myelomeningocele, especially in the Arnold-Chiari malformation.

Necrosis, subcutaneous fat: A hard, nonpitting, sharply circumscribed subcutaneous nodule that appears during the first weeks of life, grows larger over several days, and then resolves spontaneously over several weeks. Color will vary. Possible causes include trauma, cold, or asphyxia. Intervention may be necessary if the condition is associated with hypercalcemia.

Neonatal Behavioral Assessment Scale (NBAS): An examination tool developed by T. B. Brazelton to assess behavior in the term infant.

Neonatal torsion of the testis: A condition in which a testis and its tunica vaginalis rotate in the scrotal sac, inguinal canal, or abdomen. Torsion of a descended testis presents with reddish to bluish coloring of the scrotal skin and a nontender or mildly tender mass. Torsion is difficult to identify if the testis has not descended.

Nevus, pigmented: A dark brown or black macule commonly seen on the lower back or buttocks. Although pigmented nevi are generally benign, malignant changes occur in up to 10 percent of these lesions.

Nevus, port wine: A flat, nonblanching pink or reddish purple lesion with sharply delineated edges directly beneath the epidermis. The port wine nevus generally appears on the face, consists of dilated capillaries, and varies in size from small to covering almost half the body. Although usually unilateral, on occasion it crosses the midline. It neither grows in size nor resolves spontaneously. Port wine nevi located over the branches of the trigeminal nerve may be associated with Sturge-Weber syndrome.

Nevus, sebaceous: A small yellow or yellowish-orange papule or plaque consisting of immature hair follicles and sebaceous glands. It is commonly found on the scalp or face.

Nevus simplex: An irregularly bordered pink macule that blanches with pressure and becomes more prominent with crying. Found most often on the nape of the neck, the upper eyelids, the bridge of the nose, or the upper lip, the nevus simplex is composed of dilated capillaries and is seen in up to 50 percent of newborns. It is commonly called *stork bite.*

Nipple line: A reference line (used to describe the location of physical findings) passing horizontally through the nipples.

Nipples, supernumerary: Accessory nipples—raised or pigmented areas five to six cm below the normal nipples. In Caucasian infants, they may be associated with congenital anomalies.

Nodule: An elevated palpable lesion, solid and circumscribed (a papule), greater than 1 cm in diameter.

Normal variants: Minor differences in the appearance of the features between races, but that are normal for the race. Also called *minor variants.*

Nuchal chord: An umbilical cord that has become wrapped around the fetus's neck.

Nystagmus: A rapid, searching movement of the eyeballs seen in some newborns until three to four months of age. Occasional nystagmus is normal in the otherwise normal neonate; persistent is abnormal and may indicate loss of vision.

Observation: A physical assessment technique involving careful visual attention to, and notation of the status of external body parts and systems, for the purpose of forming a judgment. Also called *inspection.*

Occipital-frontal circumference (OFC): Measurement of the neonate's head taken over the occipital, parietal, and frontal prominences, avoiding the ears. This growth parameter is used, with the infant's gestational age, to determine whether the infant's head is small, appropriate, or large for gestational age. In the term infant, the normal OFC is 31–38 cm.

Oligohydramnios: The presence of less than 500 mL of amniotic fluid at term or 50 percent of normal volume at any time during pregnancy. The intrauterine compression caused by the lack of fluid may produce unusual flattening of the facial features in the newborn.

Omphalocele: Protrusion of abdominal contents through a defect at the umbilicus. A thin, translucent membrane covers the protrusion, and may rupture at delivery. Omphalocele is seen more often in male infants, especially premature males, and is usually associated with trisomies 13, 18, and 21; Beckwith-Wiedemann syndrome; or congenital heart disease.

Omphalomesenteric duct: Persistence in the newborn of this embryological duct between the ileum and the umbilicus, with seepage of ileal liquid from the opening.

Ophthalmoscope: A hand-held device, containing lenses and a mirror, that produces a beam of light for inspection of the interior of the eye. In physical examination of the newborn, it is used to assess pupillary constriction and the red reflex. It can also be used to inspect the anterior vascular capsule of the lens to determine gestational age.

Opisthotonus: Marked extensor hypertonia, with arching of the back. It may be seen with bacterial meningitis, severe hypoxic-ischemic brain damage, and massive intraventricular hemorrhage.

Orchiopexy: Surgical fixation of an undescended testis in the scrotum. Generally done between 9 and 18 months of age.

Organization: An infant's ability to integrate physiologic (heart rate, respiratory rate, oxygen consumption, digestion) and behavioral (state, motor activity) systems in response to the environment. Preterm infants show decreased organizational abilities.

Ortolani maneuver: A procedure for evaluating hip stability in the newborn. After flexing the infant's knee and hip, grasp the thigh and first abduct with a lifting motion and then adduct the leg. If a clunk is felt as the femoral head passes over the acetabulum, the infant may have congenital hip dysplasia.

Otoscope: A device used to inspect the ears. Due to the presence of vernix in the neonate's ear canal, the device is normally not used in newborn examinations.

Outer canthal distance: The measurement between the outer canthi of the two eyes.

Pallor: Paleness of the skin in the newborn may indicate compromised cardiac status. The paleness may be due to vasoconstriction and to shunting of blood away from the skin to vital organs or anemia.

Palpation: A physical assessment technique involving application of pressure to the skin with the fingertips or part of the palm to assess the condition of underlying body parts.

Palpebral fissure: The eye opening.

Papule: An elevated palpable lesion, solid and circumscribed, less than 1 cm in diameter.

Patch: A discolored, flat, nonpalpable spot (a macule) greater than 1 cm in diameter.

Patent ductus arteriosus (PDA): A cardiac abnormality marked by failure of the ductus arteriosus to close after birth. In a left-to-right shunt blood flows from the aorta to the pulmonary artery, resulting in recirculation of arterial blood through the lungs.

Patent urachus: Persistence of an embryological communication between the urinary bladder and the umbilicus, with passage of urine through the umbilicus.

Percussion, direct: A physical assessment technique involving striking the body surface sharply and listening to the sound produced, to determine the condition of an underlying body part. In *indirect (mediate)* percussion, the examiner places the middle finger of the left hand on the area to be assessed and then strikes the finger with the middle finger of the other hand. Although not generally employed in examination of the abdomen, percussion can distinguish areas of tympanic (resonant or bell-like) sound from areas of dull sound. Tympanic sounds are present over the organs that contain air; increased tympany suggests abnormal amounts of air. Dull sounds are percussed over the liver, spleen, and bladder. Extended areas of dullness suggest organ enlargement; dullness in unusual areas may indicate masses. Shifting dullness is heard with ascites. It is of limited value in examination of the neonate's chest due to its small size, but can be useful in distinguishing between air, fluid, and solid tissue in some situations. Changes in resonance indicate changes in the consistency of the underlying tissue.

Perfusion, peripheral: Cardiac perfusion to the skin.

Perinatal history: Record of occurrences in the life of the mother, the fetus, and the newborn.

Perinatal period: Definitions of the length of the perinatal period vary; it extends from about week 20 or 28 of gestation until one week to one month after birth.

Perineum: Area between the scrotum and anus in the male and the vulva and anus in the female. It should be smooth in newborns. Dimpling suggests genetic anomalies or fistulas.

Periodic breathing: A series of respirations followed by a pause of up to 20 seconds.

Periosteum: Fibrous membrane covering the bones of the skull.

PERL: A notation standing for "pupils equal and reactive to light."

Petechia (plural: petechiae): A pinpoint-sized hemorrhagic spot on the skin.

Phimosis: An irretractable foreskin. It may not be diagnosed until the infant reaches three months of age.

Pigeon chest: An abnormality of the bony structure of the chest in which the sternum protrudes. It is seen in infants with Marfan syndrome and rickets.

Pinna: The part of the ear that projects from the head. Formation, amount of cartilage present, and recoil when folded and released are considered indicators of gestational age.

Pit, ear: A slight depression anterior to the tragus. It may lead to a congenital preauricular sinus or fistula. Ear pits may be familial or associated with other anomalies.

Plagiocephaly: Asymmetrical skull shape caused by craniosynostosis (premature fusion) of the sutures on one side of the skull.

Plantar flexion: Flexing the foot toward the plantar surface.

Plantar surface: The sole of the foot. Creases appear on the plantar surface of the foot between 28 and 30 weeks gestation and cover the surface at or near term. Therefore, plantar surface creasing is one indicator of gestational age.

Plaque: A fusion or coalescence of several papules (solid, circumscribed, elevated palpable lesions less than 1 cm in diameter).

Plethora: Ruddy appearance of the skin in a newborn. Plethora may indicate a high level of red blood cells to blood volume.

Pleural cavities: Two potential spaces (left and right) within the chest cavity enclosed by a serious membrane called the pleura. A portion of the pleura called the **parietal pleura** lines the walls of the thoracic cavity; the portion called the **visceral pleura** envelops the lungs.

Pneumothorax: Accumulation of air or gas in the pleural space.

Polycythemia: A condition in which the infant's central hematocrit is greater than 65. A polycythemic infant is pink at rest but plethoric to purplish when crying. The ruddy coloring can sometimes be mistaken for cyanosis (because the unsaturated hemoglobin in the blood of the infant may mask the saturated hemoglobin, making the infant appear purplish).

Polydactyly: A congenital anomaly marked by one or more extra digits on the hands or feet. There appears to be a familial tendency to polydactyly, and it is more common in African-American infants than in those of other races. The extra digit may be only a skin tag or a floppy appendage or it may appear normal.

Ponderal index: Cube root of body weight times 100 divided by height in cm.

Popliteal angle: The angle between the lower leg and the thigh posterior to the knee. The popliteal angle decreases with advancing gestational age.

Positional deformity: A flexible deformity of an extremity with no bony abnormality involved. It is caused by intrauterine positioning and generally corrects without treatment.

Postterm: An infant born at 42 or more weeks gestation.

Precordium: The area of the anterior chest over the heart. In the full-term newborn after the first few hours of life, the precordium should be quiet; a bounding precordium is characteristic of left-to-right shunt lesions (PDA or ventricular septal defect). In premature infants, the precordium is more active due to decreased subcutaneous tissue.

Preterm: An infant born at less than 38 weeks gestation.

Priapism: Constant erection of the penis, an abnormal finding that may indicate a spinal cord lesion.

Pronation: The turning of the body or a body part face down, as of the hand so that the palm is facing down.

Prone: Positioned face down.

Proptosis: Abnormal protrusion or bulging of the eyeball. Also called *exophthalmos.*

Prune belly syndrome: A rare congenital deficiency of the abdominal muscles marked by a protruding, thin-walled abdomen covered with wrinkled skin. It occurs more frequently in males and is associated with renal and urinary tract abnormalities.

Pseudohermaphroditism: A condition in which the gonads are of one sex but one or more morphologic criteria are of the opposite sex. In **female pseudohermaphroditism,** the infant is genetically and gonadally female, with partial masculinization. In **male pseudohermaphroditism,** the infant is genetically and gonadally male, with the presence of some female characteristics.

Pseudostrabismus: The appearance of strabismus (crossed eyes) due to a flat nasal bridge or the presence of epicanthal folds.

Ptosis: Paralytic drooping of the eyelid in which the upper lid droops when the eyes are fully open.

Pulse deficit: A difference between the heart rate counted by a peripheral pulse and that counted by auscultation. A pulse deficit is frequently seen with ectopic rhythms.

Pulse pressure: The difference between the systolic and the diastolic blood pressure. For term infants, the average difference is 25–30 mmHg; for premature infants, it is 15–25 mmHg. Wide pulse pressures can indicate large aortic runoff, as in PDA. Narrow pulse pressures are seen with peripheral vasoconstriction, heart failure, and low cardiac output.

Pupillary reflex: Contraction of the pupil when the eye is exposed to bright light.

Pustule: An elevation of the skin filled with cloudy or purulent fluid.

Q-switched ruby laser: Laser used in removal of nevi or tattoos. Emits a short pulse of intense red light that is selectively absorbed by melanin located in the epidermal and dermal skin layers. The laser energy causes the melanin to break down into smaller pigment particles that are removed by the body's immune system.

Quiet alert state: A wakeful state of infant consciousness characterized by interaction with the environment. The infant focuses on stimuli and presents an alert appearance, especially in the eyes. Motor activity is minimal. In this state, preterm infants may show hyperalertness (inability to terminate fixation on a stimulus).

Rachitic rosary: In a newborn with rickets, a series of small lumps can be felt along the edge of the sternum during palpation. The lumps are enlarged costal cartilages.

Radiation: The transmission of a body sound to another location.

Rales: See **Crackles.**

Ranula: A cystic tumor, presenting as a translucent or bluish swelling beneath the tongue, caused by obstruction of a salivary duct or a mucous gland.

Recoil, arm or leg: Test used to evaluate phasic muscle tone. The infant's arm or leg is gently extended. In premature infants of 28 or fewer weeks gestation, minimal resistance is normal. Resistance increases with gestational age.

Red retinal reflex: Reflection of a clear red color from the retina when a bright light is directed at the newborn's lens. The reflex is a pale color in dark-skinned infants.

Reflex, anocutaneous: An autonomic nervous system reflex. *Stimulus:* Cutaneous stimulation of the perianal skin. *Normal response:* Contraction of the external sphincter. Also called *anal wink.*

Reflex, Babinski: A developmental reflex. *Stimulus:* Stroke the sole of the infant's foot. *Positive response:* Extension of the great toe and spreading of the other toes.

Reflex, biceps: A motor reflex that is most active during the first two days after birth and when the newborn is alert. *Stimulus:* Place thumb over insertion of infant's biceps tendon, flex newborn's arm, and tap thumb with reflex hammer. *Normal response:* Infant flexes biceps muscle.

Reflex, corneal: A peripheral sensory reflex. *Stimulus:* Blow air on the infant's eye or touch the cornea gently with a piece of cotton. *Normal response:* The infant blinks.

Reflex, Moro: A developmental reflex that is normally completely present at birth only in term neonates. This reflex may be elicited by sudden movement of surface infant is on, loud noise, or causing the head to drop approximately 30°. *Stimulus:* Hold infant supine, supporting head a few centimeters above bed, withdraw supporting hand and allow the infant to "fall back" to it. *Normal response:* As infant's head falls, infant extends and abducts arms and opens hands; then adducts and partially flexes arms, and makes fists. Infants greater than 32 weeks gestation may cry out. Premature infants do not complete the reflex by adducting and flexing the extremities, nor do they cry. Complete lack of the reflex is abnormal; asymmetric response may indicate a localized neurologic defect (such as a brachial plexus injury).

Reflex, palmar grasp: A developmental reflex that is normally present at birth in both term and preterm infants. *Stimulus:* Stroke infant's palm with a finger. *Normal response:*

Infant grasps finger and tightens grasp on attempt to withdraw finger.

Reflex, patellar (knee jerk): A motor reflex that is most active during the first two days after birth and when the newborn is alert. *Stimulus:* Tap infant's patellar tendon just below kneecap, with newborn's knee flexed and supported. *Normal response:* Infant extends knee and contracts quadriceps.

Reflex, rooting: A developmental reflex that is normally present at birth in both term and preterm infants. *Stimulus:* Stroke infant's cheek and corner of mouth. *Normal response:* Infant turns head toward stimulus and opens mouth.

Reflex, startle: Resembles Moro reflex but is more limited. See **Reflex, Moro.**

Reflex, stepping: A developmental reflex that becomes more active 72 hours after birth. *Stimulus:* Hold infant upright with soles of feet touching a flat surface. *Normal response:* Alternate stepping movements.

Reflex, sucking: A developmental reflex that is normally present at birth in both term and preterm infants. (It is weaker in preterm neonates.) *Stimulus:* Touch infant's lips. *Normal response:* Infant opens mouth and makes sucking movements.

Reflex, tonic neck: A developmental reflex that is normally present at birth only in term neonates. *Stimulus:* With infant supine, turn infant's head to one side. *Normal response:* Extension of upper extremity on side to which head is turned and flexion of upper extremity on opposite side. Lack of response or a marked response with minimal head turning is abnormal. Also called *fencing position.*

Reflex, truncal incurvation (Galant): A developmental reflex. *Stimulus:* Suspend infant ventrally, supporting anterior chest wall in palm of hand. Apply firm pressure parallel to spine in thoracic area with thumb or cotton swab. *Positive response:* Infant flexes pelvis toward side of stimulus.

Reflexes, developmental: Reflexes that do not require functional brain above the diencephalon. Those present in most newborns include the sucking, rooting, palmar grasp, tonic neck, Moro, stepping, truncal incurvation, and Babinski reflexes. Also called *primary* or *primitive* reflexes.

Respiratory distress syndrome (RDS): A condition of the newborn most often occurring in premature infants, but may be seen at term, marked by breathing difficulties and cyanosis and having as its origin a deficiency of surfactant and structural immaturity.

Retinoblastoma: A retinal tumor. Lack of a red reflex in a newborn could indicate its presence.

Retraction: A drawing in of the chest during respiration. Immediately after birth, substernal or intercostal retractions are common; if they persist, they may indicate respiratory problems. Suprasternal retraction, especially with gasping or stridor, may indicate obstruction of the upper airway.

Rhonchi: Adventitious breath sounds lower in pitch and more musical than crackles. Although seldom heard in the neonate, they may be auscultated if secretions or aspirated foreign matter is present in the large airways.

Rotation, neck: Turning of the face to the side.

Rub: Adventitious breath sound resembling the rubbing of a finger over a cupped hand held near the ear. Rubs are often heard in newborns during mechanical ventilation; they are also associated with inflammation of the pleura.

Ruga (plural: rugae): A ridge, wrinkle, or fold. Rugae first appear on the front of the scrotal sac at about 36 weeks gestation, covering the sac by 40 weeks. In the term male infant, the scrotum is fully rugated; the pre-term male has few or no rugae.

Scale: Exfoliation of dead or dying bits of skin. Scale can also result from excess keratin production.

Scaphocephaly: Long, narrow head shape caused by craniosynostosis (premature fusion) of the sagittal suture, limiting lateral growth of the skull.

Scapula: One of the pair of triangular bones at the back of the shoulder articulating with a clavicle. Commonly called the *shoulder blade.*

Scarf sign: A test for newborn gestational age involving gently pulling the arm of a supine infant across the chest and around the neck as far as possible posteriorly. The older the infant, the greater the resistance to this maneuver.

Sclera: The white portion of the eyeball.

Sclera, blue: Unusual blue coloring of the white portion of the eyeball. It is seen with a variation of osteogenesis imperfecta and certain other abnormalities.

Scoliosis: A congenital deformity of the spine in which vertebrae fail to form and/or segment. It is embryonic in origin. If unde-tected, it can affect neurologic function as well as appearance. Congenital scoliosis may be associated with genitourinary tract anomalies, Klippel-Feil syndrome, and Sprengel deformity.

Seizure: An abnormal series of movements (neurologic in origin) characterized by alter-nate muscular contraction and relaxation of unequal amplitude. The movements are less rapid than those seen in jitteriness. They do not occur in response to stimuli and cannot be stopped by flexing and hold-ing the affected limb; may be accompanied by abnormal eye movements. See also **Jitteriness.**

Sensory threshold: An infant's level of toler-ance for stimuli. Infants who exceed their sensory thresholds (are overstimulated) exhibit signs and symptoms of stress. Low sensory thresholds are generally seen in pre-term infants and in infants with neurologic impairment.

Sequence: A single defect as the cause for other anomalies (the "snowball" effect).

Simian crease: A single transverse palmar crease. It may be found in normal new-borns, but when seen with short fingers, an incurved little finger, and a low-set thumb, it is suggestive of Down syndrome.

Sinus, dermal: A posterior neural tube defect occurring along the midline of the back, frequently in the lumbar region. It may present as a dimple surrounded by tufts of hair or lipomas or may terminate in subcu-taneous tissue, a cyst, or a fibrous band. It may also extend into the spinal cord and be associated with spina bifida.

Sinus, preauricular: An abnormal channel located in front of the pinna (auricle) of the ear. If it communicates with the internal ear or the brain, chronic infection is likely.

Skin tag: A small skin outgrowth. Those occurring anterior to the tragus are thought to be embryological remnants of the first branchial arch. Skin tags may be familial or associated with other anomalies.

Small for gestational age (SGA): An infant whose weight falls below the tenth percen-tile for gestational age when plotted on a standard growth chart.

Spina bifida: The mildest form of posterior neural tube defect, with the malformation arising from lack of or incomplete closure of the posterior portion of the vertebrae. The meninges and spinal cord are normal. The defect is covered with skin (which may be dimpled), and it is most common in the lower lumbar and lumbosacral area. See also **Sinus, dermal.**

Split: Term describing a heart sound in which two components can be heard. The "splitting" is caused by the asynchronous closure of the two valves that create the sound. The rapid newborn heart rate makes splitting difficult to auscultate. In newborns splitting is usually not heard in S1. S2 is generally single at birth but is split in two-thirds of infants by 16 hours of age and in four-fifths by 48 hours of age. Wide splitting of S2 is abnormal, however.

Sprengel deformity: A congenital anomaly of the shoulder girdle, marked by some hypoplasia and malrotation of the scapula, which gives it an elevated appearance. Shoulder abduction and flexion are limited. This deformity is more often unilateral, but can be bilateral. It is often associated with congenital spinal anomalies, Klippel-Feil syndrome, and renal anomalies.

State (of consciousness): One of six levels of consciousness seen in infants. There are two sleep states *(deep* and *light),* one transitional state *(drowsiness),* and three awake states *(quiet alert, active alert,* and *crying).* Behavioral assessment evaluates the newborn's ability to control his state, move smoothly from one state to another, and maintain alertness when in an awake state. Term infants may use changes in state to control environmental input.

Stenosis, anal: Constriction or obstruction of the anorectal canal. Signs include passage of small, thin stools, progressive abdominal distention, and finally vomiting.

Stenosis, pyloric: Obstruction of the pyloric orifice of the stomach, usually presenting about 3 weeks of age, rarely before the fourth or fifth day of life. If present, it is palpable immediately after feeding or vomiting as an ovoid mass between the umbilicus and the right lower costal margin. Signs of pyloric stenosis (upper quadrant distention and visible peristalsis) in the absence of a palpable mass may indicate duodenal or jejunal obstruction in the neonate.

Sternocleidomastoid muscle: The muscle that flexes the vertebral column and rotates the head.

Stethoscope: An acoustical device used to auscultate (listen to) sounds within the body. In the neonate, these include heart, lung, venous, arterial, and intestinal sounds. A neonatal stethoscope generally has a double head composed of a flat diaphragm (for auscultating high-frequency sounds) and a bell (for auscultating low-frequency sounds). It does not magnify sound but simply eliminates environmental noise.

Stippling: A speckling of fine dots.

Strabismus: The appearance of crossed eyes in the newborn due to muscular incoordination.

Streeter dysplasia: See **Congenital constricting bands.**

Stridor: A high-pitched hoarse adventitious breath sound heard during inspiration or expiration at the larynx or upper airways. In the newborn, stridor indicates partial obstruction of the airway. It may also be heard in infants with edema of the upper airway after extubation.

Structural deformity: A fixed (or rigid) deformity involving bony abnormalities. It generally requires surgical intervention.

Subcutaneous tissue: Layer of fatty tissue underlying the dermis, which insulates the body, protects the internal organs, and stores calories.

Sucking blister: Intact or ruptured vesicle or bulla sometimes seen on the lips, fingers, or hands of the newborn. The cause is vigorous sucking, *in utero* or after birth.

Sunset sign: Eyelid retraction and a downward gaze in which the sclera is visible above the iris. The sign is often seen in infants with hydrocephalus.

Supination: Turning of the body or a body part face up, as of the hand so that the palm is facing up.

Supine: Positioned face up.

Suprasternal notch: An indentation on the upper border of the sternum.

Suture: A fibrous joint between bones of the skull. The **metopic suture** extends midline down the forehead between the two frontal bones and intersects with the **coronal suture,** which separates the frontal and parietal bones. The **sagittal suture** extends midline between the two parietal bones to the back of the head, where it intersects with the **lambdoidal suture,** which separates the parietal and occipital bones. The **squamosal suture** extends above the ear and separates the temporal from the parietal bone.

Sutures, overriding: Head molding may cause the edge of the bone on one side of a suture to feel as if it is on top of (overriding) the edge of the opposite bone. Overriding is commonly seen in the lambdoidal suture, with the parietal bone on top of the occipital. Overriding sutures must be differentiated from craniosynostosis (premature fusion of a suture).

Symmetrically growth restricted: An infant who has not grown at the expected rate— that is, who ranks at less than the tenth percentile for gestational age on standard growth charts—for *all three* growth parameters: weight, length, and occipital-frontal head circumference.

Symphysis, pubis: Midline cartilaginous joint connecting the pubic bones.

Syndactyly: Congenital webbing of the fingers and toes, frequently familial in origin. The more severe the webbing, the greater the likelihood of underlying bony abnormalities.

Syndrome: A recognizable pattern of anomalies, often of more than one system, that is historically based and leads to a diagnosis.

Systole: The period of contraction of the heart, particularly of the ventricles.

Tachycardia, sinus: A heart rate greater than 180–200 beats per minute in the newborn. Simple tachycardia, originating in the sinus node of the heart, normally occurs in response to a stimulus that increases demand on the heart. When the stimulus is removed, the rate gradually returns to normal.

Tachycardia, supraventricular (SVT): A heart rate greater than 200–300 beats per minute in the newborn. Without immediate intervention, it can lead to cardiovascular collapse.

Tachypnea: Excessively rapid and shallow respirations. In the neonate, persistent respirations of greater than 60 per minute may indicate TTN, RDS, meconium aspiration, pneumonia, hyperthermia, or pain.

Tap: A sharp, well-localized point of maximum cardiac impulse, usually associated with pressure overload or hypertrophy.

Temperament: The way in which an infant interacts with the environment. S. Chess and A. Thomas identify three categories of temperament: easy, difficult, and slow-to-warm.

Teratogenic agent: An extrinsic factor— either environmental or maternal—that causes abnormalities in fetal development. Examples include infection, metabolic disorders, and exposure to drugs or alcohol, heavy metals, many chemicals, and radiation.

Term: An infant born between the beginning of week 38 and the end of week 41 of gestation.

Testicular torsion: See **Neonatal torsion of the testis**.

Thorax: The chest. The thoracic cavity is bounded by the sternum, 12 thoracic vertebrae, 12 pair of ribs, and the diaphragm.

Thrill: A low-frequency, palpable murmur that resembles holding one's hand on a purring cat. Thrills are uncommon in the newborn.

If present, their location can aid in identification of cardiac problems.

Thrush: An oral fungal infection characterized by adherent white patches on the tongue and mucous membranes and caused by *Candida albicans.*

Thyroglossal duct cyst: A cyst on the embryological duct between the thyroid and the back of the tongue.

Tonic: Of or relating to or producing normal tone or tonus in muscles or tissue.

Torticollis: An anomaly affecting the sternocleidomastoid muscle, more often on the right side. It is not usually seen until about two weeks of age, when it can be palpated as a firm, immobile mass 1–2 cm in diameter in the midportion of the muscle. Undetected, it produces facial asymmetry and limited neck rotation.

Traction response (pull-to-sit maneuver): Tests the ability of the infant's muscles to resist the pull of gravity. When the normal term infant's hands are grasped and he is slowly pulled from a supine to a sitting position, the infant contracts the shoulder and arm muscles, and then flexes the neck, with the head lagging behind the body only minimally. The infant also flexes the elbows, knees, and ankles. When the infant reaches the sitting position, the head remains erect briefly before falling forward. Neck flexion is not seen in infants of less than 33 weeks gestation.

Tragus: A small cartilaginous flap in front of the external opening of the ear.

Transient tachypnea of the newborn (TTN): A condition of the newborn marked by excessively rapid respirations. The underlying pathology is usually retained fetal lung fluid; tachypnea subsides as fluid is absorbed or expelled.

Transillumination: A physical assessment technique involving shining light through body tissues. The area being examined is placed between the light and the observer. If a pneumothorax is suspected in the neonate, transillumination can allow comparison of the left, right, upper, and lower aspects of the chest and illuminate air pockets with a lantern-like glow. If the infant's head is an unusual size or shape or if the neurologic examination is abnormal, transillumination can help identify the reason. It is useful for identification of abnormal findings in the scrotum. Masses filled with clear fluid appear translucent with illumination; solid or blood-filled masses do not transilluminate.

Trisomy: A form of chromosomal aneuploidy characterized by the presence of 47 chromosomes. It is generally caused by nondisjunction (failure of the egg or sperm to divide the genetic material equally). The most common autosomal trisomies are of chromosome 21 (Down syndrome), chromosome 18, and chromosome 13.

Urethral meatus: Opening of the urethra on the body surface, located directly below the clitoris in female infants and at the center of the end of the penile shaft in males. Anterior displacement of the meatus at or on an enlarged clitoris suggests pseudohermaphroditism in a female infant. Hypospadias and epispadias are placement abnormalities seen in male infants.

Uvula, bifid: A split uvula. It may be associated with other congenital anomalies.

Valgus: Bent outward or twisted away from the midline of the body.

Varus: Turned inward.

Vernix caseosa: A greasy white or yellow material, composed of sebaceous gland secretions and exfoliated skin cells, that covers the newborn infant's skin. Vernix develops during the third trimester of intrauterine growth, gradually decreasing in amount as the fetus approaches 40 weeks gestation. Because vernix may be present in the newborn's auditory canal, otoscopic examination is not done immediately after birth.

Very low birth weight (VLBW): An infant who weighs less than 1,500 g at birth.

Vesicle: An elevation of the skin filled with serous fluid and less than 1 cm in diameter.

Vesicular breath sounds: Normally found over the entire chest, except over the manubrium and the trachea. During expiration, vesicular sounds are soft, short, and low-pitched; during inspiration, they are louder, longer, and higher pitched.

Weaver curve: Weaver curves are reference curves used to determine whether genetic influences account for a child's macrocephaly by comparing a reference score for the average parents' OFC with the child's reference score for OFC. A genetic cause for macrocephaly is confirmed if the child's standard score is within the range determined by the average parental score on the Weaver curve.

Werdnig-Hoffmann disease: A disorder of the lower motor neurons, causing flaccid weakness of the extremities as well as tongue fasciculation.

Wheal: A reddened, solid elevation of the skin caused by a collection of fluid in the dermis.

Wheezes: Adventitious breath sounds, usually louder on expiration than on inspiration, that are higher in pitch than rhonchi. They are usually heard only in newborns with BPD.

Whorl, hair: Spiral hair growth pattern commonly seen in the posterior parietal region of the newborn's scalp. Absence of or abnormal location of a whorl can indicate abnormal brain growth.

Witch's milk: Milky secretions engorging the breasts of some infants at birth, due to the influence of maternal estrogen. The secretions generally disappear in one to two weeks, and the enlargement subsides over several months.

Xiphoid process: Sword-shaped cartilaginous projection at the end of the sternum.

Glossary compiled and verified using the following sources:

- *Dorland's Medical Dictionary,* 29th ed. 2000. Philadelphia: Saunders.
- *Stedman's Medical Dictionary,* 26th ed. 1995. Baltimore: Lippincott Williams & Wilkins.
- *Mosby's Medical, Nursing and Allied Health Dictionary,* 3rd ed. 1990. Philadelphia: Mosby.
- Kenner C, and Lott JW, eds. 2003. *Comprehensive Neonatal Nursing: A Physiologic Perspective.* Philadelphia: Saunders.
- Polin RA, and Fox WW, eds. 1998. *Fetal and Neonatal Physiology,* vols. 1 and 2. Philadelphia: Saunders.
- Taeusch HW, and Ballard RA, eds. 1998. *Avery's Diseases of the Newborn,* 7th ed. Philadelphia: Saunders.
- Seeley RR, Stephens TD, and Tate P, eds. 1992. *Anatomy and Physiology,* 2nd ed. Philadelphia: Mosby.
- Blackburn ST, ed. 2003. *Maternal, Fetal, and Neonatal Physiology: A Clinical Perspective.* Philadelphia: Saunders.
- *Miller-Keane Encyclopedia and Dictionary of Medicine, Nursing, and Allied Health,* 5th ed. 1992. Philadelphia: Saunders.

Index

Physical Assessment of the Newborn, 4th Edition

Test Directions

1. Please fill out the answer form and include all requested information. We are unable to issue a certificate without complete information.
2. All questions and answers are developed from the information provided in the book. Select the *one best answer* and fill in the corresponding circle on the answer form.
3. Mail the answer form to: NICU Ink, 2220 Northpoint Parkway, Santa Rosa, CA 95407-7398 with a check for $90.00 (processing fee) made payable to NICU Ink. This fee is non-refundable.
4. Retain the test for your records.
5. You will be notified of your test results within 6–8 weeks.
6. If you pass the test (80%) you will earn 30 contact hours for the course, this includes 2.4 hours of pharmacology credit. Provider, Neonatal Network, approved by the California Board of Registered Nursing, Provider #CEP 6261, for 30 contact hours; Iowa Board of Nursing, Provider #189; and Florida Board of Nursing, Provider #FBN 3218, content code 2505. Neonatal Network, Provider #04-296795-A is an approved provider of continuing nursing education by the Texas Nurses Association, an accredited approver by the American Nurses Credentialing Center's Commission on Accreditation. This activity meets Type I criteria for mandatory continuing education requirements toward relicensure as established by the Board of Nurse Examiners for the State of Texas.
7. An answer key is available upon request with completion of the exam.

Course Objectives

After reading the book and taking the test, the participant will be able to:
1. List the principles of physical assessment relevant to the newborn.
2. Outline the salient information that should be recorded in the newborn history.
3. Describe the components of a gestational age assessment.
4. Describe the elements of a complete newborn physical assessment.
5. Outline the components of a newborn behavioral assessment.
6. Discuss an approach to the assessment of the dysmorphic infant.

---

1. During physical assessment of a newborn, which of the following should be palpated first?
   a. brachial pulses   c. liver
   b. femoral pulses

2. In sequencing a newborn examination, which of the following should be performed last?
   a. examination of the hips   c. palpating the abdomen
   b. eliciting a Moro reflex

3. Which of the following tests are incorporated into the examination of the newborn eye?
   a. accommodation   c. red reflex
   b. cover/uncover

4. For optimal results, the stethoscope tubing should be no longer than _____ inches.
   a. 10   c. 14
   b. 12

5. Fetal exposure to which of the following increases the risk of cardiac malformation?
   a. anticonvulsants   c. antihypertensives
   b. antidepressants

6. In an otherwise normal newborn, the most common reason for a large head is:
   a. benign familial megalencephaly
   b. Dandy-Walker malformation
   c. hypothyroidism

7. According to data from Pediatrix Medical Group, the percentage of 25-week gestational age infants who survive without severe intraventricular hemorrhage or retinopathy of prematurity is:
   a. 9   c. 48
   b. 28

8. Using Nägele's rule, the due date of a woman whose last menstrual period began on April 14, 2009, would be _____, 2010.
   a. January 21   c. March 14
   b. February 28

9. In the first trimester of pregnancy, the most sensitive fetal biometric parameter for determining gestational age is:
   a. biparietal diameter   c. femur length
   b. crown-rump length

10. In the second trimester, the most accurate estimation of gestational age is obtained by measuring:
    a. abdominal circumference
    b. femur length
    c. biparietal diameter

11. In a <37-week gestational age infant, the New Ballard Score is accurate to within _____ days.
    a. 2–4   c. 8–10
    b. 5–7

12. For optimal accuracy in determining gestational age, the anterior vascular capsule of the lens (AVCL) should be examined before _____ hours of life.
    a. 48   c. 96
    b. 72

13. Atrophy of the AVCL is accelerated in the presence of maternal:
    a. diabetes   c. renal disease
    b. hypertension

14. To obtain a score of 4 on the arm recoil test, the neonate's fist should:
    a. come in contact with the face
    b. reach the level of the shoulder
    c. pass the level of the elbow

15. To elicit the scarf sign, the neonate's:
    a. arm is pulled across the chest
    b. hand is flexed toward the wrist
    c. leg is raised toward the ear

16. The development of lanugo peaks at _____ weeks gestation.
    a. 24–26   c. 32–34
    b. 28–30

17. In a human fetus, the eyes open at _____ weeks gestation.
    a. 22–24   c. 26–28
    b. 24–26

18. In the majority of male newborns, both testes are palpable in the inguinal canal by _____ weeks gestation.
    a. 32   c. 36
    b. 34

19. Conditions known to cause asymmetric intrauterine growth restriction include:
    a. chromosomal disorders   c. maternal preeclampsia
    b. intrauterine infection

20. Melanocytes are found in which tissue layer?
    a. dermis   c. subcutaneous
    b. epidermis

21. In the term newborn, the thickness of the epidermis is _____ mm.
    a. 0.01–0.05   c. 0.1–0.5
    b. 0.06–0.1

22. Sweat glands reach adult function levels by _____ years of age.
    a. 1–2   c. 3–4
    b. 2–3

23. Lanugo first appears at _____ weeks gestation.
    a. 20   c. 28
    b. 24

24. A macule is best described as a/an:
    a. elevated lesion of <1 cm
    b. flat discolored lesion <1 cm
    c. small hemorrhagic spot

25. A 1.5 cm raised lesion with well defined borders would best be described as (a):
    a. nodule   c. vesicle
    b. plaque

26. Circumoral cyanosis should be investigated if it persists beyond _____ hours of age.
    a. 12   c. 24
    b. 18

27. A newborn with a hematocrit >65 percent is at increased risk of developing:
    a. feeding intolerance   c. renal failure
    b. hypoglycemia

28. Persistent cutis marmorata is commonly seen in which of the following syndromes?
    a. Down   c. Turner
    b. Sturge-Weber

29. A truncal rash consisting of small pustules or vesicles with erythematous bases best describes:
    a. erythema toxicum   c. pustular melanosis
    b. herpes

30. Milia are small cysts containing:
    a. eosinophils   c. sebaceous secretions
    b. leukocytes

31. Obstructed sweat glands result in the development of:
    a. miliaria
    b. scalded skin syndrome
    c. sebaceous gland hyperplasia

32. Hyperpigmented macules are most commonly found over the:
    a. buttocks and flanks   c. hands and feet
    b. face

33. Neonatal pustular melanosis is most common in infants of what ethnic background?
    a. African American   c. Native American
    b. Asian

34. Melanocytic nevi should be followed closely for the development of:
    a. bleeding   c. neurofibromatosis
    b. malignant melanoma

35. Which of the following may be a marker for tuberous sclerosis?
    a. ash leaf macules   c. pigmented nevi
    b. café au lait patches

36. Subcutaneous fat necrosis is associated with:
    a. hypercalcemia
    b. malignant skin changes
    c. skin breakdown and infection

37. Which of the following statements applies to a nevus simplex? It usually:
    a. fades after 2 years
    b. grows as the child grows
    c. grows initially then involutes

38. Sturge-Weber syndrome is characterized by port wine nevi in areas innervated by the _____ nerve.
    a. facial   c. vagus
    b. trigeminal

39. Strawberry hemangiomas are more common in which infants? Those who:
    a. have been growth-restricted
    b. have mothers with diabetes
    c. are born prematurely

40. A cavernous hemangioma associated with platelet sequestration is termed _____ syndrome.
    a. Kasabach-Merritt
    b. Klinefelter
    c. Klippel-Trenaunay-Weber

41. A rash in the groin that is moist and red with small white or yellow pustules should be treated with an:
    a. antibiotic agent   c. antiviral agent
    b. antifungal agent

42. The mortality rate of neonates with disseminated herpes is _____ percent.
    a. 20   c. 40
    b. 30

43. Infants with bullous skin eruptions and peeling skin should be treated with an agent effective against which of the following?
    a. Klebsiella   c. *Staphylococcus aureus*
    b. Pseudomonas

44. Aplasia cutis congenita is characteristic of trisomy _____.
    a. 13   c. 21
    b. 18

45. To accurately measure an infant's head circumference, the tape measure should be placed 1–2 cm above the:
    a. glabellar space   c. outer canthus of the eye
    b. helix of the ear

46. The average head circumference in a neonate of 40 weeks gestation is _____ cm.
    a. 33   c. 37
    b. 35

47. Which of the following is associated with macrocephaly?
    a. hypothyroidism   c. osteogenesis imperfecta
    b. maternal diabetes

48. The metopic suture separates the:
    a. frontal bones   c. parietal bones
    b. frontal and parietal bones

49. The anterior fontanel is usually larger in infants of what racial background?
    a. African American   c. Hispanic
    b. Asian

50. Fontanel size is correctly determined by measuring:
    a. diagonally   c. vertically
    b. horizontally

51. Fontanel fullness is most accurately determined when the infant is:
    a. side-lying   c. supine
    b. sitting

52. An enlarged anterior fontanel may be seen in infants with:
    a. congenital adrenal insufficiency
    b. hypothyroidism
    c. phenylketonuria

53. Auscultation of the fontanel should be performed on infants with multiple:
    a. hemangiomas   c. port wine stains
    b. petechiae

54. The occipital and parietal bones are separated by the _____ suture.
    a. coronal   c. sagittal
    b. lambdoidal

55. In Caucasian infants, the size of the posterior fontanel is normally _____ cm.
    a. 0.5   c. 1
    b. 0.7

56. The presence of a third fontanel is a feature found in _____ syndrome.
    a. Down   c. Turner
    b. Sturge-Weber

57. Brachycephaly results from premature fusion of which sutures?
    a. coronal   c. squamosal
    b. sagittal

58. Side-to-side head flattening, common in premature infants, is known as:
    a. craniosynostosis c. plagiocephaly
    b. dolichocephaly

59. Macewen's sign is elicited in newborns with (a):
    a. cephalhematoma   c. depressed skull fracture
    b. craniotabes

60. Subgaleal hemorrhage is most commonly seen with what type of delivery?
    a. cesarean   c. vacuum-assisted
    b. forceps-assisted

61. Damage to the facial nerve most commonly affects innervation of the muscles around the:
    a. eyes   c. lips
    b. forehead

62. In non-Asians, epicanthal folds usually disappear by _____ years of age.
    a. six   c. ten
    b. eight

63. A single continuous eyebrow may be a feature of what syndrome?
    a. Cornelia de Lange c. Klinefelter
    b. cri du chat

64. White specks around the iris may be a marker for _____ syndrome.
    a. Down   c. Turner
    b. Edward

65. An ocular finding common to osteogenesis imperfecta is:
    a. blue sclera   c. ptosis
    b. coloboma

66. Findings associated with fetal alcohol syndrome include:
    a. cleft palate   c. smooth philtrum
    b. micrognathia

67. Causes of macroglossia include:
    a. Down syndrome   c. Robin sequence
    b. hypothyroidism

68. The most common cause of a neck mass in a newborn is:
    a. cystic hygroma   c. torticollis
    b. goiter

69. In newborn infants, acrocyanosis is an expected finding for _____ hours after birth.
    a. 12   c. 48
    b. 24

70. In newborns, the primary muscle(s) of respiration is the:
    a. diaphragm   c. pectoralis
    b. intercostals

71. Compared to adults, the diaphragm in newborns is:
    a. less distensible c. more concave
    b. located lower in the chest

72. The presence of seesaw respirations in newborns is suggestive of:
    a. airway obstruction c. poor lung compliance
    b. neurologic injury

73. A vascular ring should be considered in a newborn with retractions on inspiration in which of the following areas?
    a. intercostal   c. suprasternal
    b. subcostal

74. Apnea is considered present when bradycardia or color changes accompany pauses in breathing of more than _____ seconds.
    a. 10   c. 20
    b. 15

75. In considering total pulmonary resistance, the contribution of the nasal passages is _____ percent.
    a. 25   c. 50
    b. 33

76. Causes of tracheal deviation include the presence of:
    a. atelectasis   c. pneumonia
    b. pneumomediastinum

77. In a normally grown newborn, head circumference exceeds the average chest circumference by _____ cm.
    a. 1   c. 3
    b. 2

78. Dwarfism is associated with which of the following chest shapes?
    a. barrel   c. flattened
    b. bell

79. Findings in Marfan syndrome include:
    a. flared lower ribs c. pulmonary hyperplasia
    b. pectus excavatum

80. Absence of the pectoralis major muscle is a feature of _____ syndrome.
    a. Möbius
    b. Poland
    c. prune belly

81. The breast bud in a full-term infant is usually _____ cm.
    a. 0.25–0.5
    b. 0.5–0.75
    c. 0.75–1

82. An infant who presents with lymphedema and widely-spaced nipples should be investigated for:
    a. CHARGE association
    b. Robin sequence
    c. Turner syndrome

83. Accessory nipples are more common in which ethnic group?
    a. African American
    b. Asian
    c. Caucasian

84. Snuffles are a feature of infections caused by:
    a. *Chlamydia trachomatis*
    b. *Neisseria gonorrhoeae*
    c. *Treponema pallidum*

85. Fine crackles are breath sounds characteristic of:
    a. pneumonia
    b. respiratory distress syndrome
    c. transient tachypnea

86. Fracture of the clavicle occurs in _____ percent of term deliveries.
    a. 0.9–1.8
    b. 1.9–2.9
    c. 3.0–3.9

87. Rachitic rosary is a term used to describe a clinical feature of:
    a. clavicular fracture
    b. pneumothorax
    c. rickets

88. Transillumination of the newborn's chest is more likely to yield a false negative result in the presence of:
    a. chest wall edema
    b. lung consolidation
    c. pallor

89. During high-frequency ventilation, musical breath sounds may be indicative of:
    a. air leak
    b. excessive ventilator pressure
    c. secretions

90. Compared to the general population, the risk of congenital heart disease (CHD) in infants born to mothers with diabetes mellitus is _____ times greater.
    a. 1–3
    b. 2–4
    c. 3–5

91. Infants born to women with systemic lupus erythematous should be assessed for the presence of:
    a. congenital heart block
    b. cardiac septal defects
    c. supraventricular tachycardia

92. The risk of CHD in infants born to mothers with CHD is _____ percent.
    a. 5–10
    b. 10–15
    c. 15–20

93. Maternal use of lithium is associated with which of the following heart defects in offspring?
    a. atrial septal defect
    b. coarctation of the aorta
    c. tetralogy of Fallot

94. Ventricular outflow tract defects are more common following intrauterine exposure to:
    a. alcohol
    b. hydantoin
    c. retinoic acid

95. What percentage of infants with extracardiac anomalies has CHD?
    a. 15
    b. 25
    c. 35

96. The optimal location for determining the presence of central cyanosis is the:
    a. lips
    b. mucous membranes
    c. tongue

97. Polycythemia is defined by a central hematocrit value that exceeds _____ percent.
    a. 60
    b. 65
    c. 70

98. For cyanosis to be visible, how many grams of unbound hemoglobin must be present?
    a. 5
    b. 6
    c. 7

99. In a healthy newborn, capillary refill time is normally less than _____ seconds.
    a. 3–4
    b. 4–5
    c. 5–6

100. The presence of edema only in the hands or feet is a finding in:
    a. congenital adrenal hypoplasia
    b. renal failure
    c. Turner syndrome

101. Lesions that result in bounding peripheral pulses include:
    a. aortic stenosis
    b. truncus arteriosus
    c. ventricular septal defect

102. During transition to extrauterine life, right ventricular prominence results in a visible impulse seen at the:
    a. fifth intercostal space at the midaxillary line
    b. lower left sternal border
    c. second left intercostal space

103. In neonates, the apex of the heart is normally palpated in the _____ intercostal space.
    a. third   c. fifth
    b. fourth

104. Which part of the examiner's hand is most sensitive in identifying vibratory sensations?
    a. fingertips   c. ulnar surface
    b. palm

105. Which of the following findings is associated with volume overload?
    a. heave   c. thrill
    b. tap

106. Thrills are commonly found in which of the following conditions?
    a. tetralogy of Fallot
    b. transposition of the great vessels
    c. truncus arteriosus

107. Defects involving the pulmonic valves would be best auscultated over which landmark?
    a. left sternal border   c. right sternal border
    b. midclavicular line

108. Congestive heart failure is likely to occur when supraventricular tachycardia presents for more than _____ hours.
    a. 12   c. 48
    b. 24

109. Which drug is associated with the development of premature atrial beats in newborns?
    a. caffeine   c. morphine
    b. furosemide

110. The first heart sound (S1) is best heard over the _____ area.
    a. aortic   c. pulmonic
    b. mitral

111. By 48 hours of age, up to 80 percent of newborns will have which of the following heart sounds?
    a. split S2   c. S4
    b. S3

112. Ejection clicks are heard in the presence of a/an:
    a. atrial septal defect   c. pulmonic stenosis
    b. patent ductus arteriosus

113. What percentage of newborns has a systolic ejection murmur?
    a. 36   c. 76
    b. 56

114. Which type of innocent murmur radiates to the axilla and back?
    a. pulmonary flow   c. systolic ejection
    b. Still's

115. Congestive heart failure should be suspected when the newborn's liver extends more than _____ cm below the right costal margin.
    a. 1   c. 3
    b. 2

116. A newborn infant has the following systolic blood pressure results: left upper arm 54, left leg 32, right arm 56, and right leg 35. This result:
    a. is normal
    b. likely represents coarctation of the aorta
    c. is seen in persistent pulmonary hypertension

117. What percentage of infants born following a history of polyhydramnios has major structural malformations?
    a. 10–20   c. 30–40
    b. 20–30

118. The risk of gastrointestinal abnormalities increases to 90 percent when the largest vertical pocket of amniotic fluid in the uterus is >_____ cm.
    a. 12   c. 16
    b. 14

119. In the presence of polyhydramnios, the infant should be assessed for the presence of:
    a. esophageal atresia   c. imperforate anus
    b. hiatal hernia

120. A large amount of amniotic fluid in the stomach at delivery is suggestive of:
    a. duodenal atresia   c. pyloric stenosis
    b. malrotation

121. In neonates, the abdominal circumference normally begins to exceed head circumference at _____ weeks gestational age.
    a. 34   c. 38
    b. 36

122. Characteristic findings in congenital diaphragmatic hernia include an abdomen that is:
    a. discolored   c. scaphoid
    b. distended

123. Nonbilious vomiting is characteristic of an obstruction located in the:
    a. duodenum
    b. ileum
    c. large bowel

124. Meconium ileus is a characteristic finding in which of the following conditions?
    a. cystic fibrosis
    b. Down syndrome
    c. prune belly syndrome

125. Malrotation must be ruled out in an infant presenting with:
    a. abdominal distention
    b. bilious emesis
    c. fresh blood in the stool

126. The presence of a midline ridge between the sternum and umbilicus is:
    a. associated with diaphragmatic hernia
    b. a normal finding
    c. indicative of Potter sequence

127. Umbilical hernias are more common in which group of neonates?
    a. African American
    b. Asian
    c. Caucasian

128. An infant with a thick umbilical cord may have (be):
    a. trisomy 13 or 21
    b. large-for-gestational-age
    c. postmature

129. Infants with unusual bulges in the umbilical cord should be investigated for the presence of:
    a. gastroschisis
    b. omphalocele
    c. patent urachus

130. What percentage of neonates is born with a single umbilical artery?
    a. 1
    b. 2
    c. 3

131. Which of the following is a feature of omphalitis?
    a. persistent clear drainage from the cord
    b. redness at the base of the cord
    c. yellow staining of the cord

132. A patent urachus connects the umbilicus to the:
    a. bladder
    b. ileum
    c. kidney

133. Omphaloceles are seen in infants with which of the following syndromes?
    a. Beckwith-Wiedemann
    b. Cornelia de Lange
    c. Sturge-Weber

134. Bladder exstrophy occurs:
    a. more commonly in females
    b. more commonly in males
    c. equally in males and females

135. An absent anal wink is suggestive of:
    a. central nervous system abnormality
    b. Hirschsprung's disease
    c. imperforate anus

136. In a newborn, bowel sounds are heard every ____ seconds.
    a. 10–15
    b. 15–20
    c. 20–25

137. To effectively detect the edge of the liver in a newborn, the abdomen should be depressed to _____ cm.
    a. 0.5–1
    b. 1–2
    c. 2–3

138. The length of a normal term newborn kidney is _____ cm.
    a. 2.5–3
    b. 3.5–4
    c. 4.5–5

139. Weak femoral pulses are characteristic of which cardiac anomaly?
    a. interrupted aortic arch
    b. mitral valve stenosis
    c. patent ductus arteriosus

140. When comparing newborn blood pressures in the upper and lower extremities, the difference should normally be less than _____ mmHg.
    a. 10
    b. 20
    c. 30

141. Which of the following is suggestive of oligohydramnios?
    a. barrel-shaped chest
    b. breech position
    c. positional club feet

142. In addition to renal anomalies, VACTERL association includes:
    a. anal atresia
    b. malformed ears
    c. omphalocele

143. To facilitate abdominal palpation, the examiner could:
    a. extend the infant's hips
    b. place the infant in a side-lying position
    c. provide a pacifier

144. The presence of rugae on the scrotum suggests a gestational age of at least _____ weeks.
    a. 34
    b. 36
    c. 38

145. The normal size of a testis in a term infant is _____ cm.
    a. 1.2–1.4
    b. 1.4–1.6
    c. 1.6–1.8

146. In term newborns, the average length of the stretched penis is _____ cm.
    a. 1.5   c. 3.5
    b. 2.5

147. If present, pseudomenses may persist for up to _____ days.
    a. 7   c. 14
    b. 10

148. The most common renal causes of an abdominal mass in the newborn are multicystic kidneys and _____.
    a. duplicated collection systems
    b. hydronephrosis
    c. polycystic kidneys

149. The most common midline abdominal mass in newborns is a:
    a. distended bladder   c. volvulus
    b. malrotation

150. Which of the following has been shown to cause fetal ascites?
    a. posterior urethral valves c. prune belly syndrome
    b. Potter syndrome

151. Prune belly syndrome occurs:
    a. equally in both sexes
    b. more commonly in females
    c. more commonly in males

152. Which of the following is a variant of bladder exstrophy?
    a. epispadias   c. posterior urethral valves
    b. hypospadias

153. Which of the following is a feature of cloacal exstrophy?
    a. bifid bladder c. renal hypoplasia
    b. gastroschisis

154. What percentage of newborns with a single umbilical artery has renal abnormalities?
    a. 5   c. 7
    b. 6

155. A newborn with clear discharge from the umbilical cord should be checked for the presence of:
    a. ileal-umbilical fistula   c. patent urachus
    b. omphalitis

156. The majority of infants with hypospadias also have:
    a. cryptorchidism   c. posterior urethral valves
    b. foreskin malformation

157. Epispadias is always accompanied by:
    a. chordee   c. renal abnormalities
    b. micropenis

158. Which of the following procedures should not be performed on newborns with hypospadias?
    a. circumcision   c. urinary catheterization
    b. orchiopexy

159. Which of the following predisposes a neonate to develop priapism?
    a. hypospadias   c. urinary tract infections
    b. polycythemia

160. What percentage of term neonates has an undescended testis?
    a. 2.7   c. 4.7
    b. 3.7

161. Spontaneous testicular descent rarely occurs after _____ months of age.
    a. 7   c. 9
    b. 8

162. In a newborn with testicular torsion, irreversible damage to the gonad occurs when the period of ischemia exceeds _____ hours.
    a. 12   c. 24
    b. 18

163. The average length of a newborn infant is _____ cm.
    a. 43–48   c. 53–58
    b. 48–53

164. In comparing head circumference to length, which of the following formulas provides a general guide? Head circumference in cm equals:
    a. length – 10 cm   c. length ÷ 0.5 + 10 cm
    b. length × 0.5 – 10 cm

165. Which of the following statements accurately describes the relationship between head circumference and chest circumference?
    a. chest and head circumference are about the same for nine months
    b. the difference between head and chest circumference is greater in more immature infants
    c. term infants usually have a chest circumference that is 2–4 cm greater than head circumference

166. A foot that is bent outwards away from the body is said to be in what position?
    a. dorsiflexion   c. varus
    b. valgus

167. In term infants, the ratio of upper body length to lower body length should be less than:
    a. 1.7:1   c. 1.9:1
    b. 1.8:1

168. In a term newborn at rest, mild tremors in the extremities are normal for up to _____ days after birth.
    a. 2
    b. 4
    c. 6

169. To be considered normal, a newborn's neck should rotate _____ degrees.
    a. 40
    b. 60
    c. 80

170. Which of the following should be suspected in a newborn with an asymmetric Moro reflex?
    a. fractured clavicle
    b. motor neuron lesion
    c. intracranial bleeding

171. In a newborn suspected of having trisomy 18, which of the following would you expect to see?
    a. macrodactyly
    b. overlapping index and third fingers
    c. simian crease

172. Lateral deformities of the spine can usually be attributed to:
    a. birth injury
    b. *in utero* position
    c. lordosis

173. Normal newborns usually have a hip flexion contracture of _____ degrees.
    a. 30
    b. 35
    c. 40

174. In performing an Ortolani maneuver, the examiner attempts to:
    a. assess the ease with which the hip can be dislocated
    b. move the femoral head out of the acetabulum
    c. reduce a dislocated femoral head

175. When counseling the parent of a newborn with internal tibial torsion, the nurse should be aware that:
    a. an early orthopedic consultation is recommended
    b. delayed crawling is common
    c. spontaneous recovery is expected

176. Klippel-Feil syndrome involves defects of the _____ vertebrae.
    a. cervical
    b. thoracic
    c. lumbar

177. Which muscle is affected in congenital torticollis?
    a. deltoid
    b. sternocleidomastoid
    c. supraspinatus

178. Infants with congenital scoliosis should be investigated for the presence of associated:
    a. congenital heart disease
    b. hydrocephalus
    c. renal abnormalities

179. Sprengel's deformity affects the:
    a. clavicle
    b. scapula
    c. sternum

180. Which of the following is a feature commonly associated with absence of the clavicle?
    a. large fontanels
    b. low-set ears
    c. pectus excavatum

181. Erb's palsy results from a neurologic injury at the level of:
    a. C1–C4
    b. C5–C6
    c. C7–T1

182. Klumpke's palsy presents with paralysis of the _____ arm.
    a. entire
    b. lower
    c. upper

183. What percentage of infants born in breech position has developmental dysplasia of the hip (DDH)?
    a. 16–25
    b. 26–35
    c. 36–45

184. DDH is more common in which of the following ethnic groups?
    a. African American
    b. Asian
    c. Native American

185. The risk of developing metatarsus adductus is increased in the presence of:
    a. maternal diabetes
    b. multiple gestation
    c. polyhydramnios

186. Infants of which ethnic group are at highest risk of being born with talipes equinovarus?
    a. Asian
    b. Caucasian
    c. Polynesian

187. Streeter dysplasia most commonly affects the:
    a. craniofacial structure
    b. lower extremities
    c. upper extremities

188. Polydactyly is more common in infants of what ethnic background?
    a. African American
    b. Caucasian
    c. Native American

189. Presence of a café au lait spot measuring more than 1.5 cm is a marker for:
    a. Klippel-Trelawney syndrome
    b. Marfan syndrome
    c. neurofibromatosis

190. Infants with Sturge-Weber syndrome have:
    a. arteriovenous malformations
    b. dysplastic neural tumors
    c. progressive neural degeneration

191. Which of the following skin findings is a feature of tuberous sclerosis?
    a. areas of depigmentation
    b. port wine nevi on the eyelids
    c. strawberry hemangioma

192. Which of the following is a sign of prenatal exposure to selective serotonin reuptake inhibitors (SSRIs)? A cry that is:
    a. catlike   c. weak
    b. high-pitched

193. Approximately 5 percent of infants with a brachial plexus injury also have a/an:
    a. fractured clavicle   c. phrenic nerve injury
    b. intracranial hemorrhage

194. Isolated bilateral facial weakness is characteristic of:
    a. Bell's palsy
    b. congenital myasthenia gravis
    c. Möbius syndrome

195. Widened sutures caused by abnormal ossification are seen in:
    a. infants of diabetic mothers
    b. intrauterine growth restriction
    c. large-for-gestational age infants

196. Transillumination with a flashlight of a normal neonate's skull should yield a glow beyond the flashlight of no more than _____ cm.
    a. 2   c. 4
    b. 3

197. Infants with facial hemangiomas should be examined for the presence of:
    a. bruit   c. microcephaly
    b. craniosynostosis

198. Which tendon reflex is most readily elicited after birth?
    a. biceps   c. patellar
    b. triceps

199. Postural tone is tested with the:
    a. observation of truncal tone
    b. pull-to-sit maneuver
    c. scarf sign maneuver

200. Newborns with Werdnig-Hoffmann disease have weakness of the:
    a. entire body   c. face and neck
    b. extremities

201. The Galant reflex is tested when the neonate is in what position?
    a. sitting up   c. ventral suspension
    b. supine

202. The withdrawal reflex should be present in most infants beginning in what week of gestation?
    a. 27   c. 29
    b. 28

203. In a normal newborn, turning the head to the left results in the eyes:
    a. deviating to the left   c. remaining midline
    b. deviating to the right

204. Examination of the nasolabial creases helps to assess the intactness of which cranial nerve?
    a. III   c. VII
    b. V

205. Hoarseness or stridor may be a sign of damage to which cranial nerve?
    a. accessory   c. vagus
    b. glossopharyngeal

206. Moderate encephalopathy is characterized by:
    a. hyperalertness   c. jitteriness
    b. hypotonia

207. In neonates with severe encephalopathy, the doll's eye response usually disappears during the first _____ hours after birth.
    a. 1–12   c. 24–72
    b. 12–24

208. In term infants, perinatal asphyxia most often causes injury to what part of the brain?
    a. occipital horns   c. periventricular
    b. parasagittal

209. Abnormalities seen in infants following prenatal exposure to SSRIs include:
    a. feeding intolerance   c. sleep disturbances
    b. hypoglycemia

210. The most common location for an encephalocele is in which bone?
    a. occipital   c. temporal
    b. parietal

211. Dermal sinuses are usually seen in which region of the spine?
    a. lumbar   c. sacral
    b. thoracic

212. Which area of the dura separates the cerebral hemispheres from the cerebellum?
    a. falx   c. transverse sinus
    b. tentorium

213. Traumatic separation of the joint between the squamous and lateral bones is referred to as:
  a. craniotabes
  b. occipital diastasis
  c. opisthotonos

214. A unilateral nonreactive pupil is a sign of:
  a. falx laceration
  b. rupture of the superficial cerebral vein
  c. tentorial laceration

215. The most common cause of posthemorrhagic hydrocephalus in premature infants is:
  a. inflammation of the arachnoid villi
  b. obstruction of the aqueduct of Sylvius
  c. scarring of the germinal matrix

216. By the time an infant is 72 hours of age, what percentage of PV-IVHs is detectable on ultrasound?
  a. 70
  b. 80
  c. 90

217. Stemming from delivery, the most common contributing factor in subgaleal hemorrhage is:
  a. forceps use
  b. shoulder dystocia
  c. vacuum extraction

218. The NBAS tool scores infants on _____ behavioral items.
  a. 18
  b. 25
  c. 28

219. The primary focus of the Nursing Model of the Brazelton scale is to:
  a. evaluate the neonate's developmental age
  b. identify infants needing referral to a developmental specialist
  c. promote parent-infant attachment

220. The focus of Als' Assessment of Preterm Infants' Behavior (APIB) is to assess the premature infant's ability to:
  a. cope within an NICU environment
  b. reach developmental milestones
  c. respond to parental interactions

221. Lester and Tronick's NICU Network Neurobehavioral Scale (NNNS) was designed to assess infants born prematurely and _____ infants.
  a. asphyxiated
  b. drug-exposed
  c. growth-restricted

222. The Anderson Behavioral State Scale (ABSS) was developed for use with:
  a. infants <3 months of age
  b. premature infants
  c. term infants

223. According to the ABSS, which of the following scores represents sleep states optimal for growth and recovery?
  a. 1–2
  b. 3–4
  c. 5–6

224. Irregular respirations are characteristic of which newborn state?
  a. active alert
  b. drowsiness
  c. quiet alert

225. Hand-to-mouth movements are an example of:
  a. behavioral organization
  b. motor organization
  c. time-out signals

226. Sensory threshold refers to the infant's:
  a. ability to hear
  b. level of tolerance for stimuli
  c. responsiveness to auditory and visual stimuli

227. In a newborn, approach signs include which of the following?
  a. dilated pupils
  b. finger splaying
  c. rapid breathing

228. An infant who stops turning to a shaking rattle is demonstrating:
  a. avoidance behaviors
  b. habituation
  c. sensory threshold

229. A term infant normally can track an object _____ degrees in a horizontal plane.
  a. 30
  b. 60
  c. 90

230. The pupillary reflex normally develops at _____ weeks gestation.
  a. 30
  b. 32
  c. 34

231. Premature infants are usually capable of tolerating soft sounds by _____ weeks gestational age.
  a. 26
  b. 28
  c. 30

232. A neonate who stops feeding every time someone walks by is said to have an increased level of:
  a. adaptability
  b. distractibility
  c. responsiveness

233. The percentage of infants born with a major birth defect each year is_____.
  a. 1
  b. 2
  c. 3

234. Which of the following birth defects is known to be inheritable?
  a. choanal atresia
  b. cleft palate
  c. gastroschisis

235. Thalassemia is more common in people of what ethnic background?
    a. French-Canadian   c. Northern European
    b. Mediterranean

236. Infants with hypothyroidism may display which of the following characteristics?
    a. large fontanels   c. vascular nevi
    b. peripheral lymphedema

237. A webbed neck is a finding in which of the following genetic syndromes?
    a. Edward   c. Turner
    b. Marfan

238. An infant with asymmetric crying facies is at increased risk for abnormalities of the:
    a. brain   c. kidneys
    b. heart

239. A cloudy cornea is a sign of:
    a. glaucoma   c. retinoblastoma
    b. osteogenesis imperfecta

240. In neonates with a single umbilical artery, what percentage has other major anomalies?
    a. 20   c. 60
    b. 40

241. What percentage of the normal population has a simian crease?
    a. 5–10   c. 15–20
    b. 10–15

242. Developmental dysplasia of the hip is an example of _____.
    a. a deformation   c. dysplasia
    b. a disruption

243. Retinoblastoma is an example of a disorder that is:
    a. autosomal dominant   c. X-linked recessive
    b. autosomal recessive

244. Which of the following is statistically true for parents who each carry a gene for an autosomal recessive disorder?
    a. 25 percent of their children will have the disease
    b. 50 percent of their children will have the disease
    c. 50 percent of their sons will have the disease

245. Which of the following statements is true of mitochondrial disorders?
    a. female offspring of affected women will always manifest the disease
    b. females rarely pass the disorder to their offspring
    c. males do not pass the disease to their children

246. Congenital anomalies associated with Down syndrome include:
    a. Dandy-Walker malformation
    b. imperforate anus
    c. omphalocele

247. What percentage of infants with trisomy 18 survives beyond one year of age?
    a. 0–5   c. 10–15
    b. 5–10

248. Presenting signs of Turner syndrome include:
    a. duodenal atresia   c. rocker-bottom feet
    b. edema of the extremities

249. Infants with DiGeorge syndrome have a hypoplastic or absent:
    a. adrenal gland   c. thymus gland
    b. corpus callosum

250. The most common cause of death in infants with Potter sequence is:
    a. pulmonary hypoplasia   c. sepsis
    b. renal failure

251. The incidence of Robin sequence is estimated to be 1 in _____ live births.
    a. 4,000   c. 8,000
    b. 6,000

252. The C in CHARGE association refers to:
    a. cataracts   c. congenital heart defects
    b. coloboma

253. The most common heart defect seen in newborns with fetal alcohol exposure is:
    a. coarctation of the aorta   c. ventricular septal defect
    b. pulmonary atresia

254. Features of fetal valproate syndrome include:
    a. hypospadias   c. microcephaly
    b. low-set ears

255. Facial expressions seen in "cry face" include:
    a. brow bulge   c. slack mouth
    b. nasal flaring

256. Physiologic indicators scored on the the Premature Infant Pain Profile (PIPP) scale include oxygen saturation and:
    a. blood pressure   c. respiratory rate
    b. heart rate

257. The PIPP scores an infant on gestational age, behavioral state, and how many other parameters?
    a. three   c. five
    b. four

258. Pharmacologic treatment is recommended when PIPP scores reach:
   a. 8
   b. 10
   c. 12

259. Parameters assessed in the CRIES postoperative pain assessment tool score include:
   a. gestational age
   b. need for oxygen
   c. posture

260. The CRIES tool was originally developed for infants of _____ weeks gestational age.
   a. 32–36
   b. 37–40
   c. 40+

261. The CRIES tool is more difficult to use in infants who are:
   a. already on oxygen
   b. premature
   c. receiving pain medication

262. The physiologic parameter assessed by the Neonatal Infant Pain Scale (NIPS) is:
   a. breathing pattern
   b. heart rate
   c. oxygen saturation

263. Which of the following parameters has been shown to be the most sensitive indicator of pain in newborns?
   a. cry
   b. facial expression
   c. physiologic changes

264. In ELBW infants (<1,000 g), which of the following is least sensitive in assessing pain?
   a. cry
   b. facial expression
   c. physiologic parameters

265. According to a consensus panel of pediatric pain experts, the most sensitive indicators of pain in neurologically impaired infants include:
   a. body movements
   b. facial grimace
   c. increased vital signs

266. Studies of infants exposed to SSRIs found that, compared to unexposed infants, exposed infants had fewer:
   a. arm and leg movements
   b. changes in heart rate
   c. crying episodes

267. Which of the following indicators of pain is not seen on a neonatal abstinence scoring tool?
   a. agitation
   b. crying
   c. facial grimacing

268. Chorionic villus sampling is normally done at _____ weeks of gestation.
   a. 8–10
   b. 10–12
   c. 12–14

269. Which is the earliest week from the last menstrual period that pregnancy can be detected by ultrasound?
   a. 5
   b. 7
   c. 9

270. A nuchal fold thickness of more than _____ mm is a marker for Down syndrome.
   a. 1
   b. 2
   c. 3

271. Increased fetal fibronectin in vaginal secretions predicts:
   a. chromosomal anomalies
   b. fetal hydrops
   c. preterm labor

272. In cases of severe uteroplacental insufficiency, fetal diastolic blood flow is:
   a. equivocal
   b. increased
   c. reversed

273. During a nonstress test, fetal well-being is indicated by an increase in heart rate of at least _____ beats per minute.
   a. 5
   b. 10
   c. 15

274. Triple testing includes measurements of α-fetoprotein, unconjugated estriol, and:
   a. fetal hemoglobin
   b. human chorionic gonadotropin
   c. prostaglandin

275. Low levels of placental lactogen can be found in pregnancies complicated by maternal:
   a. diabetes mellitus
   b. erythroblastosis
   c. hypertension

276. Well-controlled blood sugar is indicated by an $HgbA_{1c}$ level that is less than _____ percent.
   a. 8
   b. 9
   c. 10

277. Decreased fetal heart rate variability is commonly seen following administration of _____ to the mother.
   a. labetalol
   b. magnesium sulfate
   c. steroids

278. A sinusoidal fetal heart rate pattern is an indicator of fetal:
   a. anemia
   b. heart block
   c. sepsis

ANSWER FORM: Physical Assessment of the Newborn, 4th Edition

Please completely fill in the circle of the **one best answer** using a dark pen.

Questions are numbered vertically.

1. a. ○ b. ○ c. ○	17. a. ○ b. ○ c. ○	33. a. ○ b. ○ c. ○	49. a. ○ b. ○ c. ○	65. a. ○ b. ○ c. ○	81. a. ○ b. ○ c. ○	97. a. ○ b. ○ c. ○	113. a. ○ b. ○ c. ○	129. a. ○ b. ○ c. ○	145. a. ○ b. ○ c. ○
2. a. ○ b. ○ c. ○	18. a. ○ b. ○ c. ○	34. a. ○ b. ○ c. ○	50. a. ○ b. ○ c. ○	66. a. ○ b. ○ c. ○	82. a. ○ b. ○ c. ○	98. a. ○ b. ○ c. ○	114. a. ○ b. ○ c. ○	130. a. ○ b. ○ c. ○	146. a. ○ b. ○ c. ○
3. a. ○ b. ○ c. ○	19. a. ○ b. ○ c. ○	35. a. ○ b. ○ c. ○	51. a. ○ b. ○ c. ○	67. a. ○ b. ○ c. ○	83. a. ○ b. ○ c. ○	99. a. ○ b. ○ c. ○	115. a. ○ b. ○ c. ○	131. a. ○ b. ○ c. ○	147. a. ○ b. ○ c. ○
4. a. ○ b. ○ c. ○	20. a. ○ b. ○ c. ○	36. a. ○ b. ○ c. ○	52. a. ○ b. ○ c. ○	68. a. ○ b. ○ c. ○	84. a. ○ b. ○ c. ○	100. a. ○ b. ○ c. ○	116. a. ○ b. ○ c. ○	132. a. ○ b. ○ c. ○	148. a. ○ b. ○ c. ○
5. a. ○ b. ○ c. ○	21. a. ○ b. ○ c. ○	37. a. ○ b. ○ c. ○	53. a. ○ b. ○ c. ○	69. a. ○ b. ○ c. ○	85. a. ○ b. ○ c. ○	101. a. ○ b. ○ c. ○	117. a. ○ b. ○ c. ○	133. a. ○ b. ○ c. ○	149. a. ○ b. ○ c. ○
6. a. ○ b. ○ c. ○	22. a. ○ b. ○ c. ○	38. a. ○ b. ○ c. ○	54. a. ○ b. ○ c. ○	70. a. ○ b. ○ c. ○	86. a. ○ b. ○ c. ○	102. a. ○ b. ○ c. ○	118. a. ○ b. ○ c. ○	134. a. ○ b. ○ c. ○	150. a. ○ b. ○ c. ○
7. a. ○ b. ○ c. ○	23. a. ○ b. ○ c. ○	39. a. ○ b. ○ c. ○	55. a. ○ b. ○ c. ○	71. a. ○ b. ○ c. ○	87. a. ○ b. ○ c. ○	103. a. ○ b. ○ c. ○	119. a. ○ b. ○ c. ○	135. a. ○ b. ○ c. ○	151. a. ○ b. ○ c. ○
8. a. ○ b. ○ c. ○	24. a. ○ b. ○ c. ○	40. a. ○ b. ○ c. ○	56. a. ○ b. ○ c. ○	72. a. ○ b. ○ c. ○	88. a. ○ b. ○ c. ○	104. a. ○ b. ○ c. ○	120. a. ○ b. ○ c. ○	136. a. ○ b. ○ c. ○	152. a. ○ b. ○ c. ○
9. a. ○ b. ○ c. ○	25. a. ○ b. ○ c. ○	41. a. ○ b. ○ c. ○	57. a. ○ b. ○ c. ○	73. a. ○ b. ○ c. ○	89. a. ○ b. ○ c. ○	105. a. ○ b. ○ c. ○	121. a. ○ b. ○ c. ○	137. a. ○ b. ○ c. ○	153. a. ○ b. ○ c. ○
10. a. ○ b. ○ c. ○	26. a. ○ b. ○ c. ○	42. a. ○ b. ○ c. ○	58. a. ○ b. ○ c. ○	74. a. ○ b. ○ c. ○	90. a. ○ b. ○ c. ○	106. a. ○ b. ○ c. ○	122. a. ○ b. ○ c. ○	138. a. ○ b. ○ c. ○	154. a. ○ b. ○ c. ○
11. a. ○ b. ○ c. ○	27. a. ○ b. ○ c. ○	43. a. ○ b. ○ c. ○	59. a. ○ b. ○ c. ○	75. a. ○ b. ○ c. ○	91. a. ○ b. ○ c. ○	107. a. ○ b. ○ c. ○	123. a. ○ b. ○ c. ○	139. a. ○ b. ○ c. ○	155. a. ○ b. ○ c. ○
12. a. ○ b. ○ c. ○	28. a. ○ b. ○ c. ○	44. a. ○ b. ○ c. ○	60. a. ○ b. ○ c. ○	76. a. ○ b. ○ c. ○	92. a. ○ b. ○ c. ○	108. a. ○ b. ○ c. ○	124. a. ○ b. ○ c. ○	140. a. ○ b. ○ c. ○	156. a. ○ b. ○ c. ○
13. a. ○ b. ○ c. ○	29. a. ○ b. ○ c. ○	45. a. ○ b. ○ c. ○	61. a. ○ b. ○ c. ○	77. a. ○ b. ○ c. ○	93. a. ○ b. ○ c. ○	109. a. ○ b. ○ c. ○	125. a. ○ b. ○ c. ○	141. a. ○ b. ○ c. ○	157. a. ○ b. ○ c. ○
14. a. ○ b. ○ c. ○	30. a. ○ b. ○ c. ○	46. a. ○ b. ○ c. ○	62. a. ○ b. ○ c. ○	78. a. ○ b. ○ c. ○	94. a. ○ b. ○ c. ○	110. a. ○ b. ○ c. ○	126. a. ○ b. ○ c. ○	142. a. ○ b. ○ c. ○	158. a. ○ b. ○ c. ○
15. a. ○ b. ○ c. ○	31. a. ○ b. ○ c. ○	47. a. ○ b. ○ c. ○	63. a. ○ b. ○ c. ○	79. a. ○ b. ○ c. ○	95. a. ○ b. ○ c. ○	111. a. ○ b. ○ c. ○	127. a. ○ b. ○ c. ○	143. a. ○ b. ○ c. ○	159. a. ○ b. ○ c. ○
16. a. ○ b. ○ c. ○	32. a. ○ b. ○ c. ○	48. a. ○ b. ○ c. ○	64. a. ○ b. ○ c. ○	80. a. ○ b. ○ c. ○	96. a. ○ b. ○ c. ○	112. a. ○ b. ○ c. ○	128. a. ○ b. ○ c. ○	144. a. ○ b. ○ c. ○	160. a. ○ b. ○ c. ○

161. a. ○   173. a. ○   185. a. ○   197. a. ○   209. a. ○   221. a. ○   233. a. ○   245. a. ○   257. a. ○   269. a. ○
    b. ○   b. ○   b. ○   b. ○   b. ○   b. ○   b. ○   b. ○   b. ○   b. ○
    c. ○   c. ○   c. ○   c. ○   c. ○   c. ○   c. ○   c. ○   c. ○   c. ○

162. a. ○   174. a. ○   186. a. ○   198. a. ○   210. a. ○   222. a. ○   234. a. ○   246. a. ○   258. a. ○   270. a. ○
  b. ○   b. ○   b. ○   b. ○   b. ○   b. ○   b. ○   b. ○   b. ○   b. ○
  c. ○   c. ○   c. ○   c. ○   c. ○   c. ○   c. ○   c. ○   c. ○   c. ○

163. a. ○   175. a. ○   187. a. ○   199. a. ○   211. a. ○   223. a. ○   235. a. ○   247. a. ○   259. a. ○   271. a. ○
  b. ○   b. ○   b. ○   b. ○   b. ○   b. ○   b. ○   b. ○   b. ○   b. ○
  c. ○   c. ○   c. ○   c. ○   c. ○   c. ○   c. ○   c. ○   c. ○   c. ○

164. a. ○   176. a. ○   188. a. ○   200. a. ○   212. a. ○   224. a. ○   236. a. ○   248. a. ○   260. a. ○   272. a. ○
  b. ○   b. ○   b. ○   b. ○   b. ○   b. ○   b. ○   b. ○   b. ○   b. ○
  c. ○   c. ○   c. ○   c. ○   c. ○   c. ○   c. ○   c. ○   c. ○   c. ○

165. a. ○   177. a. ○   189. a. ○   201. a. ○   213. a. ○   225. a. ○   237. a. ○   249. a. ○   261. a. ○   273. a. ○
  b. ○   b. ○   b. ○   b. ○   b. ○   b. ○   b. ○   b. ○   b. ○   b. ○
  c. ○   c. ○   c. ○   c. ○   c. ○   c. ○   c. ○   c. ○   c. ○   c. ○

166. a. ○   178. a. ○   190. a. ○   202. a. ○   214. a. ○   226. a. ○   238. a. ○   250. a. ○   262. a. ○   274. a. ○
  b. ○   b. ○   b. ○   b. ○   b. ○   b. ○   b. ○   b. ○   b. ○   b. ○
  c. ○   c. ○   c. ○   c. ○   c. ○   c. ○   c. ○   c. ○   c. ○   c. ○

167. a. ○   179. a. ○   191. a. ○   203. a. ○   215. a. ○   227. a. ○   239. a. ○   251. a. ○   263. a. ○   275. a. ○
  b. ○   b. ○   b. ○   b. ○   b. ○   b. ○   b. ○   b. ○   b. ○   b. ○
  c. ○   c. ○   c. ○   c. ○   c. ○   c. ○   c. ○   c. ○   c. ○   c. ○

168. a. ○   180. a. ○   192. a. ○   204. a. ○   216. a. ○   228. a. ○   240. a. ○   252. a. ○   264. a. ○   276. a. ○
  b. ○   b. ○   b. ○   b. ○   b. ○   b. ○   b. ○   b. ○   b. ○   b. ○
  c. ○   c. ○   c. ○   c. ○   c. ○   c. ○   c. ○   c. ○   c. ○   c. ○

169. a. ○   181. a. ○   193. a. ○   205. a. ○   217. a. ○   229. a. ○   241. a. ○   253. a. ○   265. a. ○   277. a. ○
  b. ○   b. ○   b. ○   b. ○   b. ○   b. ○   b. ○   b. ○   b. ○   b. ○
  c. ○   c. ○   c. ○   c. ○   c. ○   c. ○   c. ○   c. ○   c. ○   c. ○

170. a. ○   182. a. ○   194. a. ○   206. a. ○   218. a. ○   230. a. ○   242. a. ○   254. a. ○   266. a. ○   278. a. ○
  b. ○   b. ○   b. ○   b. ○   b. ○   b. ○   b. ○   b. ○   b. ○   b. ○
  c. ○   c. ○   c. ○   c. ○   c. ○   c. ○   c. ○   c. ○   c. ○   c. ○

171. a. ○   183. a. ○   195. a. ○   207. a. ○   219. a. ○   231. a. ○   243. a. ○   255. a. ○   267. a. ○
  b. ○   b. ○   b. ○   b. ○   b. ○   b. ○   b. ○   b. ○   b. ○
  c. ○   c. ○   c. ○   c. ○   c. ○   c. ○   c. ○   c. ○   c. ○

172. a. ○   184. a. ○   196. a. ○   208. a. ○   220. a. ○   232. a. ○   244. a. ○   256. a. ○   268. a. ○
  b. ○   b. ○   b. ○   b. ○   b. ○   b. ○   b. ○   b. ○   b. ○
  c. ○   c. ○   c. ○   c. ○   c. ○   c. ○   c. ○   c. ○   c. ○

Physical Assessment of the Newborn, 4th Edition

Name _____
    Please Print

Address _____

City _____ State _____ Zip _____

Nursing License # _____ State(s) of License _____

Phone #_____
    (optional)

NICU Ink Books
1425 N McDowell Blvd, Ste 105
Petaluma, CA 94954

Mail a $90.00 processing fee for 30 contact hours payable to NICU Ink.®
NICU Ink,® 2220 Northpoint Parkway, Santa Rosa, CA 95407-7398.
Include an additional $10.00 for rush processing.
International Participants: International Money Order drawn on U.S. Bank only.

☐ I have enclosed an additional $10 for rush processing.

FOR OFFICE USE ONLY

RECEIVED

CHECK

GRADE

PASSED / FAILED

CERTIFICATE ISSUED

MAIL DATE IF DIFFERENT

REFERENCE #

Evaluation Directions

Thank you for taking the time to assist us in evaluating the effectiveness of this course. Using the scale below, darken the circles corresponding to your responses. If an item is not applicable, leave it blank.

①	②	③	④	⑤
Strongly Disagree	Disagree	Neutral	Agree	Strongly Agree

Objectives:

I am able to:

1. List the principles of physical assessment relevant to the newborn. ① ② ③ ④ ⑤

2. Outline the salient information that should be recorded in the newborn history. ① ② ③ ④ ⑤

3. Describe the components of a gestational age assessment. ① ② ③ ④ ⑤

4. Describe the elements of a complete newborn physical assessment. ① ② ③ ④ ⑤

5. Outline the components of a newborn behavioral assessment. ① ② ③ ④ ⑤

6. Discuss an approach to the assessment of the dysmorphic infant. ① ② ③ ④ ⑤

Presentation

1. The material presented is relevant to my practice. ① ② ③ ④ ⑤

2. The questions on the test reflected the content of the book. ① ② ③ ④ ⑤

3. The book content was comprehensive. ① ② ③ ④ ⑤

4. The test directions were clear. ① ② ③ ④ ⑤

5. I perceive the education level of this course to be: ① ② ③
   1 = Basic; 2 = Intermediate; 3 = Advanced

6. How long did it take you to complete the course? ____ hours ____ minutes

7. In what level unit do you practice? I___ II___ III___

I am a ☐ staff nurse ☐ NNP ☐ nurse manager _____ other (please state)

What subjects would you like to see offered for CE courses? _____

_____

Additional comments: _____

_____

Iowa participants may submit the evaluation directly to the Iowa Board of Nursing, 400-SW 8th St., Ste. B, Des Moines, IA 50309-4685.

Other Books by NICU Ink® BOOK PUBLISHERS

Name _____
(PLEASE PRINT ALL INFORMATION)

Address _____

City _____ State _____ Zip _____

Phone (_____) _____

Please enclose a check with your order. California residents add 8.25% sales tax, Sonoma County, CA residents add 9% sales tax. Orders received without correct California sales tax will not be filled. Please make your check payable to NICU Ink®, 2220 Northpoint Parkway, Santa Rosa, CA 95407-7398. Please allow 6–8 weeks for your order to be filled. International orders: International money order drawn on U.S. bank only. Please allow 8–12 weeks for surface delivery.

**To order by phone,
call toll free in the U.S. and Canada:
888-NICU Ink or 707-569-1415
VISA and MasterCard Accepted**

_____ Guide to Neonatal EKG book(s) x $22.95 each = _____

_____ Neonatal Medications book(s) x $59.95 each = _____

_____ Physical Assessment book(s) x $54.95 each = _____

Shipping (see below) _____

Subtotal _____

CA residents add appropriate sales tax _____

I have enclosed a total of $ _____

Shipping: Add $6.00 for the first book ordered.
Add $3.00 for each additional book ordered.
Rush fee, $5.00 per book.
For quantity orders (six or more) or foreign orders
please call for shipping charges 888-NICU Ink.

- -

Other Books by NICU Ink® BOOK PUBLISHERS

Name _____
(PLEASE PRINT ALL INFORMATION)

Address _____

City _____ State _____ Zip _____

Phone (_____) _____

Please enclose a check with your order. California residents add 8.25% sales tax, Sonoma County, CA residents add 9% sales tax. Orders received without correct California sales tax will not be filled. Please make your check payable to NICU Ink®, 2220 Northpoint Parkway, Santa Rosa, CA 95407-7398. Please allow 6–8 weeks for your order to be filled. International orders: International money order drawn on U.S. bank only. Please allow 8–12 weeks for surface delivery.

**To order by phone,
call toll free in the U.S. and Canada:
888-NICU Ink or 707-569-1415
VISA and MasterCard Accepted**

_____ Guide to Neonatal EKG book(s) x $22.95 each = _____

_____ Neonatal Medications book(s) x $59.95 each = _____

_____ Physical Assessment book(s) x $54.95 each = _____

Shipping (see below) _____

Subtotal _____

CA residents add appropriate sales tax _____

I have enclosed a total of $ _____

Shipping: Add $6.00 for the first book ordered.
Add $3.00 for each additional book ordered.
Rush fee, $5.00 per book.
For quantity orders (six or more) or foreign orders
please call for shipping charges 888-NICU Ink.